Insights Into
Lyme Disease Treatment

13 Lyme-Literate Health Care Practitioners Share Their Healing Strategies

With Bonus Articles from
Dietrich Klinghardt, M.D., Ph.D., and
James Schaller, M.D., M.A.R.

By **Connie Strasheim**

Foreword by
Maureen Mcshane, M.D.

BioMed Publishing Group
www.LymeBook.com

BioMed Publishing Group
P.O. Box 9012
South Lake Tahoe, CA 96158
www.LymeBook.com

For related books and DVDs visit us online at www.lymebook.com.

Visit the author's blog at www.lymebytes.blogspot.com.

Disclaimer

This book is not intended as medical advice. It is also not intended to prevent, diagnose, treat or cure disease. Instead, the book is intended only to share the research and opinion of the included interviewees, as well as that of author Connie Strasheim. The book is provided for informational and educational purposes only, not as treatment instructions for any disease. Much of the book is a statement of opinion in areas where the facts are controversial or do not exist. The information in this book should not be considered any more valid than any other type of informal opinion.

The physicians and health care providers who appear in this book were interviewed under informal circumstances and their statements herein do not necessarily represent their professional opinions.

The book was not written to replace the advice or care of a qualified health care professional. Be sure to check with your own qualified health care provider before beginning any protocols or procedures discussed in this book, or before stopping or altering any diet, lifestyle, or other therapies previously recommended to you by your health care provider.

Lyme disease is a controversial topic and this book should not be seen as the final word regarding Lyme disease medical care. The book should be viewed only as an unsubstantiated piece of literary work. The statements in this book have not been evaluated by the FDA.

Acknowledgements

I would like extend my sincerest thanks to all of the following people:

To God, who put it in my gut to write this book; to my family and friends, for their support during this immense and taxing project; to my publisher, Bryan Rosner, for helping to bring the book to fruition; to the health care practitioners who participated in this book, for their valiant efforts to share their sapphires of knowledge with a world that so desperately needs them; to Scott Forsgren, for reviewing this work prior to publication, and finally, to those who suffer from Lyme disease, for inspiring me to write yet another book about a subject as important as this one. May you be blessed in your journey towards health.

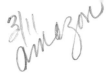

Dedication

To all the brave Lyme disease doctors who daily put it all on the line to help their patients. Your selfless actions are truly embodied by the Hippocratic Oath:

"Whatever houses I may visit, I will come for the benefit of the sick, remaining free of all intentional injustices ..."

Also by Connie Strasheim

The Lyme Disease Survival Guide: Physical, Lifestyle,
and Emotional Strategies for Healing

Available from www.LymeBook.com

Table of Contents

Disclaimer (Please Read the Disclaimer) iv

Foreword by Maureen Mcshane, M.D. 19

Preface by Connie Strasheim 25

A Note from the Publisher 30

Chapter 1: Steven J. Harris, M.D. 31

Biography 31

Healing Philosophy 32

When Lyme Disease Isn't the Primary Cause of Symptoms 33

Antibiotic Treatments for Infections 34

Typical Symptoms of Different Infections 38

Babesia 38

Bartonella 38

Ehrlichia and Anaplasma 39

Mycoplasma 39

Lyme (Borrelia) 39

Other Symptomatic Trends 40

Using Herbal Remedies to Treat Borrelia and Other Infections 40

Detoxification 41

Treatments 41

Addressing Detoxification Problems 43

Immune System Supplements 43

Healing the Gut 44

Treating Hormonal Dysfunction 44

Lifestyle Recommendations for Healing 45

Diet 45

Exercise 46

Treatments for Symptomatic Relief 46

Insomnia 46

Pain 46

Depression and Anxiety 47

Fatigue 48

Brain Fog 48

Healing Emotional Trauma 48

Who Are Those That Heal From Lyme Disease?
Who Are Those That Don't? 48

The Role of Spirituality in Healing   50

How Finances Affect Healing   50

Mistakes in Treating Lyme and Less-Than-Beneficial Treatments   51

The Biggest Challenge for People with Lyme Disease   52

How Friends and Family Can Help the Sick   52

How Long Does It Take to Heal from Lyme Disease?   53

Last Words   54

How To Contact Steven J. Harris, M.D.   54

Chapter 2: Steven Bock, M.D. 55

Biography   55

The History of My Practice   56

Changing the Paradigm of "One Disease, One Medicine"   57

Treatment Approach   58

The Lyme Healing Wheel   58

Emotional Strategies for Healing   60

The Patient as a Vessel in a Sea of Toxins   61

Healing the Body on an Energetic Level   62

Antibiotic Protocol for the Treatment of Lyme Disease Infections   62

Considerations in the Treatment of Infections   64

Clinical Diagnosis of Co-Infections   65

Considerations in Lab Testing   66

Detoxification   67

Treating Opportunistic Infections and the Immune System   68

Treating Hormonal Dysfunction   69

Treatments for Symptomatic Relief   71

Insomnia   71

Anxiety and Depression   71

Pain   72

Diet   72

Lifestyle Recommendations for Healing   73

Who Are Those that Heal from Lyme Disease and/or Chronic Illness?   74

Does Everyone with Chronic Fatigue Syndrome Really Have Lyme Disease?   75

Why Do Some People Gain Weight and Others Lose Weight When They Get Lyme Disease?   76

The Greatest Challenges of Treating Lyme Disease   76

Why I Love Treating Lyme Disease/Chronic Illness   77

Last Words   78

How to Contact Steven Bock, M.D.   78

Chapter 3: Susan L. Marra, M.S., N.D. 79

Biography   79

In the Beginning   80

First Do No Harm   82

The Art and Science of Practicing Medicine   83

Embracing the Intelligence of Nature   84

Global Warming and Global Karma   85

The Essence of the Patient   87

Listening   88

Determining Appropriate Diagnostic Tests   89

Treatment for Lyme Disease and Co-infections   91

Treating the Infections   92

Biotoxin Illness   94

Decrease the Inflammation   95

Degrade the Biofilm   96

Support the Organs   97

Intestinal Support   101

Pancreas Support   102

Liver Support   103

Joint and Muscle Support   103

Integumentary (Skin, Hair and Nails) Support   103

Brain Support   104

Insomnia   105

Headaches and Migraines   105

Mood   106

Depression   106

Attention Deficit Disorder   106

Autism   107

Energy   107

Hormones   108

Binding and Detoxifying Toxins   108

Treating Hypercoagulation and Thick Blood   109

Hypoxia   110

Management of Free Radicals, Nitric Oxide and Peroxynitrite   111

Lifestyle Recommendations for Healing Lyme Disease   112

Human Support   113

Community Support   114

Books on Lyme Disease   114

Spirit/Soul Sickness   115

Solutions to the Problem of Lyme   115

The Lessons to Be Learned   116

Closing Remarks   116

Gratitude   117

How to Contact Susan L. Marra, M.S., N.D.   117

Chapter 4: Ginger Savely, DNP 119

Biography   119

Healing Philosophy   120

Treatments for Infections   121

Borrelia   121

Babesia   122

Bartonella   123

Treating Mold, Candida and Environmental Toxins   126

Treating Insomnia   126

Nutrition   127

What Those with Lyme Disease Should Do for Proper Nutrition   128

Testing For and Treating Food Allergies   129

Supportive Supplements   129

Magnesium   130

Patient and Practitioner Challenges and Roadblocks to Healing   132

Lyme Disease vs. Chronic Fatigue Syndrome   135

Patient Roadblocks to Healing   136

Do Antibiotics Work?   136

Treating Relapses with Dr. Burrascano's Pulse Protocol   138

Profiling the Person that Heals from Lyme Disease   138

Stress Reduction and Behavior Modification   139

Strategies for Stress Reduction   140

Biofeedback   140

Cognitive Behavior Therapy   140

Humor   140

Lifestyle Adjustments   140

Financial Support — 141

Balancing Rest and Physical Conditioning — 141

Activities That People with Lyme Should Do — 142

What Friends and Family Members Can Do to Help the Sick — 142

Last Words — 143

How to Contact Ginger Savely, DNP — 143

Chapter 5: W. Lee Cowden, M.D., M.D. (H)...145

Biography — 145

Note to the Reader — 146

Dr. Cowden's Healing Philosophy — 146

Treatment Approach — 147

Testing For Lyme and Co-Infections — 148

Treatment Protocol for Infections — 149

Bartonella and Borrelia — 151

Babesia — 152

Dosing and Length of Treatment — 152

Specific and General Detoxification Strategies — 153

Addressing Detoxification Defects — 156

Treating Hormonal Dysfunction — 156

Treating Mold and Fungal Infections — 158

Treatments for Symptomatic Relief — 158

Anxiety and Depression — 158

Pain — 161

Insomnia — 163

Treating Gut Dysbiosis — 164

Healing Emotional Trauma — 165

IntegraMed Academy — 168

Profiling the Person Who Heals from Lyme Disease — 168

Strategies for Stress Reduction and Dealing with Life's Difficulties — 169

Exercise — 170

On Sunshine and the Marshall Protocol — 172

Final Words — 172

How to Contact W. Lee Cowden, M.D., M.D. (H) — 172

Chapter 6: Ingo D. E. Woitzel, M.D. 175

Biography — 175

Treatment Approach — 175

Biophoton Theory   175

How Disease Happens   176

How Bionic 880 Photons Are Transmitted Throughout the Body   177

The Cellular Effects of Photon Therapy   177

Testing for Lyme Disease   178

Problems with Traditional Tests for Lyme (Borrelia)   178

Testing for Borrelia Using Homeopathy and Energy
Medicine Modalities   179

Clinical Procedure for Treating Patients with the Bionic 880   180

The ten different treatment points   181

Using the Bionic 880 To Treat Other Health Conditions   184

Other conditions that can be successfully treated with the
Bionic 880   184

Treating For Other Infections Using Homeopathic Nosodes
and The Patient's Own Blood   186

Troubleshooting Problems in Healing   187

The Problem with Using Antibiotics for the Treatment of
Lyme Disease   188

Adjunct Therapies during Photon Treatment   189

Heal the Mind, Heal the Body   189

The Use of Immune Markers to Measure Progress in Healing   190

The Difference between North American and European Patients   191

Relative Contraindications of Photon Treatment   192

Sample Frequencies for Different Conditions   192

Recommended frequencies for conditions often found in those
with Lyme disease   193

Final Words   194

Technical Data for the Bionic 880   194

Description of the device   194

Additional Information on Photons   194

How to Contact Ingo D. E. Woitzel, M.D.   194

Author's Note   195

Translation Note   195

Chapter 7: Ronald Whitmont, M.D. 197

Biography   197

Healing Philosophy   197

Treatment Approach   200

How Many Remedies Are Required To Bring About A Cure?   203

How Long Does the Healing Process Take With Homeopathy? 204

More Thoughts on Using Antibiotics for the Treatment of
Lyme Disease 205

Are Adjunct Remedies Necessary in Homeopathy? 207

Dietary Recommendations 208

What about Treating Patients for Environmental Toxins? 208

Lifestyle Recommendations for Healing 209

The Role of Emotional Trauma in Healing 209

The Practitioner-Patient Relationship 211

Are There Herxheimer Reactions in Homeopathy? 212

The Process of Administering Remedies 216

Advantages of Homeopathy over Other Types of Treatment 217

Comparing Homeopathy to Other Types of Energy Medicine 218

Why Homeopathy Isn't Used More Widely for the Treatment
of Lyme Disease 218

Last Words 219

How to Contact Ronald Whitmont, M.D. 220

Chapter 8: Deborah Metzger, Ph.D., M.D. 221

Biography 221

Healing Philosophy 222

Sleep 223

Intestinal Dysbiosis 224

Diet & Nutrition 224

Allergies & the Immune System 225

Stealth Infections 228

Hormonal Dysfunction 228

Exercise 230

Detoxification 231

Mind-Body and Spiritual Strategies for Healing 233

Treating Lyme (Borrelia) 235

Treating Co-Infections 236

It's Not All About Borrelia 238

Other Treatments for Symptomatic Relief 240

Depression/Anxiety 240

Pain 241

Patient and Practitioner Challenges and Roadblocks to Healing 241

Mistakes in the Treatment of Lyme Disease 242

How Finances Affect Healing 243

How Friends and Family Can Help the Sick   244
Final Words   244
How to Contact Deborah Metzger, Ph.D., M.D.   245

Chapter 9: Peter J. Muran, M.D., M.B.A. 247

Biography   247
Lyme Disease: A Functional Medicine Approach   248
Environmental Inputs   250
Energy Production and Oxidative Stress   252
Detoxification and Biotransformation   253
Hormonal and Neurotransmitter Imbalances   256
Mind and Spirit   257
Structural Imbalance   258
Gastrointestinal Imbalance   260
Immune and Inflammatory Imbalance   261
Conclusion   262
Treatment Approach for Borrelia and Lyme-Related Infections   263
Other Common Infections Found in Those with Lyme Disease   266
Babesia and Bartonella   266
Dietary Recommendations   267
The Problem of Getting Patients to Change Their Diets   267
Other Uses for Amino Acids   269
The Usefulness of Metabolic Testing   270
The Role of Emotional Trauma in Illness   270
Detoxification   270
Energy Medicine Strategies for Detoxification   270
Other Detoxification Strategies   271
Healing the Gut   272
Treating Hormonal Dysfunction   274
Bacterial Behavior, Inflammation, and Hypercoagulation   277
Treatments for Symptomatic Relief   279
For Insomnia   279
For Fatigue   279
For Pain   280
Other Factors That Affect Healing   280
Philosophy on Pharmaceutical Medications   280
Less than Beneficial Approaches to Treating Lyme Disease   280

Healing Is All About Reducing the Body's Total Stress Load   281

Last words   282

How to Contact Peter J. Muran, M.D., M.B.A.   282

Chapter References   282

Chapter 10: Nicola McFadzean, N.D. 285

Biography   285

Treatment Approach   285

Treatments for Lyme and Co-Infections   286

Borrelia/Candida   286

Babesia   289

Bartonella   289

Mycoplasma   290

Ehrlichia   290

Opportunistic Viruses   290

Herbal Protocol for the Treatment of Lyme Disease   291

Supporting the Immune System   292

Treating Hormonal Dysfunction   293

Healing the Gut   294

Treatments for Symptomatic Relief   295

Insomnia   295

Pain   295

Anxiety and Depression   296

Headaches   296

Detoxification   297

Treating Detoxification Problems   298

Diet   299

Addressing Food Allergies   300

Exercise   301

Patient and Practitioner Challenges in Treating Lyme Disease   301

How Long Does It Take To Heal from Lyme Disease?   303

EFT (Emotional Freedom Technique) for Healing Emotional Trauma   303

The Role of Spirituality in Healing   303

Is Lyme Disease Always Primary in Patients' Overall Symptom Picture?   304

Hyperbaric Oxygen Treatments (HBOT) as an Adjunct to Healing   305

Beneficial Lifestyle Habits   305

How Family and Friends Can Help the Sick   306

Last Words 307

How to Contact Nicola McFadzean, N.D. 307

Chapter 11: Marlene Kunold, "Heilpraktiker" .. 309

Biography 309

How I Became Involved in Treating Lyme Disease ... 310

Healing Philosophy/Treatment Approach 314

Diagnostic Procedure 318

Hormone, Neurotransmitter and Other Types of Testing ... 319

Treating Hormonal Dysfunction 321

Treating Inflammation 323

Treating Other Infections 325

Detoxification 327

Patient and Practitioner Challenges to Healing 328

Lifestyle and Dietary Recommendations for Healing ... 330

Sleep Hygiene 330

Dietary Recommendations 330

Exercise 331

The Role of Nitric Oxide in Disease 331

Last Words 333

How to Contact Marlene Kunold, "Heilpraktiker" 333

Chapter 12: Elizabeth Hesse-Sheehan, DC, CCN.. 335

Biography 335

Healing Philosophy 336

Plant Stem Cell Extracts for the Management of Lyme and
Immune System Dysfunction 337

The Difference between Herbal Gem and PSC Plant Stem Cells ... 340

Buhner's Herbs as Stem Cells 340

Other Herbs That Are Being Used as Stem Cells 341

Detoxification 341

Using Plant Stem Cell Extracts for Detoxification 341

Other Detoxification Strategies 342

Treating Detoxification Problems 343

Diet 344

Treatments for Symptomatic Relief 345

Pain 345

Anxiety and Depression   347

Insomnia   348

Treating Hormonal Dysfunction   349

Lifestyle Recommendations for Healing   350

Therapies for Healing the Emotions and Spirit   352

Profiling the Person That Heals Fully from Lyme Disease   355

Is Lyme Disease Always the Primary Reason for Symptoms?   356

Patient and Practitioner Challenges in Treating Lyme Disease   357

How Friends and Family Can Help the Sick   359

Exercise   359

Less-than-Beneficial Lyme Disease Treatments   360

Treating Structural Problems   360

Last Words   362

How to Contact Elizabeth Hesse-Sheehan, DC, CCN   363

Chapter 13: Jeffrey Morrison, M.D. 365

Biography   365

Healing Philosophy/Treatment Approach   366

Treatment Protocol for Borrelia and Co-Infections   368

Borrelia   368

Babesia and Bartonella   369

Treating Opportunistic Infections   369

Are Lyme and Co-Infections Always the Primary Cause of
Symptoms?   369

Treating Yeast Infections   370

Heavy Metal Detoxification   370

Treating Hormonal Dysfunction   371

Treating Nutritional Deficiencies   372

Magnesium   374

Dietary Recommendations   374

Detoxification   375

Lifestyle Recommendations   376

Treatments for Symptomatic Relief   376

Insomnia   376

Pain   377

Depression/Anxiety   377

Mistakes in Treating Lyme Disease and Less-Than-Beneficial
Treatments   378

Roadblocks and Challenges to Healing   379

Friends, Family and Final Words   380

How to Contact Jeffrey Morrison, M.D.   381

Appendices 383

Why Lyme Treatments Fail, By James Schaller, M.D., M.A.R.   383

Microbes, Toxins, and Unresolved Conflicts: A Unifying Theory
Based on Interview with Dietrich Klinghardt, Ph.D., M.D.
Article by Scott Forsgren   395

About the Author 403

Lyme-Related Books & DVD's Catalog 405

Index 425

Foreword by Maureen Mcshane, M.D.

This very informative book is the first of its kind on healthcare practitioners and doctors who treat tick and insect-borne chronic illnesses with different methods. There is no single treatment answer for everyone with Lyme disease. While antibiotics may improve one person's health, the next person may need other treatments. For most, it seems that a combination of treatments works best. No matter how many hours I have spent studying Lyme disease and co-infections, I find that there is always something new to learn, so I read this book with great pleasure. It's like a window through which one can peer into other physicians' practices to see what they do to improve the health of their patients. It's a perfect addition to Connie Strasheim's first book, *The Lyme Disease Survival Guide: Physical, Lifestyle and Emotional Strategies for Healing,* which provides insights into the disease process as well as into the different approaches for treating it. The author fully understands what this illness is about and has explored it completely.

At one time, I thought that good health was the result of an excellent diet, regular exercise and rest. My perception was that this combination of strategies would keep a person healthy, no matter what happened to him or her. That attitude held me in good stead in medical school, during times when I needed endurance to complete my training. Then one day, and over the course of just one summer, all of that changed. Two weeks after construction holidays and after doing some heavy gardening in St. Donat, Quebec, I awakened one day with a headache that was accompanied by stiffness and pain in my neck and joints. I was so stiff that I had to take a fifteen-minute walk just to loosen up enough to drive to work in Chazy, NY, which was an hour south of Montreal where I lived. Over the next few days, the symptoms worsened, and I began to experience shaking chills, intense sweats, weight loss, tremors and flu-like symptoms. I couldn't eat, sleep, or think.

The Canadian healthcare system was there for me and I used it multiple times over the following ten months, yet nothing helped to return me to my former state of good health. I was met by a belief system that was unaware of Lyme disease and co-infections. During that time of my life, I saw multiple specialists, and was told that perhaps I was in early menopause. One specialist had once known someone who had experienced similar symptoms, stating that "all that she had was fibromyalgia"—as though fibromyalgia were such an insignificant disease! He then told me that I was "the healthiest-appearing patient in the office."

The usual prescription of a healthy diet, adequate rest and plenty of exercise no longer worked for me. As I became weaker, I could no longer lift weights, walk uphill or exercise. I awakened multiple times every night with pain. Long searches on the Internet became increasingly difficult for me as the initial feelings of confusion and brain fog that I had experienced led to short term memory loss just a few months later. I sent my blood to the Mayo Clinic lab, which performed a Lyme disease Western blot test on me. The results came back negative.

It's an odd feeling to be a physician, used to making decisions about other people's health and then suddenly having to depend on other physicians for your own health. I finally went to see Dr. Horowitz, an ILADS (International Lyme and Associated Diseases Society) physician who, after listening to my history, suspected that I had Lyme disease. A test through IGeneX labs confirmed this diagnosis. Dr. Horowitz, whom I later learned was part of a small but growing number of physicians deemed to be "Lyme-literate" (hence the acronym LLMD, or "Lyme-Literate Medical Doctor"), was very helpful in every way. Subsequently, I became a member of ILADS, learned more about tick-borne diseases, and was fortunate enough to be able to do a preceptorship with Dr. Horowitz, as well as with another physician named Dr. Ann Corson, in order to learn more about how to properly treat Lyme disease.

Two years of antibiotics and more years of alternative medications returned me to good health. There were many ups and downs during this time. I used alternative remedies that I would have never previously explored in my former good health. Getting over this illness can involve much more than just taking antibiotics. As you will read in this book, treatment is multi-faceted and based on the individual person's symptoms. Also, it's not just about acquiring an infection; it's about our general health at the time that we acquired the infection, as well as thereafter. It's about prior exposures to other infections, heavy metals, mold, and the mycotoxins that they produce. And, yes, regaining good health is also about eating in a healthful manner, exercising and getting rest. In fact, people that don't do these things in conjunction with other treatments don't tend to heal as well as those that do. Negative emotions adversely influence healing, as can past emotional traumas. And the list of necessary adjunct treatments goes on from there. Unless multiple areas of healing are addressed, it may be difficult to recover. Having a good support system is also important—in my case, I was fortunate enough to have a husband and family that supported me through all of the bad times. Every improvement was celebrated.

The healing journey begins when we make a conscious decision to do what it takes to return to a state of good health. This means giving ourselves permission to analyze prescription medications and different treatments, to ask questions, and be guided by others who have gone through similar experiences. Spurred on by my own poor health, I explored many different treatment alternatives during my journey back to health. There was once a time when I felt that I would never be rid of my back and leg pain. At some point, I decided to try a new healing modality, after getting lost on the Internet, and stumbling upon a NMT (NeuroModulation Technique) practitioner in Montreal. This practitioner was so skilled, that after seeing her three Fridays in a row and Herxing every weekend while being off of all medications, I woke up after the third

weekend with no back or leg pain—something that I had not expe-
rienced in three years. I then learned how to use NMT, EFT
(Emotional Freedom Technique) and TAT (Tapas Acupressure
Technique) in my own medical practice.

Over the course of my recovery, I discovered that many patients in
my practice also had Lyme disease. A significant number of them
had chronic symptoms that cleared with prolonged courses of
antibiotics. Because of the lack of Canadian doctors willing to treat
Lyme disease, Canadians began to see me for treatment. Many had
no bulls-eye rash (the supposedly "tell-tale" symptom of Lyme
disease), nor had they traveled out of the country. Up until the
previous year, I had worked for a walk-in clinic in Chazy, NY;
however, it had become increasingly difficult for me to attend to
these very ill patients in a clinic where I was supposed to see three
to four patients per hour. If I spent an hour and a half with one
patient, (which is what is required if the doctor is to take an adequate history, do a thorough physical exam and discuss the
patient's treatment plan), then the other patients would have to
wait. So I quit my job and opened my own office in Plattsburgh, NY,
in January, 2009.

I tell you my story because I want readers to understand the complexity of chronic Lyme disease. The illness can create many elusive
symptoms and therefore requires a delicate, directed, and carefully
coordinated treatment approach. The Lyme disease "complex"
involves not only Borrelia burgdorferi, which is the Lyme disease
bacteria itself, but also pathogens that are known as "co-infections,"
and which can be transmitted in the same tick bite. These co-
infections cause symptoms that may not be recognized as part of
the tick-borne illness complex by physicians who are not trained to
look for them. Testing in even the best of labs is problematic, as
some of the sickest patients may have negative test results. The
belief that there is no or little Lyme disease in Canada is an illusion
created by poor tests and ignorance of the symptoms that tick- and
insect-borne infections bring. It is all too easy to pin a meaningless
diagnosis of fibromyalgia or chronic fatigue syndrome on very ill
patients who, in reality, have Lyme disease.

The Canadian Lyme Disease Foundation (www.canlyme.org) is working with federal and provincial governments to bring about awareness of Lyme disease and co-infections to Canada. The organization is meeting with the governments of Canada, Ontario and Manitoba. However, because Lyme disease and co-infections can create multiple symptoms which become worse as time goes on and which necessitate long and expensive work-ups and multiple trips to physicians, specialists and emergency rooms, the cost to the government would be astronomical should Lyme disease be recognized for what it is and treated accordingly. Furthermore, many of the sick are no longer able to work, finish school, or support their families, which compounds the already catastrophic situation.

Regardless of the politics and money, it's time that people become aware of this problem. Many of my Canadian patients (and one from Florida who became ill while camping in Ontario) have been exposed to Borrelia in endemic areas, but were not aware of it at the time of their exposure. As a result, they did not take effective preventative measures, nor did they suspect Lyme disease after they became ill. There is not enough information out there to protect them and others like them. The Canadian Lyme Disease Foundation has been helping the public to become more aware of this health threat. It is time for our government to do the same.

Connie has produced a well-written, highly informative book for patients and practitioners alike. It's a book that I will read and re-read with interest. It's a brilliant idea to combine the approaches of multiple practitioners and their different treatment strategies into one book, and it gives readers a sense of direction and coherency when they can compare these. The book offers explanations for the different types of treatment that are out there and also gives readers new avenues of treatment to explore. I am grateful to the practitioners who generously shared their information and practice styles.

Maureen Mcshane, M.D.
American Academy of Family Practice Board Certified
Member of ILADS (International Lyme and Associated Diseases Society)
medart@sympatico.ca

Preface by Connie Strasheim

Preface by Connie Strasheim

I began researching Lyme disease in 2005, after I was first diagnosed with this devastating illness. My discoveries over the past four years have led me to try a variety of treatments, some of which have led to dramatic improvements in my symptoms. In 2007, I created a blog on Lyme disease to share the findings of my research, as well as the lessons that living with Lyme had taught me, and continues to teach me. This information can be found on the Internet at www.lymebytes.blogspot.com. In 2008, I wrote a book called *The Lyme Disease Survival Guide: Physical, Lifestyle and Emotional Strategies for Healing*, in which I share information on various Lyme disease treatments, as well as practical advice for dealing with the lifestyle and emotional difficulties of chronic illness. The latter two subjects aren't usually discussed much in Lyme books or during doctors' visits, yet I believe that addressing these aspects of illness is no less important for recovery than medical treatments.

As a result of that book, I received numerous e-mails and phone calls from other Lyme disease sufferers who shared their personal stories of suffering with me. And over the past four years, I have walked this journey alongside countless others, who, like me, have sometimes felt as though they are on a seemingly impossible quest for health. We may know that healing is possible, but we feel as though we are walking along a precipice of impossibility, because the road is long and difficult, and as long as we don't get it right, our lives—indeed, our livelihood, hangs in the balance.

While there is a lot of information out there on Lyme disease—on Internet support groups, in published conference notes and in books written by Lyme sufferers and the occasional Lyme-literate doctor—I still see many Lyme disease sufferers wandering in the wilderness, unsure of how to treat their symptoms.

These people are wondering if they are doing enough to heal; whether they should change protocol, doctor, or some other aspect of their treatment. For some, their opinions and their hope have been formed and altered by what they have read in a book or on an Internet support group, what they have seen on YouTube, or by what worked for their neighbor who had Lyme. I believe, however, that what worked for one Lyme sufferer isn't necessarily going to work for everyone else, and I have seen subtle agendas on every support group that have sometimes led people down myopic, less-than-beneficial roads. Yes, Lyme support groups can be great sources of information and comfort for those who need to learn about the disease, but my own experience has taught me that you can't stop there if you want a well-rounded perspective about how to treat the multi-faceted beast that is called Lyme. Or perhaps more appropriately, I should call it chronic illness *involving* Lyme, since treating Lyme disease is about so much more than just getting rid of infections. Neither can you stop at your neighbor who tosses out a testimonial about his own healing, attesting that X therapy is the only way to go, nor your local doctor who tells you that two rounds of doxycycline are all that you need for wellness. You might not even be able to stop at your Lyme-literate physician, who might have known more than your regular family practitioner—maybe even enough to get you out of the woods—but not enough to fix that nagging hormonal problem or fully cure you of your mysterious strain of Babesia. Or perhaps you have found answers in some of the Lyme books that are already out there, but you wonder how many people have actually been healed by these protocols, since you have tried some of them but they haven't taken you as far as you need to go.

That said, I am grateful for all of the information that has been published on Lyme disease on the Internet and in books. Without it, I would still be deep inside a dark well, wondering why my limbs and brain don't function, and just as depressed as the day when I learned that something was really awry in my biochemistry. Indeed, I am not discounting the wealth of valuable information that is already out there, but I believe that the more information that is published by Lyme-literate health care practitioners, the better off that Lyme sufferers and physicians will be.

Hence this book, and it's not only for those with Lyme, but for the health care practitioners that are treating them and who want to get deeper insights into what it really means to treat chronic illness involving Lyme. Or even what it means to treat other chronic illnesses, since the multiple dysfunctions that are found in Lyme, such as hormonal imbalances and gut dysbiosis, are also found in other chronic disease states. Because sometimes, the processes that lead to and prolong chronic illness are the same, whether you stamp them with a "Lyme" label or not.

Because I have written this book for health care practitioners and Lyme disease sufferers alike, the terminology may occasionally be difficult for, or unfamiliar to, the average layperson with Lyme. I invested a great deal of time and energy in an attempt to communicate the most difficult concepts in easy-to-understand terms for readers.

Lyme disease is one of the most complicated diseases to treat. Since no health care provider has the monopoly on treating chronic illness involving Lyme, and because other valuable perspectives exist, my goal in writing this book has been to discover and share such perspectives, with the hope of providing greater insights into healing. While Lyme-literate health care practitioners may, in some cases, have similar approaches to treating Lyme, I believe that every practitioner who has been treating this disease for any length of time has something unique to offer. That "something" may provide the missing link(s) that other practitioners need in order to help heal their patients, as well as what Lyme sufferers need to heal themselves. At the same time, by representing the perspectives of thirteen different Lyme-literate health care practitioners, the evidence of what works best for the treatment of Lyme may be silently established by the similarities, or differences, found among these practitioners' protocols.

In writing this book, I tirelessly tracked down answers to some of the more analytical questions about treating Lyme, such as: Who are those that heal, and who are those that don't? What factors play into healing besides the obvious load of infections? Questions that are asked among Lyme disease sufferers in support groups or which manifest as a vague type of wondering, but which people don't seem to be able to find answers to unless they can get into the brain of someone who has been treating Lyme patients for years.

Therefore, I wrote this book to provide insights into the treatment of Lyme disease, but in reality I am not its author. The authors are the thirteen doctors and other health care practitioners whom I interviewed and whose protocols appear in this book. I wrote down the information that they shared with me, editing and re-editing it so that it would read like a book instead of an interview. The authors then individually edited and refined their chapters upon my completion of the manuscript. A couple of them even participated in the original writing process. I am grateful for their extensive contributions. As a work involving fifteen people (when you include my publisher and editor), writing this book was an immense task, one that I did not imagine to be so labor-intensive. In the end, though, it has been worth the effort for the wealth of valuable information that I believe the book will provide to its readers. As a side note, the chapters in this book appear in no particular order; I found the information contained in all of them to be highly valuable and any attempt to organize their order would have been difficult.

As you read the book, please be aware that the information presented is not intended to provide a complete description and analysis of each practitioner's protocol, for to do so would require a separate book for each one. Instead, it is meant to provide an overview of each practitioner's healing philosophy and treatments. I do not believe this limitation to be a disadvantage, because so many with "Lyme brain" are liable to get bogged down in details. Also, the practitioners and Lyme sufferers who read this book and find the information to be useful can later focus on those ideas that are of interest to them and do further research on their own.

Furthermore, this book isn't meant to offer information on the basics of chronic Lyme disease; what it is, how it's contracted, what the symptoms are, how it's diagnosed, and so forth. For that, I encourage readers to peruse one of the other available Lyme books, or visit the ILADS (International Lyme and Associated Diseases Society) site on the Internet; www.ILADS.org, which is one of the few sites that provides accurate information on chronic Lyme disease.

Neither does this book discuss the politics of Lyme, another very important aspect of Lyme that every practitioner and Lyme sufferer should be aware of. Access to proper diagnosis and treatment has been deeply limited by political agendas, including those of the IDSA (Infectious Disease Society of America) and CDC (Centers for Disease Control). Having knowledge of the politics behind Lyme disease can make the healing journey go smoother for those with Lyme, and such knowledge is crucial for any practitioner who decides to treat cases of chronic illness involving Lyme. The treatment of chronic Lyme disease literally hangs in the balance between two diametrically opposed political positions.

Finally, while each practitioner who participated in this book offered a unique perspective, I noticed that a couple of common themes emerged as a result of the combined information. First, treating Lyme isn't just about getting rid of an infection or two; it is about addressing and treating the multiple dysfunctions or causes that led to chronic illness, Borrelia being only one of these. People don't usually just get sick because of a bacterium; they get sick because other factors contributed to the breakdown of their bodies. Secondly, when it comes to Lyme and chronic illness, there is no such thing as a one-size-fits-all protocol. Yes, it can be helpful to hear about other peoples' experiences with certain treatments, but in the end, no two people are alike, and treatment needs to be tailored to the individual. Cookbook treatments just don't work for this, or any other chronic illness.

Hopefully, this book will provide more clarity on these topics, or at least broaden the perspective of those who are seeking to learn more about Lyme disease treatments. May the book bring you, the Lyme sufferer, one step closer to the door of health, and may it bring you, the practitioner, one step closer to delivering your patients to the other side of that door.

A Note from the Publisher

This book contains a tremendous amount of information, and readers may become overwhelmed if they are not prepared to assimilate it.

When reading the book, you are encouraged to employ an "information organization strategy," so that you can keep track of the information that is most relevant and important to you.

It is recommended that while you read the book, you have at your side a highlighter marker and a notepad. You can use the highlighter to mark information that you feel is important, and that you wish to return to in the future. You can use the notepad to write down the names of treatments, tests, or procedures that you want to integrate into your treatment plan or discuss with your doctor.

• CHAPTER 1 •

Steven J. Harris, M.D.
REDWOOD CITY, CA

Biography

Steven J. Harris, M.D. has been in private practice since 2001. Dr. Harris is a medical doctor (MD), board certified in Family Practice. His private practice was operated as a sole proprietorship until 2006, after which time he formed a California medical corporation, Pacific Frontier Medical, Inc.

Since 2001, Dr. Harris has focused his practice on the diagnosis and treatment of Lyme disease and other tick-borne co-infections. He believes that chronic, persistent Lyme is an epidemic in the United States, but that there are many effective treatments available to those infected. His approach to Lyme disease incorporates strategies found in conventional, functional and complementary medicine.

Dr. Harris has taken a leadership role in CALDA (The California Lyme Disease Association), a research, patient advocate and education group which has been largely responsible for spearheading favorable legislation protecting patients' rights, expanding Lyme disease awareness and fostering continued public health education. Dr. Harris is also an active member of ILADS, (The International Lyme and Associated Diseases Society). This is a professional medical society of physicians and scientists which has become the de facto authority on effective treatment for chronic Lyme disease and is a rational counterbalance to the prevailing opinions of the IDSA (Infectious Disease Society of America), which refutes the existence of chronic Lyme disease. ILADS has focused its efforts on global physician education in order to increase the number of treating physicians available to those with Lyme.

There is currently a huge shortage of treating physicians for those with chronic Lyme disease, particularly on the West Coast. As a result, over the past three years, Dr. Harris has maintained three operating practices in various cities (Malibu, Redwood City and in Dr. Tod Thoring's practice in Arroyo Grande) in order to provide maximum geographic coverage for patients in California, Oregon and Washington. In June 2007, two new practitioners were recruited in order to increase operating efficiency and the size of the practice. Dr. Harris projects that the practice will now have more resources, with the capacity to receive twice as many patients as before.

Healing Philosophy

My healing philosophy is similar to that of Drs. Richard Horowitz, Greg Bach, Joseph Burrascano, Therese Yang and Dietrich Klinghardt. I believe that infections are a significant part of the disease process, but that (in the words of Klinghardt) "impaired physiology, biotoxin load, and immune dysregulation" are what determine the individual flavor of the disease as well as how sick people will be. I look at Borrelia burgdorferi (Bb) as one of the significant central processing organisms that make other phenomena, such as biotoxins, inorganic toxins, opportunistic infections, and the like, matter. Many people have other problems along with Bb, such as yeast, mold, viruses and metals, and while these things in themselves can make people sick, when there is no Lyme disease involved, they may not have such a profound impact upon the body. When Lyme is involved, however, these corollary factors (which are different than Lyme co-infections) begin to really wreak havoc. It's almost as if Lyme overwhelms the body to such an extent that these factors take on a life of their own. Immune surveillance and detoxification pathways in the liver, kidneys, lymphatics and skin just can't keep up. There are other infections that can cause serious illness, such as Brucella, Mycoplasmas, and maybe even mycobacterium (which causes tuberculosis), as well as others. But biotoxins, Herpes viruses, Epstein-Barr virus and people's lifestyle in general, might not matter as much if Lyme wasn't causing the body to be under so much stress.

When Lyme Disease Isn't the Primary Cause of Symptoms

There are cases of Lyme disease where Lyme isn't primary in the overall symptom picture; for example, in those who have Lyme and autism, although I am never really sure. I find that about one in four autistic kids have Lyme disease, but I don't think that Lyme is usually the primary reason for these kids' autism. It's a contributing factor, but may not be the main reason why they have autism. Also, while it may be important for people who have conditions such as ALS, Alzheimer's and rheumatoid arthritis, in addition to Lyme disease, to treat their Lyme, this doesn't mean that Lyme is their central problem or even causing the majority of their symptoms.

That said, the Borrelia organism can go dormant in the body at times, especially if one keeps pounding away relentlessly at the infection. Whenever I see this happen in my patients, I find that heavy metals, mold, a parasite or some other problem often surfaces and temporarily becomes the main (biggest) issue for them. Such issues must then also be treated.

Also, the body can only do so much simultaneous work, so as a physician, I have to pick and choose the problems that I want to treat in my patients at any particular given time. So if Borrelia is their core problem, but they present twenty different obstacles to treatment, then I might need to first address some of those obstacles, and then afterwards, focus on the Borrelia. For example, when patients have significant dental infections, or even structural abnormalities, such as bad TMJ, and if they are really sick, then I find that unless I deal with these other infections or structural problems, then it is very hard to treat their Lyme infections successfully with just antibiotics. So I may recommend, for example, that they have dental work done to deal with anaerobic infections in the mouth and which cause conditions such as osteonecrosis and osteomyelitis. Once these problems are treated, then it's much easier to treat the Lyme infections. Some physicians have an order in which they treat patients' problems, but I don't necessarily believe that there is a cookbook order in which to do things, because each person is unique. I do believe, in any case, that it is important to address those obstacles that interfere with the proper treatment of Lyme infections.

Antibiotic Treatments for Infections

I am a student of many doctors who came before me treating Lyme. I'm trying to stand on the shoulders of giants, but I sometimes think that those giants are standing so high up and doing such amazing work, that it's hard for me to top that.

I don't have a standard protocol that I use for all of my patients. My treatments for Lyme infections generally involve homeopathic, herbal, naturopathic, and sometimes even energy medicine methods, along with a strong pharmaceutical approach. I find that most of my patients need to take some pharmaceutical antibiotics to really knock out the infections. Using alternative methodologies alone makes it much less likely, statistically, that they will get over the disease.

My antibiotic approach is similar to that of Dr. Horowitz's, and includes the use of double intracellular antibiotics, along with cell-wall and cyst-busting drugs such as metronidazole and tinidazole (5-nitroimidazoles) or nitazoxanide. I might also use macrolide and tetracycline drugs, as well as third generation cephalosporins. I don't necessarily administer these all at the same time and some I will rotate.

I also aggressively treat co-infections, and while I don't believe that it is mandatory to treat co-infections first, if I have to give my patients IV antibiotics for Borrelia, then I will treat their co-infections before I treat their Borrelia. With the exception of Babesia, antibiotic regimens for co-infections must also be rotated and switched on a regular basis. For Babesia, treatments are most effective when patients start with one type of medication and stay on it for a long period of time, and then over time, "stack" other medications on top of that one. Medications for Babesia include intracellular and anti-parasitic drugs such as atovaquone (Mepron or Malarone), mefloquin (Lariam), or clindamycin, quinine, nitazoxanide (Alinia), and possibly metronidazole. Using an extracellular phase drug such as primaquin can be useful, too. The most effective way to treat the Babesia species, however, is still somewhat up in the air in the medical community.

When patients first come into my office, if I know that they have Borrelia but I'm not sure whether they have co-infections, then I will order co-infection tests. In the meantime, I will either wait to treat them or start them on a medication such as Zithromax (azithromycin). Zithromax is a good drug to start with, because if it turns out that patients have Bartonella, then Zithromax combines well with rifampin (which is used for treating Bartonella). Or if patients have Babesia, then Zithromax combines well with Mepron (which is used for treating Babesia). Or if their test results show Ehrlichia, then doxycycline, minocycline, tetracycline or rifampin can all be added to the Zithromax. If patients end up having only Borrelia, then I can combine Zithromax with a cephalosporin or tetracycline drug, or even a cyst buster if it seems that their bodies are hardy and can handle aggressive treatment right away.

I often prescribe parenteral (IV or IM) therapy to patients that have strong neurological symptoms, to those who have been very sick for more than a year, who have gastrointestinal problems, or who can't tolerate oral medications. I tend to try oral antibiotics for at least three months, before going the intravenous route. This is because if I hit patients with IV medications too fast, then they may get worse as a result of a severe Jarisch-Herxheimer reaction. This occurs when too much of a toxic load is created in the body and the organs become stressed as a result. IV medications may also perpetuate too much yeast overgrowth. For these reasons, I feel that I might be playing with fire if I start some of my patients off with IV antibiotics.

It can also be difficult to treat patients if they have a lot of co-infections, such as Bartonella, Mycoplasma, Babesia and Ehrlichia, or if they are quite ill with predominant symptoms of one or two of these co-infections. Such patients tend to get very strong reactions to treatments, which means that I can't hit their infections as directly as I would like, because they will get too sick. Doxycycline, in particular, creates this type of scenario, especially in women. So while it may be an effective medication, I don't like to use it in patients that have multiple, or severe, co-infections. Many practitioners like to start with doxycycline because it's cheap and is mostly metabolized in the colon (instead of the liver and kidneys), which means that it's fairly easy on the organs. It also has great activity against Borrelia, Anaplasma and Ehrlichia, and is somewhat effective for treating Babesia, Bartonella and Mycoplasma, but I find that people just "tank" if they take doxycycline when they have a lot of co-infections.

Doing oxidative stress, organic acid, plasma amino acids, RBC elements, mold antibody and stool tests, as well as tests for heavy metals, yeast and other environmental pollutants can help me to get an idea of what problems my patients have besides Lyme infections. Such information also helps me to determine whether they will "crash" on a particular antibiotic regimen.

Blood tests such as the C3A, C4A, CD-57, C3D, C1-Q Immune Complex and even ANA, rheumatoid factor and other immune tests of the like, tell me the amount of inflammation that patients have, which also helps me to determine the likelihood of them getting worse on a regimen. Doing a methylation panel and genetic profile can also be useful for this purpose.

A promising new test from Genelix assesses what drugs patients can tolerate, based on their genotype. As well, it measures other functions, such as how well they metabolize, assimilate and methylate. Such information enables me to determine whether my patients have liver detoxification or other problems. If test results demonstrate that they don't tolerate antibiotics very well, for example, then I might refrain from prescribing drugs and instead put them on a detoxification protocol until their ability to tolerate medications increases.

If I suspect that my patients are sensitive to medications, I will start by prescribing them a gentle medication for Borrelia, or treat them instead for co-infections, as I watch for signs of "crashing." In the past, I used to hit my patients hard with antibiotics, and they would eventually get better, but they would also have a flare-up or Herxheimer reaction for up to twelve or fifteen months following treatment, and that isn't acceptable to me. When patients already feel bad, they can't feel "more bad" for a year and a half before starting to feel good, especially if there is no promise that they are ever going to feel good in the first place! If patients do poorly on antibiotic regimens, then it means that I need to deal with other problems that they have and which are blocking the antibiotics from being fully effective. Or I might send them to a naturopathic doctor who knows a lot about detoxification, such as Drs. Claire Riendeau, Nicola McFadzean (see Dr. McFadzean's chapter later in this book for more information on her protocol), Susan Marra and Amy Derksen, where they can receive detoxification treatments before I start them again on antibiotics.

Typical Symptoms of Different Infections

Babesia

Since tests don't always reveal whether patients are co-infected, I also rely on clinical diagnoses to determine which infections, besides Borrelia, are present and causing problems for my patients. For example, if my female patients aren't menopausal, (I can check hormones to verify this) and have night sweats, flushing, severe pressure-like headaches, violent nightmares or vivid dreams, significant shortness of breath in the absence of another cause, frequent sighing or dry coughing in the absence of cardiac issues, then they may have Babesia. To ascertain the diagnosis, I might give them a clinical provocation test, especially if their lab test results are negative. For the clinical provocation, I might ask them to take herbs such as cryptolepsis or artemisia, as I observe their reaction to these. Dr. Tod Thoring in Arroyo Grande makes a cryptolepsis compound which consists of cryptolepsis, smilax, and boneset, as well as a cryptolepsis, artemisia and teasel cream, which are quite effective for this purpose. I may also use the herbal formulas Enula and Mora (NutraMedix brand), or some of the rizol oils (BioPure). Positive patient response to any of these can indicate that a parasitic infection is present. I'm not always 100% certain that the parasite is Babesia, but the tests help me to better estimate what it is. I will also sometimes do a provocation test in those already known to be infected with Lyme, using hydroxychloroquine and Zithromax, or Flagyl with Zithromax, because Babesia responds to these medications, too.

Bartonella

Typical symptoms in those with Bartonella and Borrelia (unlike the Bartonella that results from Cat Scratch disease) include ice pick-like headaches, major photophobia, anxiety or psychiatric issues, and even bi-polar symptoms. Neuropathy, reflex sympathetic dystrophy (RSD) or autism may also manifest, as well as significant cardiac or gut problems. The non-blanching "streaks" that some people find on their skin may also be a telling symptom. Some argue that plantar fascial pain is found in both Babesia and Bartonella, but I think that it is more related to Bartonella. In any case, whenever extreme anxiety is patients' overriding symptom and is found in conjunction with neuropathic symptoms, such as burning pain, then I suspect that a Bartonella-like organism is causing these symptoms.

Ehrlichia and Anaplasma

If patients have profound fatigue and severe muscle pain, especially in conjunction with high liver enzymes, low white blood cell counts and fevers, they may have Ehrlichia.

Mycoplasma

Because Mycoplasma is an intracellular organism, it's difficult to test for, but many of my patients have it. Persistent arthritis, especially in one joint that is really swollen, or a rheumatoid arthritis presentation indicate the possible presence of Mycoplasma. In children, major psychiatric problems may also indicate that the infection is present.

Lyme (Borrelia)

People with Borrelia can have all of the aforementioned symptoms, as well as many others, because Borrelia runs the gamut of symptoms. For that reason, those with this infection may feel bad in a number of different ways. Symptoms usually migrate with this infection, however, and/or tend to flare for four to seven days per month.

Also, I think that co-infections like Babesia, Bartonella, and Ehrlichia are generally not important factors in patients' overall symptom picture unless Bb (Borrelia burgdorferi) is present to give them a foothold.

I do find that some of my patients have only Bb, without any other co-infections, especially those that have been sick for more than twenty years. Such patients have been living at a lower level of functionality, and may have been suffering from symptoms of generalized pain, fatigue and cognitive issues for a tremendous amount of time. Yet, because their problems tend to be mostly related to pure Lyme disease (Borrelia), they are often easier to treat than the co-infected patients.

Other Symptomatic Trends

Another trend that I have observed is that almost all of my patients that have Lyme disease (Bb) along with rheumatoid arthritis, MS (Multiple Sclerosis), Alzheimer's or Parkinson's, are also likely to have Babesia. If I had to guess, I would say that at least a third of all Lyme disease sufferers have co-infections, and possibly more.

Using Herbal Remedies to Treat Borrelia and Other Infections

I find that I have the most success treating my patients with herbs when I use them in conjunction with pharmaceutical antibiotics. If I were to recommend only herbs for the treatment of Lyme disease, there would be frequent treatment failures. If I prescribed only antibiotics, then I would have to use more antibiotics than if I had combined them with herbs. I think that herbs really act to heighten the effects of antibiotics, and therefore, I generally formulate a protocol using two to eight anti-microbial herbs, in addition to one to four antibiotics.

Dr. Thoring, whom I mentioned earlier, has come up with a promising herbal tincture, called BLT from Clinical Response Formulas, which contains red root, teasel, boneset, black walnut, lomatium, smilax, and stillengia. I find this product to work really well for the treatment of Borrelia and Bartonella, and it may also have some activity against Babesia.

Other herbs or herbal formulas that I use in my practice include Mora, Enula, Cumanda and Banderol from NutraMedix; cryptolepsis from Woodland Essence; the rizol oils Epsilon, My, Kappa,

Gamma and Zeta from BioPure; and Dr. Zhang's herbal products Circulation P, houttuynia, allicin, artemisia and coptis. I also use a bit of noni on occasion, as well as Borrelogen and Microbogen from David Jernigan, and some of the herbal cocktails from Monastery of Herbs. I may also recommend homeopathic remedies to my patients, such as Bioresource's homeopathic molds, Notatum and Quentans and the homeopathic bacteria, Fermis and Subtilis. Stephen Buhner's recommended herbs, such as andrographis, resveratrol, stephania root, and cat's claw, are likewise important, as are chanca piedra and whole garlic. Garlic is beneficial for those who don't have trouble metabolizing sulfur-containing foods. Finally, I use olive leaf extract and monolaurin or lauricidin for viruses, oregano oil for yeast, and products from Raintree, such as Myco, Amazon C-F and A-F for various other purposes. All of the aforementioned are just the antimicrobial herbs that I use in my practice; there are others that I recommend for supporting the body in the healing process.

Detoxification

Treatments

Before I can detoxify my patients, I have to get their adrenal glands working. I recommend a broad range of adrenal supplements for this purpose, including adaptogens such as rhodiola, Cordyceps mushroom, ashwaganda and Researched Nutritional's Multiplex and NT Factor Energy. Vitamins B-5 and C, magnesium, molybdenum, and adrenal glandular formulas are likewise important. I also sometimes recommend Bezwecken's Isocort, or occasionally, hydrocortisone in low doses.

To address the drainage aspect of detoxification—that is, that which involves opening up the body's detoxification pathways so that toxins can more freely leave the body, I recommend that my patients take Burbur and Parsley from NutraMedix. These are definite staples in my practice. I also use L-Drain and K-Drain from Transformation Products, Bioresource's Mundipur, apo-Hepat, Renelix, Itires and Toxex.

For liver support, I recommend Liver Extende, which is a sarsaparilla and artichoke complex; Hepol from Projoba and Medcaps DPO from Xymogen, as well as alpha-lipoic acid, glutathione, and other glutathione precursors. Red and green clay, especially Argiletz clay and plain USP grade bentonite, are also remarkably useful. David Jernigan's CNS Neuro-Antitox II, a product called Detox Factors from Natural Partners, and sometimes concentrated fruit juices such as acai, mangosteen extract and goji berry are beneficial, too. In addition, Pinella from NutraMedix, red root, burdock root, beet juice, dandelion leaf and root, all aid in the functioning of various detoxification pathways. Finally, I may recommend that my patients use detox footpads and ionic footbaths, castor oil packs, and digestive enzymes such as Wobenzym, Vitalzym, Inflammaquel (Researched Nutritionals), as well as others.

Doing bodywork aids in detoxification. I have found therapies such as craniosacral, lymphatic and abdominal massage to be beneficial for my patients, as well as upper cervical therapy, which is a technique that increases blood flow to the brain. Dr. William Amalu performs the latter and is quite good at using it in his practice. NET (Neuro-Emotional Technique) is a physiological strategy that can also be really helpful for getting the body to release toxins. Also, I recommend stretching exercises and skin brushing techniques to all of my patients.

If heavy metals are a problem, I recommend chelation therapy using agents such as chlorella, cilantro, zeolites, DMSA, DMPS and Calcium Disodium EDTA. OSR also shows a lot of promise, especially when mixed with phospholipids. Chelex from Xymogen, Metalloclear and Ultraclear from Metagenics are also good, gentle chelation products.

Finally, I give chlorella to almost all of my patients, because I think that its uses and benefits are numerous. I may also use other toxin binders, everything from Cholestyramine to activated charcoal, Nanotech Chitosan from Allergy Research Group, glucomannan and apple or citrus pectin. Other practitioners may recommend additional or different binders.

Addressing Detoxification Problems

Compromised detoxification mechanisms in those with Lyme disease are sometimes due to methylation pathway defects. To correct this type of problem, I may recommend that my patients do the Amy Yasko protocol, and in the meantime, try to get the ammonia out of their bodies, using things like yucca root, BH4, and sometimes RNA Ammonia Support Formula. Rich Van Konynenburg has developed a simplified version of the Yasko protocol that seems to have some clinical utility. I also find that Dr. Richard's plant stem cells (Gemmo therapy) can be remarkable for fixing detoxification problems, but I tend to refer my patients out for this type of treatment.

One of the problems with patients who aren't able to detoxify well is that they are nutritionally depleted. Intracellularly, they aren't able to absorb their nutrients, so one of the things that I do to correct this problem is to order a urine and plasma amino acid profile and red blood cell elements test. I then recommend that they supplement their diets with whatever minerals and amino acids that they happen to be deficient in, according to their test results. Administering IV amino acids and minerals is sometimes necessary. I may also recommend that they take Peltier Electrolytes from Crayhon Research, which is kind of like glorified Gatorade, but which works well to replenish some of the cell's missing elements. I may also send patients out for IV nutrition, to receive different Myer's cocktails and such, to get them more nutritionally balanced.

Immune System Supplements

Various immune supplements can be beneficial for strengthening the immune system, which is another important component to healing from the Lyme disease complex. I sometimes administer intramuscular transfer factor to my patients, or I may give them Researched Nutritionals' Transfer Factor LymPlus, or Multi-

Immune Transfer Factor, the latter of which can be really useful for calming down an overactive immune system. I also use low-dose Naltrexone in my practice.

Healing the Gut

It's important for me to support my patients' physiology, to the extent that I am able, by adding the right kind of nutrition to their diets and which is easy for them to tolerate. Many of my patients are gluten and casein-sensitive, and have lots of food allergies, so eliminating these allergens from their diets is important.

In order to heal their guts and decrease Leaky Gut syndrome, I may give them substances such as Xymogen's IgG-2000 DF, which are bovine source immunoglobulins that calm the gut down. I may use this in conjunction with a product called Intestimax, which is a combination of marshmallow, butyrate, and glutamine that supports the integrity of the intestinal lining. Or I might give them rectal butyrate, which also calms the gut, or Ketotifen, which reduces inflammation and promotes healing of the intestine. Sygest, Juvecal and Roqueforti, as well as other spagyric homeopathics from Bioresource are likewise useful for this purpose.

After this, I will start treating their yeast problems. Yeast overgrowth must be controlled in order to fully heal the gut, and I use a broad range of remedies for getting rid of yeast; everything from cellulase to caprylic acid, pau d' arco, and oregano oil, to the pharmaceutical medications.

Treating Hormonal Dysfunction

Balancing hormones is a remarkably important component to healing from Lyme disease. In Lyme, the HPA (hypothalamic-pituitary-adrenal axis) is severely impaired and it's one of the more difficult areas of the body to heal. Plant stem cells seem to help the HPA-axis to some degree, but I think that hormones are one of the areas in medicine that still needs to be researched, if practitioners really want to optimize their patients' whole endocrine system.

Bioidentical hormones, when used properly, can help to restore HPA function in some with Lyme disease. Borrelia likes to destroy the body's connective tissue, and endocrine glands have a lot of connective tissue, so it is important to get antibiotics and other antimicrobials into those glands. Optimizing endocrine function is also important, but if practitioners improperly prescribe hormones, then their patients can get "out of whack." For that reason, I often refer my patients to an endocrinologist or skilled naturopathic physician who can more properly deal with this aspect of their healing.

Lifestyle Recommendations for Healing

I think that "island life" (tranquility and few toxins) is probably best for the chronically ill, although this lifestyle probably isn't realistic for most. In any case, it's important that those with Lyme get away from sources of electromagnetic stress wherever possible. Even though there may be more healing resources in cities, those who are a little more off "the grid," will fare better with their treatments. Living a slower paced life is also beneficial for healing, as is consuming a diet rich in organic food. It's okay for those with Lyme to have animal protein but it needs to be really clean, healthy meat. Basically, those who are leading really clean lives, in the absence of as many environmental toxins as possible, have greater success in their healing journey.

Diet

It is important that people with Lyme maintain a non-gluten, sugar and yeast-free diet, while keeping their body's pH up by eating foods that promote less acidic blood. For those with methylation problems, keeping sulfur-containing foods like broccoli and garlic to a minimum, as well as onions and animal protein, is a good idea. Blood type diets might be beneficial for some. I have observed that blood types A and AB have the most difficult time tolerating treatments, so such people might benefit from following a blood type diet. Eliminating dairy from the diet is especially important for those with arthritis and certain neurological conditions. Finally, those with Lyme should minimize any other food allergies that show up on their IgG and IgA blood test results.

Exercise

I think that Dr. Burrascano's approach to exercise is right on. He advocates weight training with lightweights, as well as stretching-type exercises, but cautions against doing too much aerobic exercise. I agree that people with Lyme need to stretch and do gentle exercises, and that too much aerobic exercise, too fast, will deplete the adrenal glands, decrease T-cells, and open up the blood-brain barrier so that more Borrelia can get into the brain. Anaerobic-type exercises are more important, especially when people are just starting on a new treatment protocol.

Treatments for Symptomatic Relief

Insomnia

My approach to treating insomnia is to start by giving my patients one sleep remedy at a time, and then adding others as necessary, by "stacking" them up, one on top of the other, until patients are able to sleep well. I start by recommending natural remedies such as glycine, L-theanine and GABA. Dr. Zhang has a fantastic product called Herb Som, which contains schizandra. To overcome insomnia, it is important that those with Lyme find supplements that promote their GABA pathways.

If the natural remedies don't work for my patients, then I will prescribe them pharmaceutical drugs. I will basically do everything under the sun to get them to sleep, so if the drugs don't work, then as a last resort, I will refer them out to a psychiatrist for a prescription of Xyrem, which seems to help when all else fails.

Pain

To treat my patients' nerve pain, I use everything from transdermal remedies to non-steroidal anti-inflammatory drugs. Ketoprofen cream, Kaprex from Metagenics, Kapp Arrest from Biotics, Saloxicin and Doloryx from Xymogen and UltraInflamX from Metagenics are all useful. Key and Wellness Pharmacies have transdermal neuropathy creams and gels, which are made and combined using different preparations. I also use medications such as Gabapentin and Lyrica, and occasionally, Valproic acid, Carbamazepine and Dilantin. I try to stay away from prescribing narcotic drugs, because over the long run, they increase inflammatory cytokines in the body.

If my patients' pain cannot be relieved by any of the aforementioned strategies, then I will refer them to a pain management specialist. Kids often need more pain management than adults.

Finally, curcumin from turmeric can be extremely helpful for lowering inflammation and reducing pain, as can bee venom and urine therapy (although I don't use the latter in my practice). Energetic work, stretching and detoxification strategies can also relieve pain, depending upon its source. Getting to the source of the pain is important for determining what the best remedy will be. If my patients' pain is in the morning, sometimes it's due to toxins in their bodies. If it gets worse throughout the day, then it may be that their Lyme infections are causing the pain.

Depression and Anxiety

As is true for pain, when prescribing remedies for anxiety and depression, it's important to know the cause of these symptoms. Sometimes, I find it necessary to prescribe anti-depressants, and I refer my patients to Lyme-literate psychiatrists that I know. I'm not a big fan of drugs, but sometimes people need them, at least for a short while. To help determine the underlying cause of my patients' anxiety or depression, I sometimes check their neurotransmitter levels using labs such as NeuroScience or Sanesco, and then recommend amino acids and other supplements to make up for any deficiencies. Just supplementing with magnesium or selenium can often be remarkably helpful, as can detoxifying the body of heavy metals, supporting its nutrition, and getting rid of ammonia and other neurotoxins.

Fatigue

Fatigue is one of the more difficult symptoms to treat, but it's one of the most bothersome. Like other symptoms, it is important to discover its cause, which is no easy task. Provigil, NT Factor Energy, glutathione and methyl or hydroxy B-12 can be beneficial for reducing this symptom. If patients don't have a lot of yeast, using D-ribose or even some of the Mannatech glyconutrient products may also be helpful.

Brain Fog

Thinning the blood with low dose coumadin, heparin, boluoke (lumbrokinase), serrapeptase, ginkgo or Pentoxyphylline can sometimes reduce brain fog and other cognitive symptoms. Puerarin, yucca root, NutraMedix Pinella, chlorella, and Bacopa are also good for this purpose.

Healing Emotional Trauma

Emotional trauma is a huge component of illness and can be a block to patients' healing. I think that in a sense, cells hold on to memories. Doing therapies that access the subconscious mind, such as EMDR and hypnosis, can be helpful for releasing traumatic memories on a cellular level, as can Family Constellation work and psychotherapy. Really looking deep within the self to discover the spiritual causes of illness, as well as faithfully exploring and healing past memories is important. People with Lyme often need to "go deep" in order to heal their emotional trauma.

Who Are Those That Heal From Lyme Disease? Who Are Those That Don't?

The people who tend to heal from Lyme disease are those who don't know how sick they are. They are those who are out there doing things, living life and functioning amidst all of the adversity that Lyme disease brings into their lives. They are the ones who really push themselves to get better, which means that ironically, the most adrenally-depleted people might be those who are having the most success with their recovery. Such people go out and get sunshine every day. They stretch and do all the tasks that are required of them to heal, such as daily skin brushing, colonics and keeping a good diet. They are able to focus on their symptoms but not make the symptoms the focus of their lives.

Also, people who can roll with the punches, take things in stride, adapt to adversity, self-manage symptoms as they come up and make decisions on their own, are those who heal. They are of the sort who can make the decision to stop a supplement if they no longer need it, and to research new supplements but not base their life decisions upon what others tell them about those supplements. They hunker down and stay in the healing process for the long haul, and can balance immediate gratification with deferred gratification. They are open to trying new things, don't focus on every single symptom that manifests in their bodies and don't have to know the reason "why" for everything; for example, why certain remedies work and why certain things are happening to their bodies.

I think that it is really important for those with Lyme to have a positive attitude, too. This can be taken to a fault; some Lyme sufferers might be "happy herxing" for two years, and I think that's ridiculous, but it's good if they are able to adapt to adversity and to view failures as a bump in the road, instead of as a curse.

For example, the person who is able to get over a gallbladder attack, a negative reaction to a medication or an IV line complication and say, "Okay, that didn't work, let's try something else," instead of becoming despondent and giving up, has an easier time healing. Those who don't get "stuck" in persistent thoughts of disease or who don't get post-traumatic stress from their illness or treatments also heal faster than those who do.

Toxic partners are another block to healing. It's extremely difficult for family members to understand what the sick person is going through, and it can be a huge detriment to that person's healing.

Likewise, when people harbor anger, blame others, get stuck and hung up on details, or have other forms of emotional distress, their healing becomes compromised.

Other impediments to healing include mold, yeast and other toxic chemicals in the environment.

Finally, people who aren't on the Internet all of the time asking questions about Lyme disease and getting totally despondent when hearing stories about patients who kill their pastors, have an easier time healing!

The Role of Spirituality in Healing

I think that there's a spiritual component to healing that really matters. People need to feel connected to something larger than themselves, whether that something is found within a formal religion or elsewhere. If there's a way that those with Lyme can interface with the divine, such as through prayer or meditation, then this can make a positive difference for them in their healing journey.

How Finances Affect Healing

Lyme disease is sadly, a disease for the rich. That financial resources are directly related to one's pace of improvement causes me more consternation in my treatment of Lyme patients than anything else. I can do ten thousand things under the sun for them, but if financial limitations are the main thrust of their stress, then it's really hard to get them better. If they can't pay for probiotics, for example, or some of the main detoxification supplements, then their healing becomes complicated. It's difficult to admit, but it's almost as if the wealthier patients are paving the way for the right protocols to emerge and get out there. Until a streamlined path to wellness becomes clearer, however, patients without financial resources will have a more difficult time getting better.

That said, I have some patients who, through the help of their friends, church, synagogue or family, have been able to make things happen for themselves, even when they thought that they couldn't afford a particular treatment. They have done this by going beyond in their thinking. They tell themselves things like, "I am going to do this IV treatment and I'm not going to get stuck on the details about how it's going to happen. I'm also not going to go bankrupt, or if I do, then I will refinance my house." They find a way. So I believe that those who can completely prioritize this disease and the healing process, get better. Those who say things like, "I have $2,000 and if I don't get better after I spend all of that, then I am going to kill myself," surely won't get better after spending that $2,000.

Mistakes in Treating Lyme and Less-Than-Beneficial Treatments

When health care practitioners only focus on treating co-infections, then that is a problem, as is excessively focusing on any one single aspect of healing. Having pre-defined cocktails for patients is also detrimental to their well being.

When it comes to specific treatments, I am concerned about non-frequency specific Rife machines, IV hydrogen peroxide, the salt/C protocol and colloidal silver IV's. I think that while they have their place in healing Lyme disease, and I have seen some people improve by doing them, there may be problems with such treatments.

I am also cautious about the "latest, greatest treatments" that come down the pipeline. Over the past nine years, I have seen so many treatments that patients grab onto just because they are new, but few have long-term benefits. While it may be true that the trailblazing practitioners are occasionally developing groundbreaking protocols, it is not prudent for those with Lyme to try every one as soon as it arrives. I believe that it would be more responsible for them to watch and wait for a year or so to see what complications arise and what benefits others receive as a result of such treatments. I saw problems arise with MMS and intracellular heat therapy, for instance, and do not want to be an agent of harm in a mad dash to get people well.

The Biggest Challenge for People with Lyme Disease

People with Lyme disease are generally really sick, and have been this way for a long time, but their families, doctors or friends sometimes don't believe that they are unwell and their insurance companies often won't pay for their care. As a result, they feel isolated, as if they have been living in a twilight zone, or are going crazy. So they develop mistrust of others, and even of themselves, and they start questioning whether they are legitimately sick. The second-guessing and this burden of guilt that people develop from being so pushed aside, is the number one most difficult aspect of having Lyme disease. But truly, people with Lyme are some of the sickest people on the planet, and treatment regimens are some of the most complex that I can imagine in medicine. I have had patients on up to fifty different medications and over one hundred and fifty herbs at different times during their treatment. Treatment regimens are so complex, but often, Lyme patients can't even cognitively "get it together" enough to listen to instructions about what they need to do to get better. They aren't healthy enough to manage their own care, but the only way to heal from Lyme disease is through a lot of self-management, so they are stuck in all these catch 22's, and there are just a few ways out. So it can be very beneficial to have friends and family members who can help them through it all.

How Friends and Family Can Help the Sick

Friends and family of the sick should read Pamela Weintraub's book, *Cure Unknown*, and watch the documentary, *Under Our Skin*. They should go to Lyme disease conferences on occasion and do research on Lyme. They should accompany their loved one to doctor's appointments at least some of the time, and become highly informed about what this disease is about, and realize that it doesn't just affect the patient, but the entire family.

One of the biggest problems with Lyme disease sufferers who have partners is that their libido is so low, or they hurt, so they don't want to have physical contact with their healthy partner. People usually marry one another when they are healthy, and even though they make promises to be there for each other "in sickness and in health," during times of sickness, the healthy spouse often gets "caregiver fatigue," or becomes angry and frustrated at the partner who is sick. Partners need to be aware of this and seek counseling to deal with it, so that they don't take these feelings out on their loved one, who is already suffering greatly as a result of illness. Family members and partners of Lyme sufferers need to realize that counseling is not only for the sick, but also for healthy people trying to stay healthy. That said, caregivers also need to take time off from care giving; spending occasional weekends or vacations alone can restore their capacity to help their loved one.

Finally, it's important that parents of children with Lyme disease not make their child's illness the overriding, defining characteristic of the family. Parents tend to become overwrought with stress when their kids get Lyme, but they need to remember that their kids have hopes, aspirations and desires outside of their illness. The kid is not just a sick person; there's still a lot more to him or her than the illness. Of course, parents need to ask their children how they are feeling, and if they are hurt or tired, but they shouldn't make the child's illness the central defining characteristic of their relationship. They need to find a healthy balance in their conversations and attitudes toward their child, which can be difficult.

How Long Does It Take to Heal from Lyme Disease?

Most of my patients need treatment for anywhere from nine months to three years, if they do everything right. If they comply with their treatment regimens, then most of them should get 90% or more better.

Last Words

We are coming up with new treatments all of the time. There is hope for those with Lyme disease! If current technology hasn't been able to figure it out, there are enough talented practitioners out there who care, who are researching and who are dedicated to their patients' care, and for this reason, I believe that better answers will come, in time.

How to Contact Steven J. Harris, M.D.

Pacific Frontier Medical
570 Price, #200
Redwood City, CA 94063
(650) 474-2130

•CHAPTER 2•

Steven Bock, M.D.
RHINEBECK, NY

Biography

Dr. Steven Bock has been practicing complementary and progressive medicine for over thirty years. He has treated the Lyme disease complex for over twenty-five years, utilizing the ILADS approach, by combining complementary with integrative medicine. He attended New York Medical College and received his M.D. in 1971. He became board certified in Family Practice in 1977, and holds a certification in Acupuncture, as well. Dr. Bock is Co-Founder and Co-Director of the Rhinebeck Center. He is a Diplomate of the American College of Family Practice, the American Academy of Acupuncture and the American Academy of Anti-Aging Medicine. He has been a member of International Lyme and Associated Diseases Society (ILADS) for the past twelve years, and has served for two years as a board member. Dr. Bock's medical practice merges traditional medicine with alternative and complementary medicine, and combines acupuncture, homeopathy, herbal, functional, nutritional and environmental medicine into an integrated medical model for optimal wellness. *Stay Young the Melatonin*

Way was Dr. Bock's first book, and was published in 1995 by Dutton. He has also co-authored two books with his brother, Kenneth Bock, M.D., entitled *Natural Relief of Your Child's Asthma,* published in 1999 by Harper Collins, and *The Germ Survival Guide,* published in 2003 by McGraw-Hill. Nancy Faass, MSW, MPH participated in the latter work. Dr. Bock has written for local and national newspapers, and lectured locally and nationally. He has appeared on local and national media including the ABC news show, 20/20, as well as other radio and television programs.

The History of My Practice

I started my career in family practice using traditional medicine; however, my practice quickly became more integrative, involving nutrition and the treatment of allergies and chronic conditions such as chronic fatigue syndrome and chelation therapy for cardiac issues. That was about twenty-nine years ago (I have been in practice for over thirty years). Then, about twenty-five years ago, I started using acupuncture and Chinese medicine in my practice, at the same time that I started seeing a lot more patients with chronic fatigue syndrome. These people had symptoms of joint pain, cognitive dysfunction and fatigue, as well as other typical CFS symptoms. Some of them had tested negative for Lyme disease but their symptoms resembled those of Lyme and when I would give them antibiotics, they would improve. At that time, however, I was very "anti-antibiotic", preferring to give my patients herbs and natural remedies for their symptoms, and they would often become symptom-free from allergies and other ailments with such remedies. (I now believe, however, that in the case of Lyme disease, antibiotics are absolutely necessary).

Not long thereafter, I began to treat patients for Lyme disease, and it all started with a woman who was an advocate for one of the early Lyme disease support groups. She came into my office, put her chart down in front of me, which included information from three different Lyme disease conferences, and said, "Here, read this. I have decided that you are going to be my doctor." I thought that was an interesting introduction into the field. Since then, I have treated many cases of Lyme disease.

Over the past twelve years and as mentioned in my biography, I have also been a member of ILADS (International Lyme and Associated Diseases Society). It used to be that the doctors in this organization took an antibiotics-only approach to treating Lyme disease. Now, most Lyme-literate practitioners agree that an integrative treatment approach to Lyme is necessary and that the disease can't be treated with antibiotics alone.

Finally, about seven or eight years ago, I become board certified in anti-aging medicine, so I now also utilize a lot of functional endocrinology including natural hormone replacement in my practice, which is an integral part of treating the Lyme disease complex.

Currently, my practice is about 50% Lyme disease cases and 50% other conditions.

Changing the Paradigm of "One Disease, One Medicine"

I had a very interesting case a couple of months ago. A patient who had previously been admitted to the hospital for polyarthritis came into my clinic. She was taking a medication called methotrexate, which is, I believe, a very dangerous arthritis drug that suppresses the immune system. She was also on prednisone. Suspicious that she had Lyme disease, I gave her some nutrients and started her on an antibiotic regimen. Meanwhile, her rheumatologist monitored her progress with me. After finishing the antibiotics, she was 95% better. Her doctor wrote a letter to me, stating that although he wasn't familiar with my protocol and believed that my practices were unorthodox, he was grateful that his patient was better. So whenever this sort of situation happens, I think it's good, because it makes practitioners reassess their approach to treating patients. It's really hard to change the medical community's paradigm of; "one disease, one medicine," but fortunately, it's falling by the wayside as more and more doctors realize that in cases of chronic disease, it isn't the best approach.

Treatment Approach

I like to compare my patients and their medical problems to a wheel with many spokes. The wheel represents their entire health, whether physical, psychological or spiritual, as well as their bodily stressors, including infections, hormone dysfunction, immune problems, and other issues.

The Lyme Healing Wheel

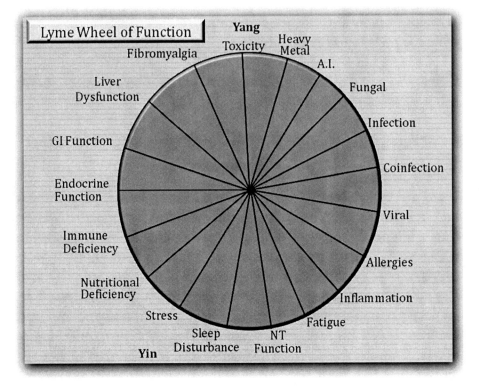

* This healing wheel is used with the permission of Dr. Bock.

The Lyme disease healing wheel can be described in terms of yin and yang, which is a concept in Chinese medicine that describes how seemingly opposite forces are interconnected and interdependent in the natural world, and give rise to one another in turn. This concept lies at the heart of many branches of classical Chinese science and philosophy, including medicine. On one side of the healing wheel is "yin" and on the other side is "yang."

To fully understand this concept requires a study of Chinese medicine, but basically, there are conditions of illness that display predominantly yin qualities, and others yang (although this is somewhat of a simplistic analogy). When formulating a protocol for a particular patient, I consider which conditions are "excessive" (yang) and which are "deficient" (yin) in that patient. This in turn provides a template that I use to determine how to get rid of the "bad" in the body, or how to add things to it that it's deficient in. The template also shows me how to prioritize these problems. So for instance, a patient might have hormone problems, insomnia, nutritional and immune deficiencies, all of which belong to one side of that person's wheel (yin), as well as fibromyalgia, toxicity, fungal infections, Lyme disease and co-infections, which belong to the other side of the wheel (yang).

In my consultations with patients, I also try to determine what the basic trigger for all of their problems was, by taking a linear history of their symptoms. I might ask them questions such as, "When was the last time that you were well? What happened five years ago when you first got sick? Were you under stress? Was your adrenal function low, or were you hiking in Cape Cod?"

People come into my practice with physical complaints, and there are many components to their illnesses, such as immune system dysfunction, inflammation and toxicity, just to name a few. I must address all of these in order to discover what they need to be optimally well in their life. So that's my treatment approach.

Lately, I have been seeing a lot of patients who have been to different specialists for their physical complaints; neurologists, internists, rheumatologists, infectious disease specialists and so on, and most have been told that their tests are negative and that nothing is wrong with them. So they are not being validated in their complaints, and as a result, I am noticing that in addition to physical problems, they have no confidence, and fear that they have mental problems or are going crazy. So I also have to support them emotionally, which might involve sending them to a practitioner to help them to deal with the emotional aspect of their illness.

Emotional Strategies for Healing

One of the practitioners that I often refer my patients to does a type of therapy called Core Energetics or "path work." The primary purpose of this therapy is to get patients to release past emotional blocks so that their truest self (their core) can emerge.

Core Energetics is based upon the idea that we have all learned to constrain our life force and inhibit our emotional and creative potential, and because of this, we have lost touch with our essence. When certain emotions have been disowned because of early life prohibitions against feeling, the energy of these emotions gets "trapped" in the body. The therapy releases these trapped feelings through different means, including physical activities that involve movement and breathing, dialogue, energy work and the power of relationship. Core Energetics works on five levels: the body, emotions, mind, will and spirit. More information on this therapy can be found on the Internet at: www.coreenergetics.org.

The great thing about Core Energetics is that the practitioner can go really deep to discover what is derailing patients' immune systems. I find this therapy to be particularly helpful when patients start sabotaging their treatment, (as sometimes happens) because Core Energetics can get them to look at the reason why they are doing this. But it isn't like talk therapy; rather, it's a psycho-spiritual discipline that gets to the root cause of emotional problems.

In addition to Core Energetics, I recommend meditation for my patients' emotional and spiritual healing, because it can help them to relax and think about the things that they want to do to heal. I may also recommend that they see a behavioral or stress management practitioner, or clinical psychologist.

The Patient as a Vessel in a Sea of Toxins

When patients tell me that they have been to a lot of doctors, and, let's say, for example, that they have headaches, fatigue, PMS and abdominal pain, the first thing that I do is try to get them to stop thinking in terms of the paradigm, "one disease, one drug." I draw a vessel on a piece of paper to help illustrate this point and tell them, "Let's say that you are a sea vessel, and the sea represents life's stressors. As you go through life, the water from the sea leaks into your vessel, affecting your physical and emotional well-being. You don't want the level of water inside your vessel to get too high over time. You want to keep your vessel strong and powerful, but if there are a lot of stressors (sea water) that build inside that vessel; toxins, infections, poor diet, etc., then the water level inside of your vessel slowly rises, until it one day reaches its limit and overflows. And then you get symptoms, such as gastrointestinal disturbances, PMS, and so on. The Western model of medicine dictates that you take a remedy to stop the symptoms, kind of like a shield, but you can't do that because at this point, your vessel is already overflowing. Instead, you must take a comprehensive, holistic approach to healing in order to lower the water level inside your vessel."

People with Lyme disease may be full or semi-full vessels, but they may also be vessels that are weak, constitutionally, as well as full, which means that they are both weak and toxic. If I attempt to detoxify such people too fast, they will "overflow" and get worse. My training in acupuncture and Chinese medicine has taught me that some people have weak constitutions, while others have strong ones, and this fact must be taken into account when treating them. Practitioners who don't understand this can be well-meaning and give their weak patients a lot of antibiotics or detoxification remedies, but when they do, it's as if they are opening up these peoples' spigots and before you know it, the vessels that are their patients are sinking.

Healing the Body on an Energetic Level

One of the therapies that I use in my practice involves the Ondamed, which is an electromagnetic pulsed biofeedback therapy device. It uses electromagnetic frequencies to balance the body. According to James Oschman, author of Energy Medicine, "Ondamed can monitor the state of one's physiology and correct imbalances as they arise." One can get to the body's underlying dysfunction with this device. It increases energy, helps sleep and relieves pain.

I recommend this therapy to my patients, because besides physical and chemical imbalances, a lot of them have disrupted electromagnetic systems. The body's electromagnetic system is based on quantum physics, where cells communicate instantly via energy, and when practitioners can tap into their patients' energy with the Ondamed, fast healing is possible. The chemical system of the body works on a slower level, through physical reactions, such as enzyme secretions, and hormone and neurotransmitter communications. So if I can tap into my patients' energy with the Ondamed, as well as through other strategies that address energy, such as acupuncture, I find that they heal better on a physical level.

Antibiotic Protocol for the Treatment of Lyme Disease Infections

When it comes to my specific antibiotic protocol for patients, I could say that A, B and C is what I do, but it wouldn't really be what I do. The information would be incomplete. I practice patient-oriented medicine. I don't treat Lyme; I treat the patient who has the Lyme.

That said, I tend to follow the ILADS guidelines when prescribing antibiotics, and follow a protocol that is similar to Lyme-literate physicians such as Drs. Joseph Burrascano and Joseph G. Jemsek.

Dr. Burrascano used to tell me that it's important to treat patients for (approximately) two and a half years with antibiotics, and while

CHAPTER 2: Steven Bock, M.D.

I now use antibiotics in my practice, the idea of giving them for long periods of time still gnaws at me. I don't like for people to be on antibiotics for two or more years, so while I may start my patients on antibiotics, at some point during their treatment, I may try to switch them to anti-microbial herbs instead. Such herbs may include cat's claw, as well as others. I also use homeopathic remedies in my practice, depending upon the patient's needs.

Patients who are really sick may require intravenous antibiotics. I may put them on a pulsed therapy regimen in which they are required to take high doses of antibiotics for three or four days per week. I vary the protocol according to the patient, however, taking into account a variety of factors. For example, it's important to know whether they have just Lyme (Borrelia), or co-infections as well; what doctors treated them with previously, and whether they have already taken a lot of antibiotics. Also, patients may have a problem that is less about Lyme and more about other issues, such as fungal infections or liver dysfunction. I don't have one single way that I treat chronic illness involving Lyme, because every patient is unique.

I always try to use herbs and homeopathy in addition to antibiotics. Sometimes, when I switch patients to herbs after they have been on antibiotics for a certain length of time, they don't respond well to the herbs. I can prescribe them a great regimen, but their illness might be so severe that I have to keep them on antibiotics for the duration of their treatment. If I use herbs, however, I don't usually give them to patients at the same time as antibiotics, unless the herbs are for treating some other aspect of healing, such as inflammation or detoxification. I use other herbs for such purposes, but not the antibiotic replacement herbs such as andrographis, because to use antibiotic herbs at the same time as pharmaceutical antibiotics would be redundant. I mean, why use a small knife to kill the bugs when you have a big gun? So I prefer to use the herbs towards the end of patients' treatment regimens when I am trying to wean them off of antibiotics.

Considerations in the Treatment of Infections

While I may prescribe intravenous antibiotics for some of my patients, as of late, I have probably been less aggressive with the IV's. Generally, I try to discover whether my patients will respond first to oral antibiotics. If they don't, then I may prescribe them IV Rocephin (ceftriaxone), Zithromax (azithromycin) or doxycycline. I may give them two to four grams of one of these antibiotics daily, on a rotating schedule of four days on and three days off. I maintain this schedule so that the body has a chance to clear the toxins that are generated by the treatments. I use a lot of pulsing therapy in my practice, whether IV or oral, especially when treating chronic conditions. I believe that putting patients on antibiotics every day can deplete them and that they can become really toxic. So I might prescribe antibiotics on Monday, Wednesday and Friday, for example, and leave the other days open so that the body has a break and an opportunity to clear the toxins that have been generated as a result of the treatments.

Another factor that I take into consideration when prescribing antibiotic regimens is the pathogen's life cycle, because the Lyme bacteria hide out in the body, and can only be killed when they are reproducing.

About five years ago, there was a biologist who gave a lecture on bacteria at the ILADS conference. He said that bacteria have been around so long that they can adapt to anything, but we tend to think too simplistically about them. And the problem with treating Lyme organisms isn't that they become resistant to antibiotics, but rather, that they develop ways to avoid antibiotics. So pulsing antibiotic regimens can also be beneficial because it's a way to surprise the bugs, because on the days when patients aren't doing treatments, the bugs tend to come out of their "holes" or hiding places, and in doing so, they become susceptible to antibiotics.

Finally, even though I now belong to the camp of those who believe in using lots of antibiotics to treat Lyme disease, I still don't like them, but I feel that they are necessary if patients are to fully heal.

Twenty years ago, I attended two conferences, one on homeopathy and one on herbal medicine. One herbalist, in his speech to over one hundred herbalists, said, "If you treat Lyme disease, I want you to know that it is important to treat this disease with antibiotics first, and then herbs later." I liked that he said this, because he was truthful and told a bunch of herbalists, who might normally have advocated herbs for everything, that they needed to use antibiotics for Lyme. Just because a treatment is "alternative," doesn't mean that it is what is warranted for a specific condition, especially when it comes to Lyme disease. And I consider myself an alternative M.D., for sure.

Clinical Diagnosis of Co-Infections

Clinical diagnosis of co-infections can be difficult, since all of the Lyme infections, including Borrelia, create symptoms such as joint pain, fatigue and headaches which overlap with those of other infections.

That said, I have noticed a few trends. For example, each of the most common co-infections tends to give people a particular type of headache. Babesia causes headaches at the top of the head; Bartonella, at the front of the head, and Borrelia, at the back of the neck. Ehrlichia tends to cause severe headaches.

Other telling signs of Bartonella include heavy night sweats, weight loss and increased neurological symptoms that are out of proportion to what Lyme (Borrelia) alone would cause. As well, those with Bartonella might have foot pain and/or enlarged lymph nodes, more so than those who have just Borrelia. I have had two patients with Bartonella who were both originally diagnosed as having lymphoma, which is a cancer of the lymph glands. One that I had treated for Lyme two years earlier and who was about to go on chemotherapy came to me for an opinion about how to treat her lymphoma. I told her that I suspected that she had Bartonella and I asked her for permission to treat it. When I did, her symptoms went away and she ended up never needing chemotherapy. So Bartonella can mimic lymphoma; it doesn't happen often, but it can happen.

Another telling sign of Bartonella is a snake-like, purple-red vascular rash on the flanks or thighs. It looks like stretch marks, which is important to know if practitioners or those with Lyme are trying to differentiate between rashes. Sometimes, however, diagnosis is intuitive and can only be confirmed after patients take a clinical trial of a remedy and practitioners observe a positive response to that remedy.

When diagnosing my patients' infections, I first examine their clinical signs and symptoms and then do laboratory testing. Unfortunately, labs are not always useful for diagnosing co-infections, so in my practice, the clinical diagnosis is primary. I also give my patients a lot of questionnaires, and ask them to rate their symptoms on scales of 0-5 or 0-10, depending upon the questionnaire. The answers from these questionnaires enable me to identify the particular symptom clusters that are present and consequently, which co-infections. Often, however, I don't fully know what is going on with my patients until I treat them, because they are dealing with so many different problems in their bodies.

Considerations in Lab Testing

Patients will often ask me whether they should do another Borrelia antibody test as they progress with their treatments, and I tell them that antibodies to Lyme can go either up or down during treatment. Follow-up testing doesn't reveal whether patients still have Lyme disease.

One test that I use that is very accurate for determining some patients' progress with treatments is the C6 peptide. It's an ELISA test that is a good, classifiable test for certain people. For those that test negative on this test but still have Lyme symptoms, the test isn't useful, but for those who test positive on it, it can be a good marker for progress during treatments. For instance, if patients score a "1" or higher on the test, then this indicates that they have Lyme disease and that the test will be useful for determining their progress on a regimen. So if a patient scores an eight on his or her test results, for example, and I successfully treat that person for

Lyme, then that value should go down within a year to normal. (A normal value is .9 or lower). And, in fact, I see this kind of thing happen. Within six months, patients' results often drop from an eight to a four, and after a year, from a four to a one. If they get a re-activation of their Borrelia, however, then that number will shoot up to a four again. Unfortunately, this only seems to be a good test for about thirty percent of those with Lyme, but for those who are responsive to it, it's a reliable test.

Detoxification

In general, I treat my patients' gastrointestinal problems first, because these need to be addressed before I can start them on antibiotics. So if they have a lot of GI symptoms, I may give them some form of bentonite medical clay with psyllium to bind up toxins, which, after a couple of days, reduces symptoms of gas and bloating. Then I will start them on a functional detoxification protocol that includes a hypoallergenic rice protein formula that contains nutrients to detoxify the liver, such as NAC (N-acetyl cysteine) and glutathione. This formula also contains watercress and raspberry to upregulate phase one detoxification and balance phase two detoxification, in addition to heavy antioxidants to neutralize toxic by-products that are created when phase two of the liver detoxification process becomes dysfunctional. I might also recommend homeopathic detoxification remedies, especially matrix and cellular remedies for the liver and GI tract, as well as Questran, which is a biliary sequestrant that takes neurotoxins out of the biliary tract into the intestines. On occasion, I may use herbs for purposes of detoxification. I also test and treat for potential problems with methylation pathways.

For the detoxification of heavy metals, I recommend substances such as chlorella, cilantro, DMSA, and EDTA, depending upon the metal and where patients are at in the recovery process. Some practitioners believe that it's important to get rid of metals before treating Lyme infections, but I don't have a set rule about it. I'm not linear in my thinking about this, or any other issue.

Mold is a major problem for some with Lyme disease and needs to be addressed, along with the other infections. Dr. Shoemaker has a biotoxin theory about mold that is useful, but mold toxins aren't the only kind of toxins that those with Lyme need to worry about. Xenobiotics, heavy metals, and other toxins can be just as, if not more, important. True, some people with a certain genetic HLA profile may be prone to mold detoxification problems, but then there are others for whom mercury, or another type of toxin, may be more important. And mercury, for example, can cause a pre-disposition to autoimmunity and make Lyme worse because of all the problems that it creates for the immune system.

Finally, other strategies that I use for detoxifying my patients include intravenous Vitamin C and glutathione. Glutathione, in particular, tends to be really depleted in those with Lyme disease.

Treating Opportunistic Infections and the Immune System

I test my patients for opportunistic infections, such as EBV (Epstein-Barr), HHV-6 (human Herpes virus six), Chlamydia and Mycoplasma, because all of these affect the immune system. Unless patients are really symptomatic, however, I don't prescribe antiviral medications, as I am not a big fan of these. I prefer natural treatments and am a big proponent of things like transfer factor for the treatment of viruses, funguses and early-stage Lyme disease. Transfer factor shouldn't be used in cases of chronic Lyme, however, because it stimulates a Th1 response, and people with chronic Lyme often already have an exaggerated Th1 response. Lyme-specific transfer factor can be used in those with chronic Lyme. To support the immune systems of those with chronic Lyme, I might also use treatments that stimulate the B-cells, such as oral immunoglobulins. Or I might work on healing patients' guts, because a lot of the body's lymphocyte (a type of immune cell) system is in the gut, and if there are problems in the gut, then the immune system is affected. So if I heal my patients' guts, I can get improvement in that part of their immune system, because problems in the gut are intimately related to the lymphatic and immune systems.

The only instance in which I might use regular transfer factor in cases of chronic Lyme is when there is strong evidence that a viral infection is also an important part of the symptom picture; for instance, if a patient has high titers of HHV-6 or EBV.

Other treatments that I recommend in general for bolstering immune system function include mushrooms and Chinese herbs.

Treating Hormonal Dysfunction

Lyme disease affects the hormones, and particularly the adrenal and thyroid glands. About ten percent of Lyme disease sufferers have autoimmune thyroiditis, and Lyme also stimulates other autoimmune processes involving the hormones.

I use a lot of hormones in my practice, because it's important that patients' hormonal systems be supported if they are to fully heal from Lyme disease. After my patient assessment that involves questionnaires and/or testing, I may start by addressing patients' adrenal and thyroid function. I may use traditional lab tests to help determine their thyroid function, but I also look at their basal body temperature, and do iodine testing to see if they are iodine deficient. Iodine plays a really important role in the body's metabolism and in fighting infections. A lot of people with breast or ovarian cysts, for example, are iodine deficient.

Other hormones that I address include pregnenolone, DHEA, estrogen and progesterone in my female patients, and DHEA and testosterone in my male patients.

I use a broad spectrum of natural supplements to treat adrenal insufficiency. I might start off by recommending Vitamins B-6, B-5 and C, and if these prove to be insufficient for restoring adrenal function, then I may recommend herbs. The herbs I use include the Chinese herb rehmannia, which is a kidney herb, as well as ashwaghanda and rhodiola, which are good for those whose nervous systems have been depleted. Cordyceps is also beneficial for the adrenals, and is an anti-aging herb, as well. If herbs don't provide satisfactory results, I may then do acupuncture, and if that doesn't do the trick, then I will prescribe physiological hydrocortisone, (not prednisone, which is pharmacological). If patients' adrenal function is low and the natural remedies aren't sufficient, I sometimes get dramatic results with hydrocortisone, if I prescribe doses of 5-10 mg, two to three times a day. With hydrocortisone, theoretically, immune suppression should only occur at higher doses, but I do think that over time, lower doses can suppress the body's innate ability to make cortisol and make it harder for patients to heal down the road. Also, one of the things that practitioners should be aware of when dosing hydrocortisone is that too much can make patients worse. It's vital not to get the dose too high. I have seen, for example, patients get worse after getting just one injection of long-acting Medrol in their backs. (An injection of Medrol lasts two weeks). It makes their Lyme infections go crazy. If practitioners are just boosting their patients' cortisol levels to normal, however, then the cortisol is beneficial to the body, but if the doses bring the levels to above normal, then patients will get worse.

Also, some people are allergic to their own hormones, especially women, who tend to be allergic to their body's estrogen and proge-sterone. I don't see allergies happen as often with cortisol. To determine whether hormonal allergies are present, I test my patients using allergic extracts of estrogen, progesterone, LH and FSH. For example, I recently had a patient who would get bad PMS and headaches before her menstrual cycle, and when I gave her progesterone, she had a crazy reaction. So I checked her FSH (follicle-stimulating hormone) and LH (luteinizing hormone), which are pituitary hormones. I also tested her progesterone and estrogen and then made up different allergy serums based on that information, for her to take during her cycle whenever she has symptoms. The serums neutralize her body's reactions to her own estrogen and progesterone, thereby facilitating normal immune-hormonal balance.

Treatments for Symptomatic Relief

Insomnia

I often recommend melatonin for the treatment of insomnia in those with Lyme. Ten years ago, I wrote a book on this hormone and I tend to advocate it because it is physiologic and natural. Other people might just need minerals, such as calcium at night, to help restore their sleep patterns. Yet others might benefit from taking 5-HTP if they are depleted in serotonin and suffer from symptoms of depression. If none of these remedies work, then I might recommend herbs, acupuncture or treatment with the Ondamed device, the latter of which has a sleep program that works really well. If women are perimenopausal, then I may give them progesterone, because it's a relaxing hormone that aids in sleep.

I don't have a set protocol for treating insomnia, however. Instead, I have an extensive menu of remedies, starting with natural substances and which go all the way down to pharmaceutical drugs. So if my patients have tried five or six natural remedies for their insomnia and none have worked, then I might suggest that they try Ambien, for example, and take that for two or three weeks while the other parts of their therapy are taking effect. Doing this keeps them from worrying about being fatigued and unable to sleep. When it comes to insomnia, there is a time for natural remedies, and there is a time for drugs.

Anxiety and Depression

I often recommend neurotransmitter replacement for the treatment of anxiety and depression in those with Lyme, so instead of giving my patients SSRI drugs to increase their serotonin levels, I might give them 5-HTP, or if they have anxiety or agitation, GABA or L-theanine. I may also use homeopathic remedies, Chinese herbs, acupuncture, or Ondamed frequencies to treat these symptoms.

Pain

For the treatment of pain and inflammation, I often do acupuncture on my patients. I also use a variety of different nutritional and herbal remedies to decrease this symptom.

Lately, I have been giving my patients injectable homeopathic remedies for their cervical and spinal pain. I inject these remedies into different points on their bodies, where they work to relieve nerve and muscle pain. Such remedies are also beneficial for relieving arthritis symptoms.

If my patients are taking a lot of antibiotics, I might also compound pain medications in a gel, to save their stomachs from having to endure the effects of too many drugs. One gel that I use has anti-analgesic, anti-inflammatory and muscle relaxant properties, and is made in a lecithin-based ointment that patients can rub on painful parts of their bodies.

Finally, I find that low dose Naltrexone is quite effective for pain relief and for improving immune function. There are a lot of different options for treating pain, and sometimes even analgesics and medications such as Neurontin and Lyrica are necessary.

Diet

I have used nutrition in my practice for over thirty years. Nutrition is the cornerstone and basis for the effective treatment of most conditions that I treat in my clinic, including Lyme disease. Determining the most appropriate diet and supplements for a particular patient is accomplished clinically and through laboratory testing.

First, I test my patients for gliadin antibodies, the presence of which indicates sensitivity to gluten. Gluten can cause innumerable problems in the body, including GI disturbances, fatigue, and peripheral neuropathy. My training and experience have taught me a lot about food sensitivities, and I think that practitioners have to be careful about saying that all people with Lyme disease need to be on the same kind of diet, which is why tests for sensitivities and allergies can be important.

Also, I have noticed that the more practitioners restrict their patients' diets, the more frustration and stress that these patients have to manage. This in turn wears them out and negatively impacts their immune systems, so practitioners should take this factor into consideration when prescribing a diet for their patients.

All Lyme sufferers should avoid refined sugar though, because sugar can raise insulin and leptin levels, which in turn can create leptin or insulin resistance. When either of these conditions is present, then people with Lyme have an increased susceptibility to inflammation, which makes their Lyme disease worse.

That said, I think it's important for Lyme sufferers to be able to cheat on their diets every once in awhile. Those who are doing well with their healing might be able to get away with having a dessert once a week, while those who still have a long way to go in their recovery might only be able to indulge in a piece of cake at the occasional party.

Also, drinking coffee taxes the adrenals and also causes inflammation, but if my patients are drinking three cups of coffee per day, I don't want them to get withdrawal headaches to complicate their symptom picture while healing. So I might suggest that they slowly decrease the amount of coffee that they drink every day, until they don't need it anymore. Abrupt withdrawal is not good. I don't want to make patients feel as though they are in a no-win situation.

Lifestyle Recommendations for Healing

I have a patient who can't get emotional or financial support from her loved ones. She has to go through this healing journey all by herself. She works fifteen hours a day, doesn't sleep, periodically stops medications and vitamins, and comes in to my clinic every three to four months, with her body crashing and Lyme disease going crazy. So I recently had a conference with her, her significant other, and her parents, to bring up the problems in her life which are preventing her from healing. I told her loved ones that they needed to help her to deal with her disease and the unhealthy decisions that she is making if she is to fully recover. Addressing unhealthy habits is important for healing, as is accessing and dealing with the deeper issues that prevent patients from getting well, such as a lack of emotional or financial support from family members.

Obviously, getting enough rest, doing moderate exercise and getting oxygen into the cells, taking supplements, doing mild physical therapy and eating well are other lifestyle habits that help the body to heal.

Those with Lyme should involve and educate their family and friends about their disease. Most people don't know about Lyme, and patients always come back from doctors' visits with tons of things to do. They have a supplement schedule and therapies that they need to start, but there's always this kind of stress that they are subjected to from friends and family members which makes it difficult for them to carry out their obligations. For example, family members might not believe that their loved ones are sick, or that they really have to do all of the treatments that their doctors have told them that they need to do. They may think that their loved ones can heal in just a few weeks, or they may make unhelpful comments such as, "How is it possible that you can't work?" To friends and family members, the sick person's symptoms are just symptoms, but they don't realize how intense and disabling these can be.

Who Are Those that Heal from Lyme Disease and/or Chronic Illness?

This is a complicated question. I would say that people who have a lot of trauma (and I don't necessarily mean as a result of past abuse) and who are working through a lot of problems have a harder time healing. Their trauma could be related to any number of causes, but in any case, they may be receiving some secondary benefit by being sick or in pain as a result of the trauma. The motivations for these benefits, as well as the trauma itself, must be addressed if such people are to fully heal.

Also, those who have had Lyme for a long time and who have low mitochondrial and/or adrenal function as a result may not respond well to treatments. It's hard for me to know whether such factors will be a problem for my patients, however, until I try out and monitor different treatment programs with them to see how they respond.

When I look at the Lyme wheel (as described earlier) and consider the people who have a lot of deficiencies and excesses, or just a lot of "stuff" going on their bodies, then I think that such people might have a harder time healing, too.

Finally, if patients have mold sensitivity and/or a decreased genetic ability to get rid of toxins, this may also hinder their ability to heal.

Does Everyone with Chronic Fatigue Syndrome Really Have Lyme Disease?

First of all, I don't like labels that pigeonhole people into having chronic fatigue syndrome or Lyme disease. I look at illness like the wheel that I described previously, which illustrates that there are a lot of components to disease. Thirty percent of a patient's dysfunction might be due to adrenal problems, for example, or eighty percent of it might be due to immune problems, or twenty-five percent due to infections. In chronic illness, it always seems that there is a certain element of this or a certain element of that involved in a patient's overall symptom picture, but it's not always clear how much each one of those elements is contributing to the breakdown of the body. Our bodies are more complex than just a diagnosis, and sometimes, the only way to know how much Lyme disease is contributing to a person's overall symptom picture is to treat that person.

Why Do Some People Gain Weight and Others Lose Weight When They Get Lyme Disease?

Metabolic testing can reveal whether a person's extracellular water components, such as the lymphatic system or the air outside of their cells, is overburdened with toxins. People who have too many toxins in these areas are those who are prone to weight gain. I put these types of patients on a strong detoxification protocol, in addition to antibiotics.

Those who lose weight tend to be in what I call a "deficiency" category (referring again to the concept of deficiencies and excesses in Chinese medicine). These people tend to have weak adrenals and conditions such as functional hypoadrenia, and hence, are also weak overall. They also tend to have problems with electrolyte balance, and they lose weight because they don't metabolize their food properly. Effectively helping these types of people requires supporting their adrenal glands.

The Greatest Challenges of Treating Lyme Disease

I often tell other health care practitioners that it's their experience with patients which enables them to determine down the road what their patients' problems will be and how to treat these. I coach doctors at conferences, and during these conferences, the doctors learn a lot about how to treat Lyme disease, but then when they go to treat their patients, a lot of different scenarios start happening with their patients' symptoms. Then these doctors, if they have dived deeply into treating Lyme, suddenly don't know what to do next, because there are so many twists and turns with this disease, as well as possible treatment outcomes. They know that their patients have the Lyme disease complex and they may have a general idea about how to treat it, but it's when they really start "going downstream" with their patients that things really start to get tricky. For example, their patients might end up with a certain kind of Herxheimer reaction that requires special attention; they might have thyroid or adrenal problems that suddenly turn up a month down the line, or neurotransmitter imbalances that need to be dealt with. A couple of years ago, I gave a lecture called, "Road-blocks in Chronic Lyme", and discussed the roadblocks that practitioners stumble upon when treating patients with chronic Lyme, so that they might know what to do when certain problems or issues surface during treatment.

Why I Love Treating Lyme Disease/Chronic Illness

One thing that I love about practicing in the areas of complex Lyme disease and chronic illness is that every person who comes in to see me each day is unique, and has an entirely different spectrum of problems, and I enjoy the challenge of treating and helping them to heal from these. My patient visits tend to last for an hour and a half, and often, during those visits, the patients will get a little weepy, because they are grateful to have finally found a doctor who will really listen to them. And I appreciate being able to spend this time with them so that I can help them. Most doctors only get seven minutes with their patients, but my theory is that you can't make a diagnosis when you only spend seven minutes with a patient.

Not long ago, I had a patient with a lot of symptoms, including headaches, joint pain, and weight gain. Lyme affects metabolic function so it isn't uncommon for people to gain weight with this disease. This patient had been to a rheumatologist, who took her medical history on the computer for about five minutes before prescribing her a weight reduction medicine. After that, she went to an internist, who recommended that she do gastric bypass surgery. So when she came into my office, I listened to her, and learned that she had a lot of other problems besides Lyme disease, and that the treatments that the other doctors had recommended that she do were simply "off the wall" and absolutely crazy. Sometimes, I wonder what Western medicine is coming to! In any case, during this patient's visit with me, she was crying with relief because someone was actually listening to her for the first time.

For me, it is awesome to be in the presence of people who suddenly realize that they are not crazy, and that they don't have to be subject to this patriarchal health care system that hands you a drug and says, "Just take this. That's all I can do. Bye, bye." I love that I am making a difference for people. Do I have more success than some practitioners? Yes, I think so, but medicine is an art. There are difficult cases, and patients can have some healing block that I can't address, but the thing is, no doctor knows how to fix everything.

When I lecture to doctors, I sometimes draw a circle in my presentations to represent medical information. I then make pie slices in that circle to illustrate what we doctors know and don't know about medicine. So let's suppose that twenty or thirty degrees of the pie represents what we know, and another thirty degrees represents what we know that we don't know. So what does the other 300 degrees of the pie represent? It's what we don't know that we don't know!

There is always going to be a part of the pie that represents information that we don't know that we don't know, but I like to practice medicine "being in the question." Patients bring me new information all of the time, and I tell them, "Thanks. I'm going to do research in that area now." So my energy isn't stagnant; it's always flowing because I am always learning.

Last Words

In summary, I consider it an honor to practice medicine, and to deal with people's most intimate and complicated issues. In my attempt to make a difference in the practice of treating chronic Lyme disease, this feeling is magnified.

How to Contact Steven Bock, M.D.

Steven J. Bock, M.D.
sbock@rhinebeckhealth.com
Tel: 845-876-7082

•CHAPTER 3•

Susan L. Marra, M.S., N.D.
SEATTLE, WA

Biography

Twenty five years ago, Dr. Marra began her professional journey to discover the intricacies of the mind/body connection and how their interplay relates to disease development. She graduated from Guilford College in Greensboro, NC, with honors in Psychology and then received her Master's of Science degree in Psychology at Bucknell University in Lewisburg, PA. While there, she won several state and national awards for her academic and research achievements.

Soon thereafter, she was employed at the National Institute of Mental Health working under Thomas R. Insel, M.D. as a research psychologist in the Department of Brain and Behavior and while there, developed an appreciation for the scientific process of information gathering and reporting. However, her interest in the mind/body connection and medicine was not fully actualized until she enrolled at Bastyr University in Seattle, Washington. There she worked closely with Alan R. Gaby, M.D. studying clinical and therapeutic nutrition.

In addition, while attending Bastyr University, she opened the first Natural Health Research Clinic with Dr. Carlo Calabrese and Dr. Leanna Standish and worked as the United States liaison for Murdock Madaus Schwabe, a German phytoceutical company that specialized in the production of Echinaguard. In 1999, after receiving her degree in Naturopathic Medicine from Bastyr, she moved to Connecticut and opened a private practice that centered largely on environmental medicine and tick-borne infections.

Over the next eight years, in addition to operating her private practice, Dr. Marra trained with world leading experts in Lyme disease, including pediatric Lyme disease specialist, Charles Ray Jones, M.D., in New Haven, CT, and adult Lyme specialist Richard Horowitz, M.D., in Hyde Park, NY.

Dr. Marra's training in Lyme disease treatment and diagnosis is extensive. She maintains a professional interest in integrative medicine and attends meetings that foster knowledge in this area. She is a member of several professional organizations including ILADS (International Lyme and Associated Diseases Society).

Dr. Marra currently lives and works in Seattle, WA with her yellow lab Saxon and "labradoodle" puppy, Mielle. She hopes to bring greater awareness about tick-borne infections to the public through her private practice and community lectures.

In the Beginning

In 1999, as a recent Bastyr graduate and novice clinician, Dr. Marra moved to Westport, CT and initially began practicing environmental medicine with an emphasis on sublingual immunotherapy to treat food, air-borne, inhalant, and chemical allergies. While interviewing her patients about various allergies, she realized that there were salient symptoms among them which included more than just the classic rhinitis, cough and weeping eyes. She began to take note of these symptoms and developed a patient intake form that had sections devoted to each organ system (e.g., nervous system, musculoskeletal system). After documenting her patients' symptoms on this form, she realized that most of them had significant muscle and joint pain, as well as brain fog, poor ability to concentrate, odd paresthesias, headaches, tinnitus, neck pain, insomnia, multiple chemical sensitivities, gluten and casein sensitivities, photosensitivity hyperacusia, irritable bowel, extreme disabling fatigue, night sweats, dysmenorrhea, and a plethora of other symptoms that seemed to traverse many, if not all, of the organ systems. Up until that point, she had suspected that their allergies were simply a symptom of an "irritable immune system" that was disturbed at a much deeper level, and that food, water, or the environment was perhaps poisoning them, because so many had intolerable chemical sensitivities accompanied by severe headaches and fatigue. Many of these patients lived in and around New York City and after further reflection, she concluded that the pollution from the city was the causal factor underlying this odd symptom constellation. But something still did not fit. She believed that something systemic was going on but had no idea what it was. She called other physicians in the area and asked them for their opinions and finally came upon Dr. Bernard Raxlen, a psychiatrist in Greenwich, CT who had a reputation for being an open-minded medical doctor. He also believed in orthomolecular medicine, which was a particular area of interest for Dr. Marra. They had lunch, and when she discussed her patients' clinical presentations with him, Dr. Raxlen was quick to inform her that they had "Lyme disease" and that her practice was located at the epicenter of an epidemic. Dr. Marra had briefly learned about Lyme disease in naturopathic school, but at the time was unfamiliar with the ramifications of such a diagnosis. Additionally, having vacationed on Martha's Vineyard during her summers as a child, she knew that Lyme disease was present but was unaware of its vast prevalence or infectious danger.

She contacted Dr. Nick Harris, president and CEO of IGeneX, Inc., in Palo Alto, CA and discussed her clinical observations with him, as well. He also concluded that most of her patient population had likely been exposed to Borrelia, the bacterium that causes Lyme disease, but that adequate testing was necessary for documentation purposes. Startled by this information, she soon realized that her entire practice might be comprised of infectious disease patients and began testing them through IGeneX. Amazingly, nearly 90% of them tested positive for at least one of the tick-borne infections. Stunned by the significance of this revelation, she started to travel to Dr. Charles Ray Jones' office in New Haven, CT once a week for the following six years to learn how to properly diagnose and treat Lyme disease and co-infections. The body of new information that she received there was daunting at the time, but she knew that she simply could not heal her patients until she determined the root cause of their symptoms. This marked the beginning of her training as a naturopathic Lyme disease specialist.

First Do No Harm

One of the oaths that students of naturopathic medicine take is to "first do no harm to the patient." To a naturopathic physician of course, this means, "try not to use pharmaceutical intervention", and instead, work with patients' diet, lifestyle, and other stressors in order to maximize their health and well being. Adequately treating Lyme disease, however, significantly challenges the naturopathic perspective on health. I had every intention, upon graduating from naturopathic medical school, of employing a holistic, alternative approach to health care, until I clinically met Borrelia, Babesia, Bartonella, Anaplasma, Ehrlichia, Mycoplasma, Tularemia, Brucella, HemoBartonella and Agrobacteria (the latter is believed to be the causative agent of Morgellons Disease). I frequently refer to these players as the "21st century chain gang bugs" whose intent is to occupy and monopolize the "streets" of the human body. They are malicious, clever, resilient, cunning, employ camouflage techniques and are adaptable to an ever-changing micro- and macro-environment. Not unlike most other living beings, they have one goal—proliferation. So to "first do no harm" would mean allowing them to proliferate in the patient's body. Hence, as a naturopathic physician, I needed to change my definition of what it meant to "do no harm" so that I could be at peace with my diagnoses and treatments in medicine and continue to provide high quality individual care to my patients. As a practitioner, I am constantly reminded of how I need to re-define the term "first do no harm" to "first regain health", because the latter is the primary premise by which I approach all of my patients' problems. In the continued refinement of the way in which I practice medicine, I am cognizant of doing as little harm as possible, which has always been my intent. I have learned over the years, however, and especially when treating the tick-borne infections, that I must take the lesser of two evil roads. Therefore, it may be necessary to prescribe a course of antibiotics to decrease the body's pathogen load.

The Art and Science of Practicing Medicine

As a naturopathic physician, I feel particularly fortunate to be able to embrace both the art and science of medicine, just as I recognize the value of both the left and right brain functions in humans. One cannot operate without the other and therefore I believe that the application of both art and science in medicine is particularly important in the diagnosis and treatment of Lyme disease. Clearly, the classic scientific method of double blind, safety and efficacy studies, as well as others, allows us to examine the facts that comprise the body of knowledge on treating tick-borne infections. Sophisticated studies can often provide a unique perspective on underlying disease pathophysiology that may not be readily observed clinically. However, I believe that understanding the depth and complexity of zoonotic diseases (those diseases which are transmitted from animals to humans) probably requires a paradigm shift where physicians and scientists lend more credence to individual case reports and anecdotal evidence. This is important because the clinical presentations of these diseases are often variable and changing over time as the infections proliferate and the immune system becomes tolerant and compromised.

Herein lies the need for an appreciation of the art of medicine. The ability to observe similarities, make cognitive leaps, draw inferences, utilize intuitive hunches, note patterns, plan tailored treatment strategies and use holistic information gathering techniques serve the clinician treating tick-borne diseases well. In the same way that the human brain utilizes the strengths of each hemisphere, with the left being logical, rational, mechanistic, and analytical, and the right, holistic, artistic, intuitive, and creative, physicians and scientists may benefit from using information that is gathered in various ways. I personally find it necessary to use both my scientific background and my artistic propensity to problem solve when trying to make sense of these complicated infectious diseases. My intent is to use information from a variety of different reputable disciplines in order to achieve optimal health for my patients. In science, facts are the fuel for further inquiry, but in art, color, texture, size, and hue are the factors for further understanding of disease. Using both allows for a rich interpretation of the disease process as well as for the diagnosis and treatment that ultimately benefits the patient.

Embracing the Intelligence of Nature

As a naturopathic physician, I chose to follow a professional path that embraced the intelligence of nature. In graduate school, I studied primate animal behavior and the work of evolutionary biologists such as E.O. Wilson, Ph.D., Konrad Lorenz, Ph.D., and Stephen Jay Gould, Ph.D. who largely shaped my appreciation for the natural world. Little did I know that later in my career I would use the general principles of evolution, adaptation and survival of the fittest to understand the complex nature of the microbes that are responsible for tick-borne diseases. Jeremy Narby, Ph.D. in his book, *The Intelligence of Nature*, describes chapter after chapter the ways in which plant and animal species have evolved particular traits in response to specific selection pressures that have allowed them to successfully proliferate. For example, in one chapter, Narby describes a Macaw bird in South America that feeds on berries that contain toxic alkaloids that can be lethal. But the Macaw species has evolved a way to rid itself of these toxins by feeding on a clay that binds to the toxic alkaloids, which are then excreted from the body. I find it remarkable that Macaws exhibit specific behaviors that allow them to feed on potentially toxic food without being harmed. Arnot Karlen, in his book, *The Biography of a Germ,* describes the "brilliance" of spirochetes in their ability to mutate relatively quickly, to morph based on environmental nutrient availability, and to evade the host immune system by dwelling deep within tissues in order to survive. These invaders are clever little beasts with a long history of evolutionary success. It is my belief that in order to understand Lyme disease and the co-infections, we need to carefully examine the environments where these "bugs" live and have lived, so that we can understand their full capacity to perform "tricks" which ensure their survival. As human beings, we may be somewhat "egocentric" in our view of life simply because we employ consciousness, read books, drive cars, and engage in spirituality. But when we disregard the elaborate behaviors of plant, animal and microbial species that have allowed for their evolutionary success, then we miss the "intelligence of nature."

Global Warming and Global Karma

Over the last five to ten years, researchers and scientists have emphasized how global warming is impacting various wildlife species' habitats as well as our own. Former Vice President Al Gore, in the DVD, *An Inconvenient Truth*, does a superb job of outlining the various reasons for the planet's three to five degree temperature increases over the last twenty years, and most notably, over the last ten years. Increasing levels of carbon dioxide in the atmosphere as a result of global pollution cause a "green house effect" which substantially warms the earth. Leonardo DiCaprio, in his DVD, *The 11th Hour,* emphasizes the urgent need to curb our energy expenditure in order to protect the earth from any further destruction due to global warming. One needs only to look out the window in February to see blooming flowers that once blossomed in April or May to realize that in fact, something has changed. Clearly, an intelligent nature that has resulted from millions of years of natural selection has orchestrated life on earth so that it prospers in a particular way and at particular times, so that species may co-habitate, share limited resources, capitalize on particular niches, and compete intelligently for habitats. Weather has certain-ly been a natural force that has shaped selection pressures, affecting all of life on earth. When human energy consumption and expenditure alter climate over the course of forty to fifty years, natural selection simply can't keep up and aberrations in microenvironments occur. This may be one of the reasons, among others, why we have seen an astronomical rise in the number of ticks and tick-borne diseases over the last decade. Increases in global temperatures change the microenvironment, allowing for the continued proliferation of species that carry infectious microbes (e.g. ticks, mosquitoes, sand flies, lice, mites, etc.). All of life is a web, and when one variable is altered, the effects are felt elsewhere and can be devastating.

The phenomena of insect proliferation can also be explained by "global karma." The notion of karma, which means basically, "what goes around comes around," is illustrated perfectly by the case of the rapid rise in Lyme disease. We have been notoriously "unconscious" in our evolution of energy use and waste management, as evidenced by the fact that we have now altered our natural macro- and micro-ecosystems to such a degree that we are now being directly and adversely affected by our own behavior. I can think of no better example of "global karma."

Joseph Jemsek, M.D., an infectious disease specialist in South Carolina, notes that the global Lyme disease epidemic is a "tsunami" that is about to hit the human species in a devastating way. We are about to reap the consequences of our past cavalier behavior in regard to maintaining a balance with the natural environment. Andy Abramson Wilson with Open Eye Pictures in Sausalito, CA describes the current state of affairs for Lyme disease patients in a brilliant DVD entitled *Under Our Skin*. This DVD can be purchased on the Internet at: www.openeyepictures.com. I highly recommend this video for anyone affected by Lyme disease (including family members). It illuminates the chain of events that have led to the current state of affairs for Lyme disease patients.

The Essence of the Patient

In my practice of medicine, it is most important for me to obtain a clear understanding of the "essence" of each one of my patients. Essence is a term not generally used in traditional medicine, but is frequently used in homeopathic medicine. Essence refers to the "feel" or "totality" of a patient including his or her genetic and environmental pre-dispositions, personality, energy, likes and dislikes, temperament, character, ambition, goals, interests, responsibilities, concerns, weaknesses, strengths, diet, lifestyle, sensitivity, creativity, and so on. In my initial two-hour appointment with patients, I try to get a "feel" for them beyond their symptoms, so that I can determine the most appropriate tests to run and develop a tailored treatment plan that works specifically for them.

This, of course, is an ongoing learning opportunity for me. Every patient that I meet enriches my knowledge about the human condition and how that interfaces with the tick-borne disease process in an individual. Arriving at an accurate "portrait" of a patient is critical for developing a treatment plan that will work for him or her. For example, some people are uncomfortable being treated for tick-borne diseases using antibiotics. This is important for practitioners to understand because patients' belief systems must be in sync with their treatment plan. Otherwise, cognitive dissonance can develop and an underlying "angst" might prevent them from accessing their own healing abilities. Practitioners have belief systems as well, and effective physicians will restrain their personal belief systems in order to allow patients to access their own innate healing abilities. I continue to perfect my skills in this area, as it is one of my greatest challenges as a practitioner. I do have an opinion about which treatments are best, but because I don't occupy my patients' bodies or psyches, I need to be particularly sensitive to their individual needs in order to provide an optimally effective treatment plan for them. To the person with Lyme, I would say: "Beware of the controlling physician!"

Listening

Perhaps one of my greatest challenges as a practitioner is to *really* listen to my patients. As I mature as a person and physician, I realize that it is an act of arrogance to not listen to patients. They may not have a medical background, but they live in their bodies and daily experience the effects of disease upon their bodies, which means that they can provide valuable information to their practitioners. Under no circumstance does this fact become more important than when diagnosing and treating tick-borne illness, because frequently, patients infected with zoonotic diseases report very odd symptoms. For example, they will report the feeling of being "shocked", or experiencing sensations of "cold water running down their face", or "a metal taste in their mouth", or perceptual/visual disturbances like "halos around lights", "floaters" in their eyes or bells ringing in their ears. Admittedly, these are strange symptoms, which is one of the reasons why Lyme disease patients are frequently diagnosed with psychosomatic illness. However, if practitioners look more closely at the symptom pictures of such patients, they will likely find more clues about which microbial infections are present. For example, people that complain about a feeling of being electrically shocked may be suffering from a borrelia infection in the central nervous system. Borrelia is known for its neurotropic behavior and it gravitates to areas in the body where high-density fatty acids are present. The brain and peripheral nerves are coated with myelin, which is largely composed of fatty acids and which increases the conductive capacity of an electrochemical event. The feelings of electric shock may be related to the fact that as the Borrelia organisms drill their way through the myelin sheath of nerve axons, they disrupt the electro-conductivity of nerves and cause unusual firing of those nerves, which the brain, in turn, interprets as an electric shock.

I am not certain if this is a correct interpretation of the symptom but in all cases that I have seen where electric shock was noted, the patient was infected with borrelia. When practitioners pay close attention to their patients' symptoms and carefully consider the source of these, it leads to testing and diagnosis of the proper infections. Cold hands and feet, for example, are generally the result of poor circulation, but there may be more to it than that. Bartonella, otherwise known as "Cat Scratch Fever" is known to have an affinity for the vascular endothelium, and it may be that when patients are infected with Bartonella, they experience cold hands and feet because the microbe is interfering with blood vessel vasoconstriction and vasodilation. Again, I don't know if I am interpreting the etiology of this symptom correctly, but nearly all of my patients that exhibit this symptom test positive for Bartonella. My point is that symptoms are clues to the disease puzzle and if you, the practitioner, can use them to help you navigate towards a proper diagnosis, you will have greater success in treating your patients. So let the patients tell you their story so that you may use their symptoms as clues to the larger puzzle. Obviously, this process gets incredibly challenging when it comes to treating patients who have multiple co-infections and secondary infections. Such people are extremely ill and have many, many debilitating symptoms.

Determining Appropriate Diagnostic Tests

The diagnosis of tick-borne diseases is a complicated task involving a multitude of variables that must be examined. Often it is difficult to "pinpoint" a particular microbe as being the causative agent for particular symptoms and this is especially true when it comes to tick-borne infections. Fever, malaise, joint pain, headache, and fatigue can be symptoms of many different infections and therefore, it is critical for the practitioner to do a careful diagnostic work-up on the patient. Several diagnostic laboratories specialize in tick-borne infections; however, I choose to use IGeneX, Inc. in Palo Alto, CA for most of my testing, and Fry Laboratories in Scottsdale, AZ. Stephen Fry, M.D. has perfected the giemsa stain, which is a type of test that identifies a yet unknown pathogen tentatively called HemoBartonella by its epierythrocytic characteristics. In my practice, I have found these labs to be the most reliable. If I suspect that patients have seronegative test results, which often happens as a result of long term pathogen exposure, then I use either a poly-anti-microbial challenge or a poly-phytoceutical challenge to aid in the discovery of the infectious agents. Generally, a two to four week challenge is necessary in order for patients to seroconvert and for their results to come out positive; however, on occasion, I have needed to do a two month challenge. Some gestational Lyme disease cases will take as long as a year to seroconvert using this challenge. Practitioners can contact IGeneX, Inc at 1-800-832-3200 for challenge protocols.

Obviously, it is important for practitioners to perform many other types of blood tests on their patients as well, including immune system, thyroid gland, and adrenal gland status tests. As well, tests that have to do with genetic predisposition (HLA's) markers, homocysteine and folic acid synthesis, autoimmune and coagulation markers, detoxification pathway status, heavy metal and chemical exposures, allergies, Vitamin D and Vitamin B-12 levels, female and male hormone levels, DHEA sulfate, intracellular minerals and intracellular glutathione levels, are important. And there may be many others that are needed, too. For example, Lyme disease and co-infections can affect many different organ systems and patients may therefore require organ-specific tests as well (i.e., EKG, EEG, brain MRI, PET scan, chest x-ray, abdominal ultrasound). As you can see, the picture can quickly become complicated. To make matters worse, many patients have secondary infections that need to be documented, such as Mycoplasma pneumoniae, Chlamydia pneumoniae, Herpes viruses 6 and 8, Cytomegalovirus, Epstein-Barr, and so on. It's important for practitioners to be aware of these infections because they provide an indication of their patients' pathogen load. The more infections that are present, the more the immune system is taxed. Lastly, Raphael Stricker, M.D., a hematologist and Lyme disease specialist in San Francisco, CA, has noted three other tests that are abnormal in chronic Lyme disease patients. These include the CD-57 count, (which measures natural killer cell activity and indicates the number of natural killer cells present), and the C3a and C4a inflammatory markers, which indicate infectious or autoimmune inflammation.

I use laboratory tests to discover patient abnormalities that I wouldn't ordinarily be able to identify by just taking a thorough history or doing a physical exam alone. Practitioners who are interested in learning more about the ancillary tests necessary for doing a complete tick-borne disease work-up on their patients should join ILADS at www.ILADS.org and sign up for a preceptorship. My preceptorship with Dr. Richard Horowitz in Hyde Park, NY, as well as my training with Dr. Charles Ray Jones in New Haven, CT, have been invaluable to me in this regard. There are no classes or books that can afford practitioners the same experience that can be obtained by watching a Lyme disease practitioner perform his/her skills. A preceptorship allows practitioners to obtain clinical insights that will be immediately applicable to their practice. It's the epitome of hands-on learning. Another invaluable clinical tool is Dr. Joseph Burrascano's *Lyme Disease Treatment Guidelines,* which can be downloaded from the ILADS website. Practitioners will find themselves frequently referring to this comprehensive manual. Additionally, they can order a CD from the ILADS website entitled, *The Nuts and Bolts of Lyme Disease,* which provides an excellent comprehensive review of the treatment for tick-borne infections.

Treatment for Lyme Disease and Co-Infections

Treating co-infections is perhaps my favorite part of practicing medicine because it requires an application of the art of medicine. In my practice, I apply some salient treatment guidelines that I learned along the way from Drs. Jones, Burrascano and Horowitz. In general, the following are important components of all of my treatment plans:

1. Treating infections and biotoxin illness

2. Decreasing inflammation

3. Degrading biofilm

4. Supporting the organs

5. Binding and detoxifying toxins

6. Thinning the blood

If I suspect that my patients have heavy metal poisoning, then I add chelation to their treatment plan, or if I suspect that they have abnormal detoxification pathways which are unidentified by lab tests, then I support these pathways through various means. I find that by addressing all of the aforementioned, I can develop a comprehensive treatment plan that supports areas of particular concern for my patients.

Treating the Infections

I generally use a combination of antibiotics, antimicrobial herbs, and vitamins to treat infections, depending upon the patient and his or her suspected infections. I tailor the treatment plan specifically to the "bug" that is currently taking center stage in the patient's symptom picture, because it is my belief that these microbes actually work together and that in patients with multiple infections, each bug takes a turn at being "center stage". This often makes treatment confusing, especially when laboratory tests indicate one conclusion, but clinical presentation indicates another. Therefore, experience is helpful for teasing out the prominent infection. There are times, however, when more than one infection is dominant and in such cases, the application of multiple remedies may be necessary. For more information on treatment for tick-borne infections, refer to Joseph Burrascano MD's treatment guidelines. For more information on herbal treatments for Lyme disease, refer to Stephen Harrod Buhner's book, *Healing Lyme: Natural Healing and Prevention of Lyme Borreliosis and Its Coinfections.*

Rife machines may also be helpful for the treatment of Lyme disease. To date, I have not seen Rife machines cure patients, but I have seen them aid in the dissolution of pathogen load. Scientists and physicians are not certain as to the mechanism of action of the Rife machine, but it appears to me that all living things are influenced by electromagnetic fields and tick-borne pathogens are no exception. I have often wondered how EMF's may affect these microbes. I suspect that the electric current (negatively charged moving ions) somehow destabilizes the pathogen's biofilm by binding to positively charged elements such as calcium, zinc, magnesium, mercury, lead and cadmium, whose function may be to secure the biofilm lattice. This may also be the reason why chelation therapy often helps chronic Lyme patients. Removing heavy metal ions probably also destabilizes the biofilm macro-environment, rendering the microbes more vulnerable to antibiotics and antimicrobial herbs. I am not aware of any scientific studies that elucidate this idea so this is simply my conceptualization of the relationship between "bugs, biofilm and ions." For more information on Rife machines, check out Bryan Rosner's book, *Lyme Disease and Rife Machines*.

Light therapy may also be a valuable means of decreasing pathogen load. I am unaware of any studies on this subject but light is a form of energy and all living things respond in some fashion to energy. Perhaps with high enough frequencies, light can alter the electromagnetic signature of certain microbes and thereby decrease their vital force and pathogenicity. Certainly more research in this area is needed.

Ozone therapy has also been used by many with Lyme, and provided some with notable beneficial effects. Ozone is an allotrope of oxygen, a triatomic molecule found in nature. Its name is derived from the word *ozein,* which means "to smell"—ozone has a very distinct smell that is, for example, noticeable after a thunderstorm. It is a powerful oxidizing gaseous agent that can transfer electrons to a substrate, due to its volatility. This means that it may neutralize the deleterious effects that spirochetes and neurotoxins have upon the body. Many different applications of ozone exist, including ozone saunas, ozonated water beverages, ozonated olive oil colonics and ear, rectal and vaginal insufflations. Ozone oxidizes and thereby neutralizes substrates such as neurotoxins, while reducing free radical damage caused by chronic infection. Certainly this has, at the very least, an adjunctive therapeutic value in the treatment of Lyme disease.

Ultraviolet blood irradiation and autohemotherapy are two adjunct therapies that must be considered with caution. Essentially, these techniques cleanse the blood of impurities that accumulate as the result of chronic infection, but those with Lyme should make certain that they are overseen by qualified and experienced physicians, as the potential for harm is not an insignificant consideration with these treatments.

Eliminating secondary viral and fungal infections is critical for reducing the immune system's pathogen burden. Herbs such as licorice (*Glycyrrhiza glabra*), oregano (*Origanum vulgare*), aloe (*Aloe vera*), and astragalus, as well as Vitamins A and C and the amino acid lysine are good for treating viruses. For fungal problems, plant tannins, oregano, pao d'arco *(Tabebuia species)*, garlic, licorice, tea tree *(Melaleuca)*, black walnut *(Juglans nigra)*, chamomile *(Matricaria recutita)*, goldenseal *(Hydrastis Canadensis)* or turmeric *(curcumen longa)* may be useful. For more aggressive antiviral treatment, Valtrex or Valcyte can be used, and for more aggressive fungal treatment, Nystatin, Diflucan, Sporanox, or Amphotericin B may be appropriate. For nasal fungus, sprays of Diflucan or Amphotericin B, the latter of which is compounded by a specialty pharmacy, are good. Lamasil or Zim's Crack Cream, which can be purchased at www.crackcreme.com, can be beneficial for treating topical funguses.

Biotoxin Illness

Richard Shoemaker, M.D. in Potomac, MD, first recognized "biotoxin illness" when he realized that many of his patients, poisoned by the ciguatera toxin, remained severely ill after their treatment. Further research revealed that these patients had been exposed to a biotoxin, either through mold, food, water, air or insect bites, and did not have the requisite immune system genes to handle the toxic load. These genes are known as HLA DR genes. People with a certain HLA pattern develop inappropriate immunity and produce antibodies to myelin basic protein, gliadin and cardiolipin. The alternative complement pathway of these people's immune systems may be activated and they may have increased levels of C3a and C4a. Hence, they produce excessive inflammatory cytokines and cannot properly rid their bodies of biotoxins, which inevitably renders them severely ill.

Biotoxins bind to a surface receptor on adipocytes (cells that primarily compose adipose, or fatty tissue) which activates cytokines. Increased cytokines also damage leptin receptors in the hypothalamus and decrease the production of melanocyte stimulating hormone (MSH). Increased cytokines in the arterial vasculature probably attract white blood cells and fibrin molecules, which leads to decreased blood flow and decreased oxygen levels in the tissues (a state of tissue anoxia). Additionally, reduced vascular endothelial growth factor (VEGF) may lead to fatigue, shortness of breath and muscle cramping. Therefore, those with biotoxin illness must take toxin binders in order to heal.

Finally, decreased MSH probably causes a myriad of other effects upon the body including: sleep disturbances, chronic pain, gastrointestinal malabsorption, ADH (antidiuretic hormone) insufficiency, decreased sex hormones and elevated levels of stress hormones. It may also allow the proliferation of MARCoNS (multiple antibiotic resistant coagulase negative staphalococci) in mucosal tissues. In my practice, MARCoNS seems to be a particular problem for my patients with chronic sinusitis and I prefer to use a combination of Quercenase nasal spray, intranasal Rifampin and intranasal Diflucan or Amphotericin B to treat it.

Decrease the Inflammation

Inflammation is an integral part of any infection. When tissues become infected with pathogens, the immune system sends a variety of chemical molecules such as cytokines, chemokines, and other cells to aid in the battle against further invasion by these pathogens. Pro-inflammatory cytokines probably play a significant role in the pathogenicity of tick-borne diseases. I view inflammation as a considerable barrier to treatment because in the same way that an angry person is unable to hear and receive the perspective of another, angry or inflamed tissues can't properly receive nutrients, water or antimicrobial agents. Inflammation interferes with the receptivity of tissues. Therefore, I use a variety of supplements and techniques to decrease inflammation in my patients, including hydrotherapy, fish oil, curcumin, proteolytic enzymes, massage, acupuncture and diet. Limiting dietary intake of pro-inflammatory foods such as gluten, casein, and sugar is a practice that perhaps everyone, not just those with Lyme, should engage in. Dr. Kenneth Singleton's book, *The Lyme Disease Solution*, contains a detailed anti-inflammatory diet that includes recipes. I recommend this book to all of my patients. It is easy to read and is written in large print. Everyone responds to treatment interventions differently and for this reason, it's good for practitioners to have a good sense of their patients' essence, so that the most appropriate therapies can be administered, in accordance with their patients' specific needs.

Degrade the Biofilm

Alan MacDonald, M.D., a New York pathologist and pioneer in spirochete microscopy, was the first physician to recognize and document the presence and importance of biofilm production among tick-borne pathogens. However, Dr. William Costerton, Ph.D., has been studying the elaborate microenvironments of biofilm in many microbial species for most of his professional life and has published extensively in this area. His book, *The Biofilm Primer*, is particularly useful for understanding these complex matrices. Eva Sapi, Ph.D., at the University of New Haven, collaborates with Dr. MacDonald on Borrelia biofilm research. In their research, they have noted several environmental conditions that contribute to spirochete biofilm formation including cell density, nutrient depletion and penicillin administration.

The National Institutes of Health have estimated that as much as 80% of all chronic infections (i.e., sinusitis, otitis media and bronchitis) may be due to the presence of biofilm. Biofilm is composed of mucopolysaccharides and DNA and its formation begins as a few organisms attach to one another and to a substrate. This results in the formation of a lattice-like structure that functions to promote microbial communication, house microbes, provide nutrients to the dwellers and protect the microbes against invasion and destruction by the host's immune system and antibiotics. Multiple microbial species may live in a single biofilm community and this may foster intraspecies as well as interspecies exchange of DNA, yielding "hybrid- like" bugs. This may add another level of complexity to the treatment of tick-borne diseases. I have found addressing biofilm to be particularly important in the treatment of patients infected with Bartonella. This is just my clinical observation, but when I use enzymes such as Boluoke, Nattokinase, Zyactinase and so on, in combination with N-acetyl-cysteine and lactoferrin to degrade the biofilm, patients seem to respond to antimicrobial agents much better. Admittedly, the Herxheimer reactions are a little more severe but Dr. Jones trained me "to appreciate the Herx, since it is indicative of bug decimation." Using either Benadryl or Alka Seltzer Gold, in combination with quercetin and other bioflavanoids can minimize Herxheimer reactions. Warm lemon water and a diet rich in alkaline foods also helps to mute the Herxheimer reaction.

Support the Organs

Organ support during antimicrobial treatment of tick-borne infections is a broad area of treatment that requires careful consideration. The very name "antibiotic" means "against life" and although antibiotics are directed against microbes, they also inadvertently affect other tissues. Generally, antibiotics are very drying to tissues, so it is critical that patients remain hydrated while undergoing treatment. Drugs and herbs can tax the liver, kidneys, and a variety of other organs, so appropriate nutrient and herbal support should be considered throughout treatment. Practitioners need to pay careful attention to their patients' symptoms in order to properly support their organs that are most affected by treatments. Obviously, this varies from patient to patient. Additionally, tick-borne infections can target a particular organ (i.e., the brain, heart, lungs, muscles, joints, and intestines) and specific nutrient support may be required for these organs. I try to review this issue during every patient appointment as well, and perform routine blood tests to assess how the organs are withstanding the stress of rigorous treatment.

Spirochetes are destructive microbial predators and can really "do a number" on the hypothalamus, which ultimately affects the entire endocrine system. Therefore, endocrine organ support may be necessary throughout treatment. Again, practitioners should assess this on an individual basis during every follow-up visit that they have with their patients. By doing so, they can be certain of making any necessary interventions to their healing process. Treatment plans can include herbs, vitamins, homeopathy, energy medicine, acupuncture, massage, hydrotherapy, colonics, Reiki, counseling, meditation, saunas, high dilutional medicine, German biological medicine, immunotherapy, ozone therapy, IV nutrients, especially high dose buffered Vitamin C, and just about anything that promotes holistic wellness.

Lastly, I have been finding that most people with chronic Lyme disease and/or co-infections need immune support. However, providing immune support can be a double-edged sword. Because Lyme disease is also known to initiate a host of autoimmune reactions, it's important that practitioners test for these, to ensure that any immune support therapy won't exacerbate a previously existing autoimmune disorder. For example, if a patient exhibits a low CD-57 count but also has a positive ANA test, or evidence of thyroid antibodies, then the practitioner might consider using Vitamin C to support that person's immune system, since this treatment is unlikely to worsen the autoimmune disorder. Vitamin C is an excellent water-soluble antioxidant, and in high enough doses, can saturate the tissues, remove destructive free radicals and then be easily excreted through the kidneys. I am cautioning practitioners about autoimmunity because I have inadvertently overlooked it in the past, and I feel it is important to address.

Natural immune support products can also include any of the following: thymic protein, shitake and maitake mushrooms, Vitamin D, arabinogalactans, specific transfer factors, lactoferrin, colostrum, *Ecklonia cava*, green lipped mussels, astragalus, echinacea, Vitamin C, zinc picolinate, trace minerals, onion *(Allium cepa)*, garlic *(Allium sativum)*, licorice *(Glycyrrhiza glabra)*, or oregano *(Origanum vulgare)*, to name a few. One of the strengths of naturopathic medicine is that it emphasizes immune support. A large body of information on this subject can be found at the Bastyr University bookstore in Kenmore, WA.

Supporting the immune system also includes managing histamine. Histamine is a substance that mediates the body's allergic response and which is stored and released from blood basophils, mast cells and nerve endings. Histamine is also a neurotransmitter and influences many physiological functions such as body temperature, sleep, metabolism, mood and even the ability to think. Abraham Hoffer, M.D. and Carl Pfeiffer, M.D., both orthomolecular physicians, were pioneers in examining histamine imbalances in patients with schizophrenia. As a naturopathic medical student, I spent several years studying their work, not knowing then how applicable this information would be to my practice later, during my clinical years.

Many of my patients have high histamine levels, as evidenced from their dermatographia tests, allergies, and red pinna (Winter's ear). Practitioners can analyze their patients' blood histamine levels through the Princeton Bio Center in Princeton, NJ, although in my practice, I generally trust my clinical instincts when it comes to diagnosing this problem. Reducing histamine levels, especially in the brain, is very important, particularly in children with brain allergies and neuroborreliosis, but also in adults. Histamine stimulates the release of serotonin, dopamine, and norepinephrine in the hypothalamus, and conversely, dopamine and epinephrine modulate histamine release. Therefore, it is reasonable to assume that chronic Lyme disease patients have an increase in histamine production as the end result of an overburdened immune system. I find that decreasing histamine with the use of herbs such as nettles, quercetin, and andrographis, or in more severe cases, Ketotifen or Benadryl, often helps to relieve some of the brain fog and congestion that patients experience during treatment.

Drs. Hoffer and Pfeiffer also noticed that their patient populations often had pyroluria, a condition characterized by elevated urinary levels of kryptopyrrole (a mauve-colored substance). Pyroles (kryptopyrrole means hidden pyrole) are used primarily in the formation of porphyrin, which is the major constituent of hemoglobin, a molecule responsible for carrying oxygen to tissues. Kryptopyrrole binds irreversibly with pyridoxine (Vitamin B6), which is important because many neurotransmitter pathways use B-6 as a co-factor. The kryptopyrrole-B6 compound then combines with any available zinc, and is excreted from the body, ultimately depleting the body of both B-6 and zinc. This is relevant to Lyme disease patients because B-6 is important for proper brain function and zinc is equally important for proper immune function, and where deficiencies of both are present, patients have a more difficult time recovering. Hence, supplementing with zinc picolinate and pyridoxine may be important. More information about pyrole testing can be obtained from Vitamin Diagnostics in Keyport, New Jersey, at: 732-583-7774. I have always wondered if Dr. Hoffer and Dr. Pfeiffer were treating Lyme disease patients and didn't know it, especially since Dr. Hoffer practices in Victoria, BC, a known tick endemic area. In fact, I have also wondered whether orthomolecular medicine (high dose nutritional medicine) was borne out of the observation that Lyme disease patients are often severely depleted in nutrients. And I have wondered if the alternative medicine movement, which grew so rapidly in the 1980's and 1990's in the United States, came about because those with undiagnosed Lyme disease and who had a myriad of odd symptoms, were unable to find help through the "traditional" system. This may have then forced them to seek care through other healthcare providers, hence fostering the growth of the alternative medicine movement.

Intestinal Support

Naturopathic physicians are taught that the gut is "God", and that intestinal dysbiosis is the root of all illness. While I have modified my beliefs in this regard, I do emphasize optimal intestinal health in my practice. Clearly, a "leaky gut" sets the stage for a host of immune and autoimmune problems, and often, the gut may need to be healed before people with Lyme can embark on antimicrobial treatment. On the other hand, infection may be the root cause of their gut dysbiosis. I continually educate myself on the subject of intestinal health because most of my patients, at one time or another, will have problems with this organ system. Abdominal pain, gas, bloating, diarrhea and constipation are some of the common symptoms exhibited by those infected with tick-borne infections. I use a Comprehensive Digestive Stool Analysis test (from Genova Diagnostics) to examine my patients' digestive abnormalities and to help detect which problems are directly caused by infection. For example, a low secretory IgA, which is commonly seen in Lyme disease patients, is usually indicative of infection occupying the mucosal layer of the intestine. In my practice, Bartonella appears to be the biggest culprit here and often, treating patients with antimicrobial herbs, along with aloe, glutamine, marshmallow root, and the Syntrion product, SyRegule, can clear out some of the infection.

That said, I believe that the most important component to any anti-infectious treatment plan in the gut is the strategic use of probiotics. My patients know that taking probiotics is just as important as taking antimicrobial herbs or antibiotics. The intestinal microflora is extremely complex and contains over 400 distinct microbial species in delicate balance. This balance not only allows for proper nutrient absorption and assimilation, but also permits proper drug absorption. If there are "holes" in the intestine, as is so often seen in the leaky gut syndrome that accompanies Lyme disease, then drug molecules may not be metabolized properly, which in turn puts significant stress on the gastrointestinal system. Additionally, it may facilitate the build-up of toxins and debris along the mucosal lining of the intestine, which further complicates healing. Therefore, proper probiotic supplementation is critical. In my practice, I like to use a combination of Theralac or Prescript Assist Pro and saccharomyces boulardii. I also encourage my patients to do a colonic once a month and use coffee enemas as needed. Periodic and continued cleansing of the bowels ensures healthy mucosal tissues maximally prepared for nutrient absorption.

Constipation is another problem that needs to be addressed and rectified in those with Lyme prior to the initiation of any antimicrobial therapy. Eliminating toxins is a crucial component of any treatment plan designed to combat tick-borne illnesses. Those with Lyme should excrete fecal matter on a daily basis. If they don't, then they should use any of the following to mobilize the stool: triphala, psyllium *(Plantago ispghula),* magnesium solution (excepting those with *Bartonella),* aloe *(Aloe vera),* cascara *(Rhamnus purshani cortex),* senna *(Casia senna),* dandelion root *(taraxacum officinale),* fenugreek *(Trigonella foenum graecum),* chlorophyll or flax seed oil. Maintaining a diet that is low in gluten and casein is also helpful, as is light to moderate daily exercise, which aids in peristalsis.

Pancreas Support

Many chronic Lyme disease patients develop insulin resistance as the result of the multiple biochemical perturbations that are caused by spirochete tissue invasion. Low MSH, for example, causes leptin resistance, which is frequently seen in those with biotoxin illness. Serum leptin levels rise, causing rapid weight gain, which then affects the ability of insulin to reduce blood sugar levels. The biochemistry involved here is not well understood and I may be making several cognitive leaps, but clearly a relationship exists among these endocrine molecules that seem to be altered in Lyme disease. The use of chromium picolinate and *Gymnema sylvestre,* niacin, pancreatin, billberry, and vanadyl sulfate may help to stabilize blood sugar levels.

Liver Support

Liver support is particularly important for those who choose to use antibiotics, because many antibiotic medications are metabolized through the liver. In particular, the liver's cytochrome P450 system is affected by pharmaceutical drugs and therefore, proper support is essential. Artemisinin in prolonged high doses also stresses the liver. Oral liposomal glutathione, lipoic acid, selenium citrate, taurine, *Silymarin* (milk thistle), artichoke, Liv 52 (an ayurvedic herbal combination), licorice root or *Phyllanthus amarus,* may be used to support the liver. Additionally, delivering some antibiotics in a "pulse-like" fashion can keep the liver from becoming over-taxed. Physicians and practitioners should check with a pharmacist before pulsing any antibiotics, as some of these, such as Rifampin (which can cause serious thrombocytopenia), can produce delete-rious effects when used improperly. Additionally, herbal and antibiotic combinations for Lyme disease should be formulated by a knowledgeable practitioner, as many drug/herb interactions are not therapeutic.

Joint and Muscle Support

Clearly, one of the places towards which spirochetes gravitate is the collagen layer of muscles and joints. Inflammation ensues in these regions, resulting in an arthritic condition. Certain foods, such as wheat, dairy and piperine-containing foods may exacerbate the inflammatory process. Nightshade vegetables such as potatoes and tomatoes typically have high concentrations of piperine and are known to cause joint inflammation. Removing these foods will significantly reduce joint pain, as will supplementing with glucosa-mine sulfate, niacinamide, Vitamin E, selenium citrate, Vitamin C, boron, S-Adenosyl-L-methionine, Boswellia, and Curcumin, all of which can be found in oral supplements.

Integumentary (Skin, Hair and Nails) Support

The skin provides a large surface area for detoxification. Many chronic Lyme disease patients suffer from a variety of irritating and painful skin lesions, particularly when they are undergoing detox-

ification. Avoiding sugar and carbohydrates is likely to be necessary in order to minimize the occurrence of these. Colonics or an
intestinal cleanse may also be beneficial to those with severe skin
eruptions. Brushing may be used to slough off old dead skin, which
hinders detoxification. Supplementation with zinc picolinate,
niacinamide, pyridoxine, essential fatty acids, pancreatin, and
Vitamins A and C may provide some relief from pruritus. Topical
Vitamin C and Azelaic acid may also be useful. As previously noted
in this chapter, histamine management will aid in reducing the
inflammatory component of detoxification.

Brain Support

For those with neuroborreliosis, brain nutrient support may be
important. The use of omega 3, 6 and 9 essential fatty acids can be
helpful for decreasing inflammation, although there is debate
among physicians about whether these feed the spirochetes since
they do not manufacture their own fatty acids. Also, the use of IV
phosphatidylcholine per Dr. Patricia Kane's protocol may be helpful, but I caution patients to use intravenous therapies sparingly in
order to preserve the integrity of their veins. Veins can become
sclerosed and fibrotic from repeated needle pricks. This becomes
particularly important if patients need to go on IV antibiotics after
having received many nutritional IV's.

Supplementing with all of the B vitamins is also important because
those with tick-borne infections tend to have low levels of these,
particularly pyridoxine (vitamin B-6). Vitamin B-6 is a cofactor in
the production of many neurotransmitters, so maintaining adequate levels throughout treatment is necessary. Methylcobalamin
may also be important, but blood levels should be monitored. I like
to give taurine to patients who have an irritable nervous system, as
it tends to have a calming effect upon the brain, as does GABA
(gamma-aminobutyric acid). Ginko biloba, Vinpocetine, and
arginine can be useful for increasing blood flow to the brain.
Finally, many amino acids are depleted in people with infections so
supplementation with these may also be important. *The Brain*

Chemistry Diet by Michael Lesser, M.D. is a helpful resource for learning more about brain nutrition.

Insomnia

For the treatment of insomnia, I recommend tri-methylglycine, GABA, 5-Hydroxytryptophan, taurine, theanine, or melatonin to my patients. Fresh lavender placed inside the pillowcase can also help to induce sleep as it has calming effects upon the brain. In most cases, one or many of these supplements/herbs can "kick start" the body's sleep cycle so that its natural rhythm eventually takes over. However, prolonged or treatment-resistant insomnia is a symptom that I take very seriously because I believe that sleep is the "silent nurse"; a time when the immune system, in particular, regenerates. Prolonged sleep deprivation and failure to properly enter REM sleep can have detrimental effects upon the brain and body. For severe cases of insomnia, Ambien, Lunesta and even a benzodiazepine may be necessary. Patients often express concern about the addictive qualities of the benzodiazepines, and I encourage those that live in Seattle to see Dr. Linda Williams, who is a Lyme-literate psychiatrist, skilled in the clinical application of these medications. I personally believe that achieving deep, restful sleep is on balance more important than developing an addiction that can be dealt with at a later time when optimal health is regained. Sleep is indeed the "silent nurse," and "chief nourisher in life's feast."

Headaches and Migraines

For the treatment of headaches and migraines, I use intranasal Vitamin B-12 or a standardized, patented extract of butter root, Petadolex. Hydration and bowel movements will also help to alleviate headaches. For migraines, patients can use a topical combination of DMSO, magnesium and emu oil. This will often mute a migraine. Some patients also find relief from migraine headaches by using Imitrex. Chronic Lyme disease patients should avoid the use of prednisone for migraines or rebound headaches, as it is immunosuppressive.

Mood

Many with tick-borne diseases will experience mood lability or even rage. This is often difficult for them and their family members to manage and may require special treatment and perhaps even counseling. Again, I refer patients with these symptoms to a Lyme-literate psychiatrist that I know, who uses medications such as Lamictol, Topimax, Depakote and others, to stabilize mood. I believe that it is extremely important, however, to involve a Lyme-literate psychiatrist when treating these symptoms with medications, because there are specific "cocktails" of medications that work well for neuroborreliosis and neurobartonellosis.

Depression

Most people with Lyme disease go through a "depressive phase" during their illness and treatment. This may be due directly to the infection(s), or it may be secondary to their illness and due more to circumstances. Many with Lyme have lost their jobs, homes, spouses, friends, insurance and dignity, by virtue of the fact that they have been undiagnosed for long periods of time. This is extremely unfortunate but again, proper nutrient and perhaps pharmacological intervention can help lessen the effects of depression, whether due to infections or circumstances. I take depression very seriously and, again, refer my patients to a Lyme-literate psychiatrist. I believe that depressive tendencies interfere with the body's capacity to heal and need to be dealt with throughout treatment if patients are to achieve optimal wellness. The "dark night of the soul" is not a particularly healing place for those with Lyme to dwell for long periods of time.

Attention Deficit Disorder

Neuroborreliosis patients often have poor attention spans, a diminished ability to focus and "brain fog." Proper nutritional support and management of neuroinflammation and brain allergies can help to mitigate these symptoms. One technique, which involves decreasing "heat" in the head, is accomplished by placing a cool rag on the patient's forehead and his or her feet in a warm tub. This sets up a circuit that pulls heat out of the head. Avoidance of foods that cause brain symptoms, most notably wheat, is critical. William Philpott, M.D. and Carl Pfeiffer, M.D., physicians who practice orthomolecular medicine, suggest that inefficient gluten digestion produces exorphins, similar to endorphins, that readily cross the blood brain barrier and induce rage and chaotic behavior. Perhaps the most beneficial diet for those who are undergoing treatment for tick-borne illness is the "Paleolithic diet" as proposed by Melvin Konner, M.D. in his book, *The Paleolithic Prescription*. This diet consists largely of fruits, vegetables, nuts and meat. Finally, decreasing histamine levels with the use of an antihistamine herb like nettles or the anti-oxidant quercetin can be helpful for reducing symptoms of ADD. In more severe cases, the use of Benadryl or Ketotifen may be required.

Autism

Tami Duncan, the founder of the Lyme-Induced Autism Foundation (www.lymeinducedautism.com), and Robert Bransfield, a New Jersey psychiatrist, were the first people to initiate further inquiry into the relationship between Lyme disease and autism. Their work has led to the development of an annual conference on Lyme disease and autism. Outstanding speakers and state-of-the-art alternative treatments for autism are always present at these conferences. While there is no question that Lyme disease can cause an autism-like syndrome, probably due to excessive inflammation in vulnerable developing brain tissue, among other factors, further research into this phenomenon is necessary. Lyme sufferers and physicians interested in this particular aspect of Lyme disease may also find the "Defeat Autism Now" conferences to be beneficial.

Energy

The long-term effects of chronic infection take a toll on the mitochondria, which are the "power houses" found in most cells of the body. Poor energy and endurance are hallmark symptoms of tick-borne infections and to combat these symptoms, I initially prefer to give my patients herbs such as ashwaganda, rhodiola, or eleuthercoccus (Siberian Ginseng) because they also function as adaptogens and support adrenal gland function. Ribose may also be helpful and for those with severe cases of fatigue, physiological doses of cortisol (Cortef) may be necessary. I have also found that daily mild to moderate exercise helps to increase energy and stamina.

Hormones

Those with tick-borne illnesses often have a myriad of hormonal imbalances due to disturbances in their hypothalamic, pituitary and end organ feedback systems. To determine the specific problems that are present, it may be necessary for practitioners to perform laboratory tests on their patients, including those which measure thyroid and adrenal gland function, male and female hormones, DHEA sulfate, pregnenolone, insulin, growth hormone, and even vasopressin. I manage some of my patients' hormone imbalances myself with herbs and nutrients, while others I refer to a specialist. I have a "comfort zone" when it comes to treating hormones and if I feel the slightest bit uncomfortable with the severity of symptoms that my patients are exhibiting, then I will refer them to a specialist who is more knowledgeable in endocrinology. Hormones are secreted in micromolar to nanomolar concentrations throughout the body and therefore, careful manipulation of these potent bio-chemical substances is critical for healing to take place. Furthermore, cancer (another anaerobic disease) is often associated with endocrine dysfunction, which is why I generally refer my patients to an endocrine specialist for treatment of certain hormon-al issues.

Binding and Detoxifying Toxins

Healthy human beings take for granted their normal patterns of urination, defecation and sweating, but these avenues of toxin release are often compromised in the chronically ill. It is important that such avenues remain open and functional throughout patients' treatment programs, which means that practitioners must often provide their patients with detoxification support during their treatment for infections, if they are to fully heal. Tick-borne pathogens are known to release endotoxins into the blood, which can then bind to the body's cells, and especially fat cells. The brain is particularly vulnerable to the effects of toxins such as quinolinic acid, which can contribute to symptoms of "brain fog and cloudy thinking" in chronic Lyme disease patients. IV glutathione is known to cleanse liver detoxification pathways but one can also use artichoke, dandelion root, lipoic acid, selenium and a host of other natural products. I like to use chitosan, chlorella, charcoal, bentonite clay, apple pectin, or zeolite in my treatment protocols. Detox footbaths or pads, infrared saunas and/or sweat lodges may also be helpful. Most essential, however, is getting patients to do some form of aerobic exercise for ten to twenty minutes daily. This gets their blood moving and mobilizes waste for excretion. For heavy metal detoxification, I prefer chlorella, DMSA 30mg/kg or humic acid. Detoxification pathway support can also include folinic acid, and B-12 supplements (see Richard Van Konynenburg, Ph.D.'s presentation at the 9th International IACFS/ME Conference, Reno, Nevada, 2009).

Finally, many people with Lyme find detoxification diets to be helpful. These can include whole foods and up to thirty-six ounces of fresh vegetable juice per day, especially carrot juice. Carrot juice is believed to cleanse the body's extracellular matrix where many toxins reside. In my own healing journey, I drank sixteen ounces of fresh carrot juice daily, which made me feel much better. Carrot juice may also alkalize the blood, which is important for healing.

Treating Hypercoagulation and Thick Blood

Hypercoagulation (thick blood, blood stagnation or chi stagnation) as it relates to tick-borne infections, is an area of treatment that particularly interests me. David Berg, MS at Hemex laboratories has noted that many with chronic Lyme disease exhibit abnormal coagulation values. A thorough laboratory test work-up, which includes PT, PTT, INR, fibrinogen, lipoprotein, homocysteine, plasminogen activator inhibitor - 1, tissue plasminogen activator, d-dimer, and fibrinogen degradation products, can be helpful in assessing the state of patients' blood. If they have hypercoagulation, the use of Boluoke and other enzymes can aid in fibrin degradation. It may also be necessary to use sublingual heparin to thin the blood. Medical doctors may instead choose to use subcutaneous injections of heparin. In my practice, I have found that patients with multiple co-infections have the thickest blood, especially those who are infected with Bartonella. Bartonella seems to have a particular affinity for vascular tissue and may influence blood flow, especially to the extremities. Cold hands and feet are common symptoms in those with Lyme disease and co-infections, which suggests that they have poor peripheral circulation. Additionally, poor circulation indicates that the tissues are oxygen deprived, and anaerobic microbes covet this type of environment. Poor circulation can also affect the degree to which nutrients, water and medication reach diseased tissues. Chi and blood stagnation are conditions that Chinese medicine has treated for centuries with acupuncture. The maintenance of proper "flow" in every respect is a critical component to the healing of all tissues. For a detailed description of coagulation factors that are involved in disease, visit: www.hemex.com, or call David Berg, MS at Arizona Coagulation Consultants, Inc. (602-997-9477). Patients and practitioners may be able to join one of his informative workshops to learn about this new and exciting area of medicine as it relates to tick-borne infections. Finally, chronic Lyme disease patients often bruise easily, which suggests capillary fragility. Vitamin C and proanthocyanidins can be used to support vessel integrity. Certain foods that are high in salicylates can also help thin the blood. These include peppermint, oregano, turmeric, paprika, cinnamon, thyme, cayenne, curry, ginger, dill and licorice.

Hypoxia

Many patients with chronic Lyme disease complain of chest pain, shortness of breath, and exhaustion. These can be symptoms of Babesia, but they can also be symptoms of hypoxia, a condition in which tissues don't receive enough oxygen. Patients with "thick blood" and coagulation defects seem to be at the greatest risk for developing this problem. In chronic infection, somehow the body coats the arterial vessel walls with fibrin. This causes vessel wall rigidity, creates an anaerobic environment for pathogens and allows the bugs to evade the host's immune system. In addition, this fibrin barrier prevents oxygen, water, nutrients and medications from reaching the tissues in appropriate concentrations. Hypoxia can result, which leaves patients feeling depleted. I like to use nebulized glutathione and oxygen to relieve my patients of the feeling that they aren't getting enough oxygen. Lincare, Inc, is a national company that supplies portable oxygen, and generally I prescribe four liters per minute, for twenty to thirty minutes, two to four times a day. The treatments are taken either through a nasal cannula or through a re-breather mask. These methods of administration are not good for those with multiple chemical sensitivities or latex allergies, however, as the tubing on the devices may cause allergic reactions.

Management of Free Radicals, Nitric Oxide and Peroxynitrite

Free radicals (usually oxygen) are molecular species that increase in response to infection. As the concentration of free radicals in the brain increases, the tissue loses its integrity and function and essentially becomes toxic and unable to perform its normal duties. This is particularly evident when peroxynitrite (an oxidizing and nitrating agent which can damage a wide array of molecules in cells, including DNA and proteins) contributes to the degradation of the blood-brain barrier so that selective permeability to nutritive substances becomes impaired. Neural toxicity manifests symptomatically as cognitive and sensory impairment, brain fog and mood lability.

Martin Paul, Ph.D., at Washington State University, has spent many years researching the role that nitric oxide (NO) plays in the development of neurodegenerative diseases. Nitric oxide is known to play an essential role in the modulation of vascular tone, neurotransmission and immune system function. When certain brain cells become activated as the result of an infection, they release inflammatory cytokines, which promote the release of nitric oxide. Through an elaborate series of chemical reactions, nitric oxide combines with free radical oxygen to form peroxynitrite, which is highly toxic to the brain.

This situation can be rectified through the strategic supplementation of high dose antioxidants. Nutrients such as Vitamins E and C, ginkgo biloba, lipoic acid, selenium, green tea and various bioflavinoids essentially "scavenge" the free radicals and neutralize the effects of peroxynitrite on the tissues. When these nutrients are given, tissue function seems to return to some degree in many people with neurodegenerative diseases such as Parkinson's, Alzheimer's, ALS and perhaps Autism, and even when the etiology of the toxicity is infectious. Therapeutically, I address various biochemical pathways in my patients in order to decrease the effects of free radical toxicity upon their brains and increase the likelihood of restoring normal brain function. This requires the calculated and strategic use of various antioxidants, which function synergistically to provide protection to the brain.

Lifestyle Recommendations for Healing Lyme Disease

It's no secret that lifestyle significantly affects the speed and degree by which those with Lyme disease recover. I have found that when in the throes of illness—when patients find it difficult to get out of bed—having a soft, soothing environment can be beneficial for healing. Soft colors, textures, foods (pureed), music, and so forth, set a vibrational tone that is conducive for deep healing. Loud music, bright colors, etc., although vibrant, are not helpful for healing the body. Rudolph Steiner, an early 20th century Austrian philosopher, educator, architect and esotericist, founded a spiritual science movement called Anthroposophy. He has written volumes of books on the subject of healing and lends some interesting insights to the process. Those with Lyme can access his information by visiting the A. Waldorf school bookstore or by ordering his books on the Internet at: www.steinerbooks.org. His manuscripts provide pearls of wisdom on the subject of one's healing environment. Some with Lyme might find his work interesting and helpful, as they design their own path toward recovery.

Also, nature is perhaps one of the most healing environments that there is, since, for example, the sound of wind, water, rain and rustling trees, and the sight of trees, flowers, ocean and mountains, are therapeutic in and of themselves. As nature is also the abode of ticks, however, I caution my patients to protect themselves against tick bites when out in woods, fields and grasses. In any case, frequently visiting nature can have a profoundly positive effect upon the speed of recovery.

Human Support

Sadly, one of the things that those with Lyme disease often suffer from most is a lack of human contact. The disease often leaves them bedridden, which then isolates them from friends and family. This is not conducive to healing, as human beings are social animals and thrive in extended social settings. Support groups can therefore be beneficial for those who are sick, and meetings with a counselor can lessen the effects of illness isolation. Book groups, coffee/tea social hours, lunch dates and/or a simple walk in the park, can also have dramatically positive effects upon their well being.

It's important for family members to include their loved ones with Lyme in all activities so that they can maintain their place in the social organization of the family. Unfortunately, family members sometimes become distant due to not being able to identify with the loved one who has Lyme. Whenever I encounter this problem in my practice, I bring up the subject of cancer to family members of the sick. I tell them that if their loved one had cancer, there would be an immediate show of support for that family member and which would be felt immediately by him or her. But because Lyme disease is a "mysterious illness", often those with Lyme are left to fend for themselves. This can have catastrophic consequences for them because people need contact with other human beings. They need to been seen, heard and appreciated, especially when they're sick and even more so when they have Lyme disease. Chronic Lyme patients are often misinterpreted as being hypochondriacs and malingerers so that they may have a heightened need to be listened to and heard by others. And rightfully so, I might add.

Community Support

There are a variety of Lyme disease support groups in many states. Information on these can be found by doing an Internet Google search. Also, the Lyme Disease Association has a website that provides access to resources (www.lymediseaseassociation.org) and the California Lyme Disease Association (CALDA) publishes a quarterly journal which can be purchased by visiting: www.lymedisease.org. This journal generally contains a very informative group of articles written by physicians and Lyme sufferers who disperse new and interesting information to the Lyme disease community. Time for Lyme, Inc., in Greenwich, CT is another non-profit organization that has a tremendous amount of information on all aspects of Lyme. More information can be found on the Internet at: (www.timeforlyme.org). This organization also awards money to researchers to further investigate Lyme disease and new treatments. Finally, Turn the Corner Foundation (www.turnthecorner.org) in New York City is another non-profit organization that donates a considerable amount of money to educate physicians about Lyme disease through its support of the ILADS preceptorship training program. A significant amount of money is directed towards research as well, which supports ongoing efforts on all fronts to find a cure for Lyme disease. The above-mentioned support groups are probably the most established, but are by no means the only ones. Those with Lyme should search the Internet to find a group that best suits their needs.

Books on Lyme Disease

Both physicians and patients with Lyme have written an array of books on Lyme disease. I encourage people to visit the Internet site: www.amazon.com and type "Lyme Disease and Co-infections" into the search engine in order to find the literature that is sold there (which includes used books). I cannot recommend a "best" book because people search for different information. Many want information on alternative medicine, while others, on traditional treatment approaches or both of these. So it's best for people to do a search themselves in order to find books that meet their specific needs. Visiting the local library to check out their collection of Lyme disease books may be a good idea, as well.

Spirit/Soul Sickness

As a practitioner, the most disheartening thing to witness in people with chronic Lyme disease is a loss of spirit. This occurs in many with Lyme and is characterized by a loss in one's vitality for life and/or an inability to experience joy. At present, it's not clear to me whether this is a result of the difficulty in receiving proper diagnosis and treatment, or if the spirochetes actually "eat away" at the spirit. These microbes appear to be so calculated and cunning that it wouldn't surprise me if they actually purposefully eroded away at the spirit in an attempt to weaken their host. The antidote for this involves those with Lyme surrounding themselves with the things and people that make them the happiest. Activities such as journal writing, artwork, playing music, singing, macramé, sewing, puzzles and building projects feed the spirit and soul. I tell my patients, "Don't give in to the bugs. Don't let them take your power. Don't let them steal your joy."

Solutions to the Problem of Lyme

Time for Lyme, Inc. and the LDA (Lyme Disease Association) have helped to fund the first Lyme disease research facility at Columbia University, which is directed by Brian Fallon, M.D. This facility is devoted to furthering society's understanding of tick-borne diseases. Recent heightened interest by many universities and private companies has been promising, as well. As scientists and physicians begin to acknowledge the Lyme disease epidemic across the globe, I suspect that more and more research on this issue will be initiated. My hope is that a cure is in sight.

The Lessons to Be Learned

It's no surprise to most people that life is nothing but a string of lessons that we all need to learn. Everybody's set of lessons is different and those learned through illness are no exception. During the 1980's and 1990's, when alternative medicine first became popular, Jean Shinoda Bolen, M.D., Deepak Chopra, M.D., Mona Lisa Schultz, M.D., Thomas Moore, and Louise Haye, all wrote books regarding the "gifts" that illness unveils. When in the throes of chronic illness, it's difficult for the sick to see anything good about their situation, but if they take the time to reflect upon it, such introspection may yield different and interesting results. For example, perhaps it teaches them that they need to slow down and engage in more self-care, spend more time with family, cultivate hobbies or their spiritual life, have more free time, or perhaps simply learn more about the process of introspection! Wisdom is crystallized pain and pain is felt anytime we're asked (or forced) to make a significant life change. I encourage all of my patients to avoid falling prey to a "victim" mentality and instead look for the gifts in their healing journey. If they are able to do this, then they are sometimes amazed at what they find. Meeting remarkable and interesting people and developing a talent or interest that they didn't know that they had are examples of such gifts which in turn provide areas for rich personal growth and the discovery of new gifts and pleasures in their lives.

Closing Remarks

Perhaps what concerns me most about those with chronic Lyme disease is their propensity to enter a state of desperation and despair. Such a state is dangerous because it robs them of their personal power, the very attribute that is needed to continue on a healing journey. I encourage all of my patients to embrace an attitude of patience and perseverance in order to deal with the daily challenges inherent in chronic Lyme disease. I tell them to keep learning, trying new things (safety matters here) and meeting new people to the best of their ability, and certainly some good will come of those efforts. I also tell them to look for coincidences and synchronicities in their healing journey, as these are often clues that they are on the right track. In addition, I tell them to keep their spirits alive, to laugh if they can and as often as they can, because Norman Cousins believes that laughter is the best medicine that there is. And lastly, I tell them to remember that, "It's not what happens to you in life, but how you handle it" that matters. To all those who are suffering from Lyme disease: I wish you good fortune on the lengthy and arduous journey to recovery.

Gratitude

To all my mentors, friends and family who have helped to shape my world: thank you for your guidance and support: Ari Preuss, Jackie Ludel, Ph.D., Thomas Insel, M.D., Alan Gaby, M.D., Charles Ray Jones, M.D., Richard Horowitz, M.D., Nick Harris, Ph.D., Stephen Fry, M.D., Aristo Vojdani, Ph.D., Lauren Montgomery, Ph.D., Bonnie Friedman, and to my parents, Bruce and Janet Marra, who helped to edit the first draft of this chapter. A special thanks also goes to my ILADS colleagues who continually demonstrate courage under fire, and a steadfast belief in the truth about Lyme disease and co-infections. You are inspirational and have truly taught me that if "you don't stand for something, you'll fall for anything."

How to Contact Susan L. Marra, M.S., N.D.

Susan L. Marra, M.S., N.D.
Tailored Care
4500 9th Avenue NE, Suite 300
Seattle, Washington 98105
Ph: 206-299-2676 / Fax: 206-547-0925
Website: www.drsusanmarra.com

• CHAPTER 4 •

Ginger Savely, DNP
SAN FRANCISCO, CA

Biography

Dr. Ginger Savely is originally from Maryland but has lived in Austin, TX since 1979. In 2005, she opened her practice in San Francisco and currently resides there two weeks per month. She has Bachelor's degrees in Psychology, Music and Nursing. She graduated number one in her Bachelor's in Nursing program at U.T. Austin and was awarded the Outstanding Graduating Senior Award. Dr. Savely holds Master's degrees in Educational Philosophy and Nursing (specifically, the Family Nurse Practitioner program at U.T. Austin). She received her doctorate degree in nursing practice from Case Western Reserve University. She also holds advanced certification as a menopause clinician and as a master psycho-pharmacologist. She is fluent in Italian and conversant in French and Spanish.

Before entering the medical field, Dr. Savely worked for ten years as a performing singer/keyboardist/songwriter. She also worked for fifteen years as a Lamaze childbirth instructor.

Prior to treating tick-borne diseases, Dr. Savely had a special interest in fibromyalgia and chronic fatigue syndrome and gave professional presentations on these topics, including co-presentation of original research at the 1996 chronic fatigue syndrome conference in San Francisco.

In 1999, Dr. Savely started to gain expertise in the diagnosis and treatment of tick-borne diseases. She is now recognized as one of the top Lyme disease specialists in the country and patients come to her San Francisco office from all over the United States. Dr. Savely is an active member of ILADS (International Lyme and Associated Diseases Society). She also serves on the advisory boards of both the California Lyme Disease Association and the Charles E. Holman Foundation for Morgellons Research.

Healing Philosophy

It is unlikely that any treatment for Lyme disease can completely eradicate the pathogens responsible for tick-borne infections. Unfortunately, the pathogens have too many survival techniques. Instead, the goal should be to control the infections by reducing the body's bacterial/parasitic load and by strengthening the immune system so that it can take over the job of keeping the infections under control.

Antibiotics are the essential cornerstone of treatment but are not all that is required to get well. In order to facilitate the body's ability to heal, those with Lyme must do everything possible to strengthen their immune systems.

Getting one's health back is a full-time job. The chronically ill need to become aware of how everything affects their heath, including their environment, diet, habits and attitude. Even once the infections are under control, those with Lyme will need to live the rest of their lives making healthy lifestyle choices so that their immune systems will remain strong and able to keep the "bugs" at bay.

Treatments for Infections

Borrelia

When treating Lyme disease, I see two types of patients. While each type may have symptoms of the other, overall, patients resemble one type more than the other. These two types are: 1) patients with primarily musculoskeletal symptoms which resemble syndromes such as fibromyalgia and 2) patients with primarily neurological symptoms that resemble syndromes such as chronic fatigue syndrome or Multiple Sclerosis. I call those with musculoskeletal symptoms the "pain" people. I do an exam during my patients' first visit to determine which type they are, and to what degree. For example, I look for affected reflexes; are they hyper or hypo? Also, I test their pupil reaction to light, and perform balance and other neurologic tests.

For treatment of the musculoskeletal patients, I tend to start with oral antibiotics, such as high dose doxycycline, a combination of clarithromycin and cefdinir, or a combination of Ketek and high dose amoxicillin.

For the neurological patients, if I see that they have a lot of neurological signs and symptoms, the first thing that I will do, if they are not allergic to penicillin, is give them Bicillin (penicillin G) injections. I prefer Bicillin to intravenous therapy because it is less expensive, less risky and requires less intervention. Rocephin (ceftriaxone) is another good medication that can also be given in shots but it has a short half-life so patients must receive injections often, which can be painful. Because Bicillin has a longer half-life, it can be given only once or twice per week. I prescribe Bicillin LA (and it must be the LA form), 1.2 ml, or 2.4 ml intramuscularly every three to four days, depending upon how aggressive patients want to be with their treatment. I find Bicillin to work really well, and it's good to try first, before intravenous antibiotics, because some patients get just as beneficial an effect with the shots as with an IV.

If I then pair up Bicillin injections with Ketek, and pulse Flagyl (metronidazole), two weeks on, two weeks off, I find this to be my best "killer" combination for my patients. So for neurological types, my protocol is basically one or two oral medications, along with Bicillin injections.

Of course, everyone with Lyme disease has neurological symptoms to some degree, but in some people they are more pronounced than others, especially in those with MS-like symptoms, early-onset dementia, Parkinson's or fulminate psychosis.

I would actually give intravenous antibiotics to every Lyme patient, if it weren't for the expense and inconvenience. Intravenous treatments work better and faster, no matter what kind of Lyme disease patients have. Unfortunately, though, we (the patient and I) have to consider a lot of things in treatment, including cost.

Babesia

When it comes to Lyme co-infections, I will sometimes treat my patients' Babesia right off the bat with the tried and true combination of Mepron (atovaquone) and Zithromax (azithromycin) or Biaxin, along with Flagyl. This combination of remedies integrates two different Babesia treatment approaches and also kills Borrelia. However, I use this three-drug protocol only if patients can tolerate it. Not everyone can tolerate Flagyl early on in their treatment.

In addition, I include artemisinin at a dose of 800-900 mg (300 mg, three times per day) in the antibiotic protocol. I find that using high doses of artemisinin makes a huge difference in treatment outcomes. In the past, I used lower doses of this herb but over the years have realized that it's important to use higher doses and to pulse it, four days on, three days off. It's an important part of the treatment protocol for Babesia.

When patients' insurance plans won't cover payment for Zithromax, I will prescribe Biaxin, or Ketek. The unfortunate thing about medicine these days is that patients' health care choices often have to do with finances; with what their insurance plans will cover or what they can afford. It's a sad state of affairs.

While Mepron, Zithromax and artemisinin are often an effective combination for some types of Babesia, they don't always get rid of Babesia duncani, or Babesia WA-1, as it is sometimes called. Babesia WA-1 is extremely hard to get rid of. I don't always see patients improve with the aforementioned combination of antibiotics, even after months of use. With Babesia microti, I have found that patients can sometimes get well in as little as four to six months of treatment, but Babesia duncani is an entirely different matter.

Patients with this strain can often treat until kingdom come; indeed, after two years of treatment, some witness no change in symptoms. So I have to try other combinations of medications for patients with Babesia duncani, such as Lariam (mefloquine) and plaquenil, or chloroquine and primaquine. The drawback of the latter medications, however, is that they aren't well tolerated by patients so they aren't usually used as the first line of defense against the infection. I also use Malarone, and sometimes that works when Mepron doesn't, but we (in the medical community) don't know why, since Malarone, like Mepron, is atovaquone, but with proguanil added to it. But treatment usually means trying different things to see what works. Practitioners sometimes have to run through the mill of options. My approach is to start with the medication that has the best combination of being both effective and well tolerated, although sometimes the most effective drug is the one that is the least well tolerated, which means I sometimes end up leaving the most effective one for later.

Bartonella

Take Bartonella, for instance. I used to start patients on a quinolone antibiotic such as ciprofloxacin or Levaquin (levofloxacin) to treat this infection, and wait before giving them the rifampin and doxycycline, because the latter two are not as easily tolerated as the former two. But the longer I treat Bartonella, the more I tend to lean towards using the least tolerated and most effective medications first, because I often end up using them anyway, when the others just don't work well enough. So for the treatment of Bartonella, rifampin and doxycycline generally work the best, in my experience. Note that patients in different geographical locations may respond better to different antibiotics.

Bartonella requires treatment for a minimum of four months, but some patients need to take antibiotics for much longer than that. In general, Bartonella is easier to treat than Babesia microti, but not necessarily easier than Babesia duncani.

If there's one thing that I have learned from treating Lyme patients for so many years, it is that the more antibiotics that they are able to take and tolerate, the better off they will be. It's important to flood the system with antibiotics. Therefore, intravenous therapy, if tolerated, would be my first choice of treatment for patients, because it's the best way to get the most antibiotics into the body at the fastest rate. Intramuscular antibiotics would be my second choice, and oral antibiotics, third. That said, if patients have a cast iron gut, it may be possible for them to take five to six antibiotics at once, and in this case, oral dosing may be just as effective as intramuscular or intravenous dosing.

I think that you can tell how long a practitioner has been treating Lyme disease by how aggressive their treatment is. The newbies tend to be wimpy. Those who have been treating this disease a long time, like Drs. Burrascano and Jones, will give up to five or six antibiotics at once. The longer that I have been doing this, the more aggressive I have become with my treatments, too. Dr. Jones tells me, however, that I should use the term "appropriate" instead of "aggressive", when referring to treatments! So I keep adding antibiotics into patients' protocols as long as they can tolerate them, and I find that this approach works better.

Interestingly enough, on several occasions, I have found that after my patients have been on two antibiotics, and I switch them to two new ones, instead of just taking the new antibiotics, they accidentally take all four—the former two plus the new two. They then come back a month later and say, "Wow, I am so much better! This was the best month I ever had!" They got confused in their protocol, but taking the extra antibiotics actually resulted in them taking giant leaps forward in their healing.

But then again, there are so many factors that come into play when it comes to healing, and as a practitioner, you can't just say, "This is what you *have* to do," because everyone's needs are different.

So what should patients be able to tolerate in terms of antibiotic doses? Well, this is one of the biggest controversies in the world of Lyme. There are two camps of practitioners in the Lyme disease world. First, the "ramping up" camp, and then the "blast 'em hard" camp. The "ramping up" camp believes in slowly increasing antibiotic doses and the number of medications that patients take over time, so that they can avoid horrendous Herxheimer reactions. The concern with this approach to treatment is that the bugs get a warning of sorts from the lower dose antibiotics and can then hide from subsequent treatments. Conversely, the advantage of hitting the bugs hard right off the bat is that they are caught by surprise. The downside of the "blast 'em" approach is that patients get stronger Herxheimer reactions. So deciding upon which approach to take can be a tough decision for practitioners. In my practice, I tend to start out with the latter one. However, if I notice that my patients' Herxheimer reactions are so severe that their ability to heal is being hampered by the creation of a cytokine storm that could be damaging the body, then I will back off on their dosing. As a practitioner, you can't know in advance which patients are going to be more intolerant of treatments. About 10% of my patients don't Herx at all! I wish all of them could be this way, but unfortunately, that's not the way it is. Others Herx so badly that they think they are going to die. So initially, I try to hit the bugs hard first, to see if my patients can weather the storm, while supporting them the best that I can along the way.

Treating Mold, Candida and Environmental Toxins

I treat my patients' Candida towards the end of their treatment regimen, because the antibiotics for Lyme cause yeast, so there's no point in treating for yeast as long as patients are taking antibiotics. When I do treat them for yeast, I also treat them for mold, using Cholestyramine (as advocated by Dr. Ritchie Shoemaker, M.D.) to bind the mold's biotoxins. I think that mold is a huge problem for Lyme disease patients, too. For some, it may even be the main reason why they got sick, and is the reason why they stay sick. Recent work by Dr. Ritchie Shoemaker has also shown that Lyme patients who are continually exposed to environmental mold will not get well.

Besides Candida and mold, heavy metals and other toxins can potentially affect recovery from the Lyme disease complex. As a practitioner, I have to look at everything that could be impacting my patients' immune systems. So I must do two things at once: get rid of their infections, and empower their immune systems, which means getting rid of everything that drags the system down. Eliminating patients' allergies and sensitivities, for instance, such as wheat or milk, can lift tremendous burdens from their immune systems. Also, reducing their exposure to different environmental toxins, such as mold (as mentioned above) and heavy metals, can help. Some of my patients have heavy metal toxicity, but since I don't specialize in heavy metal toxicity removal, I refer them to a heavy metal detoxification specialist. I haven't had the time to learn how to treat this aspect of illness in depth. I already have too much to do as it is. I'm taking care of my patients' hormones, blood pressure, infections and many other things. There are so many aspects of treatment to consider, and I just can't cover all of the bases.

Treating Insomnia

Sleep is restorative and necessary for the body to heal. Sleep dysfunction is one of the most significant and debilitating aspects of Lyme disease. Unlike the insomnia that is experienced by the average person due to stress, Lyme disease insomnia is a central nervous system problem and can't be treated with the same methods that are used for the average person, such as a warm bath or glass of milk before bed.

If patients' sleep cycles are turned around, then it's important to get them back to sleeping when it's dark. Taking melatonin at doses of 0.5-3.0 mg at 9:00 p.m. can help to regulate their sleep cycle, while taking three teaspoons of Natural Calm magnesium powder in the evening can help them to relax. If frequent urination prevents them from sleeping through the night, then avoiding fluids a few hours before bedtime can be helpful. If this doesn't work, then some may require DDAVP, a prescription hormone that prevents frequent urination.

Whenever I give my patients a prescription sleep medication, I tell them to take it every night right before they get ready for bed. If they wait too long to get to bed after taking the medication, it may not be effective. I also advise them to start by taking the lowest dose necessary and gradually increase it each night, until they are able to sleep soundly through the night without feeling groggy the next morning.

Nutrition

Anyone can benefit from good nutrition, both for feeling good and for maintaining a healthy body over the long run. A body that is under physical and/or mental stress has nutritional needs that are above normal. Those with tick-borne diseases have specific, and above normal, nutritional needs due to abnormal body processes. B-12 and magnesium, for example, are two nutrients that those with Lyme tend to need more of than the average person. Also, free radicals are thought to be more abundant in Lyme sufferers, which makes anti-oxidants an important nutritional requirement.

What Those with Lyme Disease Should Do for Proper Nutrition

1. Avoid drinking alcohol and smoking. Limit caffeinated beverages.

2. Drink eight to ten glasses of water per day.

3. Those with tick-borne illnesses crave sugars due to faulty carbohydrate metabolism, but indulging in these makes the situation worse, leading to hypoglycemic fatigue. Limit simple carbohydrates such as potatoes, pasta, rice, and white bread to one small serving at lunch and dinner. Avoid sweets but if you feel that you must have them, it should always be after a healthy meal and never before noon.

4. Double protein intake to 90-100 grams per day, stressing low-fat proteins such as fish, skinless chicken, lean cuts of beef and pork, fat-free milk products, egg whites, seitan loaf and soy powder. Snack on roasted soy nuts, which are packed with protein.

5. Aim to get at least 25 grams of fiber per day. One-third cup of Kellogg's All-Bran Buds can be added to your morning cereal, which will provide half of the recommended daily requirement for fiber. (By the way, these are tasty and don't get mushy!) Eat lots of veggies, four servings of fruit per day, and always choose whole grains.

6. Since it's difficult to get enough dark greens in the diet, try buying a product like Kyo-Green or Green Magnum and add a tablespoon of this to a smoothie. It's a tasteless powder, but has the same amount of nutrients as a pound of spinach!

7. Add ground flaxseeds to smoothies, cereals, rice, casseroles, etc. Flaxseed provides many benefits to the body, including high amounts of fiber and omega-3 fatty acids, which are natural anti-inflammatory substances. Start with a low dose, as too much may initially cause gas or loose stools. Flaxseeds should be kept in the refrigerator to avoid rancidity.

When formulating a diet plan for their patients, it's important for practitioners to discover what their patients' food allergies are and eliminate those. I test all of my patients for gluten sensitivity, but whether or not they test positive to the gliadin protein, they are yet likely to feel better on a gluten-free diet, and invariably, most all of them do. I also recommend that they eat a "no white" diet, which means avoiding foods that have white flour or white sugar in them. So that means no white rice, no white potatoes or white bread. Instead, I encourage low-fat proteins, vegetables, fruits, brown rice (I don't believe that brown rice feeds infections) and complex carbohydrates. These are pretty much my standard dietary recommendations, but I also think that when it comes to diet, patients get a feel for what their bodies need.

Testing For and Treating Food Allergies

People with allergies have hyperactive immune responses to many substances that the body recognizes as harmful. Their immune systems switch into overdrive when exposed to minor insults such as dust, pollen, healthy foods, and so on. This constant activation of the immune system leaves it drained and exhausted so that when bacteria that really need to be dealt with (Borrelia for example), come into the picture, the immune system is not as strong as it needs to be. Many people with Lyme disease have problems with allergies, even though they may not realize it. They especially tend to not recognize food allergies, because they consume the offending foods on a daily basis and their bodies have learned to mask the negative effects of the foods. It isn't until they remove such foods from their diets and then re-introduce them back in that they are able to perceive their negative effects. Those who wish to learn more about food allergies should read the book, *Detecting Hidden Food Allergies* by William Crook.

Supportive Supplements

Vitamins and Minerals

To make sure that my patients are getting the nutrition that they need, I strongly urge them to schedule a consultation with a nutritionist or naturopath who specializes in helping people with chronic or debilitating health problems, and who can help them with this aspect of treatment.

It's a good idea for patients with Lyme to invest in a few plastic seven-day pill holder containers, so that they can organize their medications, including vitamins, at the beginning of each week. This can help those with brain fog remember if they have taken their supplements!

Magnesium

Magnesium tends to be very deficient in Lyme disease sufferers. Some symptoms of magnesium (Mg) deficiency include:

1. Accelerated heart rate

2. High blood pressure

3. Neuromuscular irritability

4. Headaches

5. Hyperactive reflexes

6. Muscle cramps

7. Joint pain

8. Irritability, anxiety, depression

Lyme disease is one of many illnesses that cause magnesium deficiency. The Borrelia burgdorferi bacteria (Bb) is unique from other organisms because it "goes after" magnesium in the host's body, whereas most microbes go after iron. Researchers have been surprised to find that Bb does not seek iron from its host, but that it does need magnesium. Many Lyme disease symptoms, including those that involve the muscles, joints, vision, appetite and heart, as well as inflammation and immune deficiencies that manifest in specific symptoms such as cramping and headaches, are often classic magnesium deficiency symptoms. Taking a good magnesium supplement often decreases these symptoms.

Preliminary research on Morgellons disease shows that the disease fibers are coated with minerals, which are presumably leached out of the body by illness. So Morgellons patients need to supplement with magnesium and other minerals, as well.

Magnesium is involved in an extraordinary range of functions in the body. By restoring proper magnesium levels, the immune system's ability to target pathogens improves. There is a hypothesis within the Lyme disease community that if we can keep adequate levels of magnesium in the body, we will also enable the body's immune system to regain its ability to target and attack the Bb organism itself. (It is also thought that magnesium might incite Borrelia to come out of hiding to get the magnesium).

A person's response to magnesium doesn't depend solely upon the amount of elemental magnesium in a particular supplement, however. It depends more upon the amount that's absorbed and bio-available to the body, and the amount needed to correct the deficiency. The gut (the jejunum and ileum) absorbs the majority of ingested magnesium, so the solubility and absorption of a particular type of magnesium across a range of pH's are important to consider when correcting deficiencies. Some magnesium supplements, for instance, have low solubility and are poorly absorbed in the intestine. Common magnesium salts, such as sulfate (Epsom salts), hydroxide (milk of magnesia), and oxide are poor supplements due to their low bioavailability. Also, magnesium chloride may present unwanted side effects due to its hygroscopic (readily absorbing moisture) properties.

I recommend Peter Gillham's Natural Calm for correcting magnesium deficiencies because my patients have had good experiences with it (www.petergillham.com).It comes as a flavored powder that can be mixed with water, or as a plain powder that can be mixed in juice or a smoothie.

When dosing magnesium, patients should increase their nightly amount until their stools become comfortably soft. Too much magnesium will lead to diarrhea. If my patients don't like taking magnesium in powder form, I recommend MagTab SR or Mag Malate.

Patient and Practitioner Challenges and Roadblocks to Healing

One of my greatest challenges as a practitioner is getting my patients to keep plugging away at their treatments, because they get very frustrated and want to give up. It's really hard, because when they don't see any change in their symptom picture, it's as if they can't "see the forest for the trees." If I can help them to get through their treatments, they are often then able to look back and realize that they are getting better, but in general, it's very hard for them to "hang in there." Providing reassurance is one of the best things that practitioners can do for Lyme disease patients, however, and a great majority of their job involves being cheerleaders or psychologists.

Another challenge that I have is coming up with individualized treatment plans for my patients, because they are all so different and I never know what's going to work for them. For instance, I have some people for whom artemisinin makes all the difference in the world, and other people for whom it doesn't do a thing. There is so much that we as practitioners don't know about treating Lyme disease. Further complicating things is the fact that there are so many different strains of Borrelia and other infections going around that we don't know about, which means that we don't necessarily know how or what we are treating.

Patients don't always understand this, either. Occasionally, they will get really angry with me because they think that a treatment that worked for another person should have worked for them, and it didn't. Lyme sufferers are constantly talking to one another and giving advice over the Internet, too. They are desperate and are constantly coming in to my office and telling me things like, "I heard on the Internet that this is the best method for treating Lyme, so I want you to do this treatment." This can sometimes complicate things because what works best for one person doesn't always work best for another.

So when patients write me angry letters and say things like, "You withheld this treatment from me. It would have helped me!" I want to tell them that they might be the one in million that that particular treatment would have helped. Interestingly enough, some of these people are intelligent and well-educated, and they do end up finding things that work better for them than antibiotics. Problem is, they end up accusing me of being incompetent, even though, as a health care provider, I am making decisions based on statistics all of the time. I have to first give patients the treatment that works the best for the majority. I can't know whether the next person that I am treating is going to be part of the minority of people for whom a treatment isn't going to work, but some people get angry over this issue, anyway. Of course, when people are sick, they aren't at their best.

Really, though, it's so hard treating Lyme disease! It's no wonder that most doctors don't want to touch this disease with a ten-foot pole. It's a very iffy, wishy-washy disease, and most doctors are more comfortable with conditions that they know exactly how to treat, and in fact, the treatment approach to other maladies is often more standardized. I'm always telling nurse practitioners at national conferences that we (nurse practitioners) are actually the perfect type of practitioner for treating Lyme because our style of taking care of people is much more individualized and holistic than that of physicians'. It's a good area for us. We are more comfortable with this type of thing, whereas medical doctors tend to dislike situations where they are not sure what's going on.

If I knew of a remedy that was the "key" to everyone's healing, then yes, I would be shouting about it from the rooftops. This is the thing that drives me so crazy, though. Every time I think that I've found something that is "it" for everyone, I find patients for whom it doesn't work.

For example, I sometimes recommend the mushroom Coriolus to my patients, because I notice that it raises CD-57 levels like crazy. Some of my patients take it and say, "I feel so much better on this!", whereas it doesn't seem to help others at all. It's always interesting how people respond differently to things. As another example, I have patients who use an herbal treatment called burbur, and some will swear that it ameliorates their Herxheimer reactions, while others claim that it doesn't do anything to improve their symptoms. For those that it helps, I don't know how much of it is the placebo effect, but I'm never going to tell people not to try something if it makes them feel better. I have a few things that I would always say "No" to, such as intravenous hydrogen peroxide, but for the most part, if patients ask, "Should I try this?" I will tell them, "Sure, go ahead, try whatever works."

I find that my patients almost always respond positively to my Lyme disease treatments, but the question is, how much? For those that only improve somewhat, the reasons are multiple. They might have a resistant strain of the organism, a genetic predisposition that blocks their healing, or other infections that are primary in their symptom picture. As well, there may be other unknown factors involved and which keep them from healing fully.

Patients often ask me about the importance of treating viral infections, and if I were to check viral titers on most of my Lyme patients, I would find that they all have high titers for other infections, but I think that such infections are opportunistic. That is, they are infections that show up in test results and become active because of Lyme disease. I then tell my patients that these will tend to go away once we treat their Lyme.

Lyme Disease vs. Chronic Fatigue Syndrome

There is some debate in the chronic fatigue world about whether Lyme disease itself may be the primary cause of chronic fatigue syndrome. The question is very hard to answer. Sometimes, a person may have chronic mold, or another issue that is causing their symptoms, even if Lyme is present as a background problem.

On the other hand, I used to be very involved in the chronic fatigue world, and at some point, I began to realize that CFS was caused, in many cases, by Lyme disease, and for that reason, I became more involved in treating Lyme disease.

Those who present with classic CFS symptoms such as chronic fatigue and brain fog are often the most difficult to treat. There is sometimes very little response to treatment in this type of patient, so who knows what this really means?

In the end, however, I'm a big proponent of presenting every treatment to my patients as though it was going to work, even though I have colleagues who disagree with this approach. They say that doing this is akin to "pulling the wool over someone's eyes," and think that it's better to be frank with patients, but I look at the matter differently. I think that patients' healing is aided significantly when they believe that they are going to get better. A practitioner who says, "Do this, and you will get better" will have patients who tend to get better. A practitioner who tells patients: "You have a 50/50 chance of healing" might end up discouraging them. Besides, what's the worst that can happen if the person doesn't get better? People don't tend to come back and scream, "You said this was going to work!" So in my practice, I look my patients in the eye and tell them, "We're going to do this treatment and you are going to get better." And I can do this and say with all honesty that I feel they are going to get better, because most of the time, they do, and in hindsight, they will often say, "That is the best thing you could have said to me." People need hope, and I don't believe in false hope. You have to give people hope. That's what gets them through this.

Patient Roadblocks to Healing

I find that my toughest patients are those with PTSD (post-traumatic stress disorder). There's a lot going on with them emotionally and their healing is complicated. Sometimes they don't seem to get well, and I don't know how much of this is tied into their emotions. All Lyme doctors have patients that don't seem to get better, but in reality, these are few. It is unfortunate, though, because I hear about a lot of negative conversation on the Internet Lyme disease support groups. People ask, "Is it worth it to treat Lyme? I have read that people don't get better, anyway."

Are you kidding? I wouldn't treat this if people didn't get better—it would be cruel and unfair to take their money and time! Not to mention depressing. The fun and wonderful part of treating Lyme disease is seeing people get their lives back. It's a very exciting and powerful thing, and I think that's what keeps me doing this (fighting the regulatory boards and administering difficult treatments) because I get to watch my patients come back to life before my very eyes.

So people do get better. As for healing and my protocols, I find that those who have been sick for less than a year tend to get better after about a year. Most of my patients with chronic Lyme disease, however, need two years, at minimum, to heal, and on average, two and a half to three years, occasionally a little longer. A very small percentage, perhaps 5%, as well as those who have been sick for twenty years or longer need more time, sometimes five years or more, to heal. But those who have been sick that long do get better. It just takes time.

Do Antibiotics Work?

There is a perception on the Internet that people don't get better with antibiotics.

It seems to me, however, that the people on the Internet support groups are the ones who don't get better. They get a skewed view, or perception of the Lyme world. Those who heal from Lyme disease aren't on the Internet, because they move on with their lives once they get better. I often tell my patients that Internet chat rooms are beneficial in some ways, but they can also be depressing. Those who tend to linger there are those rare people who don't get better. Some are cynical and/or depressed, and so tend to bring others down. They are not a fair representation of those who heal from Lyme—perhaps they represent a number as small as 1% of the Lyme disease population.

Again, all of us who treat Lyme disease wouldn't do it if patients didn't get better. I mean, how depressing! Imagine treating and treating and your patients never getting better. We do this because people do get better. It's unfortunate that those with Lyme who are just learning about the disease and trying to find answers on the Internet, get discouraged by what they learn.

It's true, though, that there are some people who can't take antibiotics. These people might be "permanent Herxers." Their Herxing never stops and so they have to find other solutions for healing.

Also, no amount of treatment can bring people with irreversible damage in their bodies, such as those with ALS, back to full health. I must tell them that yes, it is possible that they have Lyme disease, and maybe Lyme was the initial trigger for their ALS, but the damage to their bodies has already been done. We may be able to halt progression of the disease temporarily, but we can't bring them back to full health.

I am, by the way, intimately involved with this disease. I have had Lyme, as have my two daughters and my mother. Also, my son has gestational Lyme and my sister died from Lyme and ALS. I have found that those practitioners who have had personal experience with this disease are more empathetic, and tend to "get it" more than those who haven't—and it turns out that most Lyme doctors or their family members have in fact dealt with Lyme disease themselves. They may not admit it, but most of them have. That is why they are so ahead of the curve of conventional medical knowledge.

Treating Relapses with Dr. Burrascano's Pulse Protocol

Every now and again, my patients will relapse after I stop their antibiotic treatments. If they do, I apply Dr. Burrascano's pulsing protocol, which involves pulsing antibiotics for six to eight weeks. If patients are going to relapse, it is usually six months to a year after stopping treatments. Whenever that happens, I hit their infections again with another pulse treatment, but I must wait until they completely "crash", because Burrascano's theory is that patients have to wait until they hit rock bottom before practitioners can "hit" them again with another pulse treatment. They can't just have beginning signs of returning symptoms, or else the protocol won't work well; they must crash entirely. After my patients have gone into remission, if they relapse, I usually have to do only one pulse, and occasionally, two. Dr. Burrascano says that three is the maximum number of pulse treatments that are usually required for patients to get completely well and I have never had to do more than two of these pulses, because after that, I find that my patients are absolutely better.

Profiling the Person that Heals from Lyme Disease

Smokers will never get better. It's amazing how many Lyme sufferers drink, smoke and do drugs. When my patients do things that tear down their immune systems, they don't tend to heal. Those who do what it takes, eat the right food, adhere to treatments and so on, are the ones who get better.

Also, I have consistently seen that people who are able to get rid of their anger heal. Those who are eaten up with anger and resentment, as well as those who get depressed and ask questions like, "Why me?" don't tend to heal. Those that have a calmer, less fatalistic perspective and say things like, "I know this happened for a reason. I may not know that reason, but I accept it", tend to do better. I have patients who are sick as dogs, but they maintain their sense of humanity and humor. They crack jokes and they laugh. They are the ones who heal. People go through grieving stages when they first get sick, and it's not until they finally arrive at a place of acceptance of their illness that they really start to heal. Those who are angry, those who are kicking, fighting and screaming, and living their lives as though the illness wasn't there, tend to be hindered in their healing. They push through their activities and think, "By golly, this isn't going to get me down". They continue to work full time and ignore their symptoms, but their symptoms don't go away. It's surprising how many people just keep pushing themselves in their daily activities, and yet they are sicker than dogs. It blows my mind. It's like they are in denial and running away from the disease. Teenagers are very much this way. They refuse to let it stop them. Those who accept their new situation, and say, "Okay, this is the new me. What can I do in this situation?" get better. Once patients are able to relax and accept their illness, then they start to heal.

Stress Reduction and Behavior Modification

Western medicine is beginning to realize that it isn't possible to separate the mind from the body in the healing process. People have often been told that their illness is all in their head, and in a way, it is! Tick-borne diseases infect the brain and cause malfunction in the limbic system, a part of the brain that receives all kinds of inputs from the external world (emotional, physical and otherwise) and "translates" them into body functions. To say that stress reduction and behavior modification will help patients' physical condition does not mean that part of their problem is psychosomatic. It means that their limbic system is highly sensitive to stress, and, as is the case with many physical problems, will have a better chance of healing itself when the burdens of stress are removed from it.

Strategies for Stress Reduction

Biofeedback

This therapy teaches those with Lyme to identify when and where their bodies are reacting to stress and how to let go of that stress. Mental health provider networks have information on practitioners and places where this type of therapy can be done.

Cognitive Behavior Therapy

This therapy helps those with Lyme to identify the unrealistic thought patterns that cause them stress and anxiety and to adopt new mind sets that enable them to be easier on themselves. It can also teach them to set limits, let go of guilt, blaming and the need to be in control, as well as how to accentuate the positive aspects of their lives, and so on. Patients can call therapists in their insurance plan to see if any of them specialize in this type of therapy.

Humor

It has been said that laughter is the best medicine. It's good for those with Lyme to surround themselves with light-hearted people, to find humor in their current situation and to not take themselves or their illnesses too seriously. It's also beneficial for patients to watch funny TV shows or movies, while avoiding the "heavy" ones.

Lifestyle Adjustments

Those with Lyme should analyze their life situation and list all of the things in their lives that are causing them stress, and then decide to eliminate as many of these things as possible. If they can reduce their work schedule to part-time, for example, this can be beneficial, as can quitting their job if they are financially able to (See below).

Financial Support

For many people with Lyme, financial worries are at the top of their list of stressors. It can be beneficial for them to file for disability payments through their employer's disability insurance program (if the employer has one) or file for disability benefits under the Social Security Disability Income program (SSDI). The SSDI process is difficult and there are many roadblocks. I highly recommend that those with Lyme enlist the help of a disability counselor if they decide to apply for this income. The standard fee charged by disability lawyers is 25% of what the client wins in back pay, with a maximum fee of $5,300. This is the standard fee for all disability lawyers and counselors and is regulated by the Social Security Administration. There is no fee charged to clients if they don't win their case, except for a small service fee because the lawyers work on a contingency basis.

Balancing Rest and Physical Conditioning

People with Lyme are often perplexed because they feel as though they're getting two opposite messages from their health care provider: rest, but get up and move! The fact is, they need to find a balance between both. Too much rest can lead to de-conditioning of the body, which will make them feel even weaker, as well as more tired and depressed. Too much activity, however, will lead to an exacerbation of their symptoms and longer recovery time. Ideally, those with Lyme should try to do some form of mild to moderate exercise every day. Some Lyme disease sufferers who are reading this might be thinking, "I barely have enough energy to get through the day, let alone exercise!" The idea is to do daily reconditioning, but starting off slow and easy, and progressing so gradually that they never become frustrated or exhausted. They should never exercise aerobically, but research has shown that those with Lyme improve by doing other forms of mild to moderate exercise.

Activities That People with Lyme Should Do

1. Every day, take a half-hour (no more!) nap in the afternoon. More than a half -hour leads to grogginess, due to the body coming out of a deeper sleep.

2. Pay attention to the body! Learn to recognize signs of fatigue and then get some rest before becoming drop-dead tired.

3. Plan a regular time every day to do "movement therapy". (I don't use the "E" word!). People should do this even if they can only manage a few stretches, and they should make it a habit. Also, it's important that they keep their expectations low, and forget the motto, "No pain, no gain!" They should start their first week of "movement therapy" with a very low goal in mind (i.e.; walking to the mailbox and back). It's also beneficial to do some mild stretching before the "movement therapy", as well as afterwards. Beginning yoga is great for those with Lyme, but they shouldn't sign up for a challenging class! I taught myself to do yoga with Richard Hittleman's, *Yoga 28-Day Exercise Plan*. Swimming is also an ideal, gentle exercise to try.

Other activities that those with Lyme can do for their daily "movement therapy" include walking, Pilates, working with light hand weights, and cycling on flat surfaces at a slow to moderate pace. They should avoid running, jogging, aerobic classes, heavy weights, or any sport that increases the heart rate.

What Friends and Family Members Can Do to Help the Sick

While it's important for loved ones to be there for sick friends and/or family members, it's also important for caretakers to be supported because it's really hard to be a parent or spouse of someone who has Lyme disease. They suffer, too. For instance, one thing that's hard about taking care of Lyme patients is that they are so sensitive to everything. You want to hug your loved ones with Lyme, but they are so hypersensitive that it hurts for them to receive a hug or be touched.

Also, it would help if loved ones could try to learn as much as they can about Lyme disease, so that they know what their sick family members are going through. Because the biggest problem with this disease, unlike any other illness such as cancer, for instance, is that people wonder, even if it's just a little, if the Lyme sufferer is really sick. People think, "Well, c'mon, can't you just snap out of it? Can't you just push yourself a little?" I see relationships break up over this and I see dissention in families, because family members refuse to believe that there is anything wrong with the sick person. He or she just looks so normal!

Last Words

While treating Lyme disease is a great challenge, for me, it's so exciting to watch people get their lives back. There's nothing like it. Watching the transformation of those who once lost it all, were in the dumps, couldn't function and who felt like their lives were over, is wonderful and what makes my job worth the sacrifice.

How to Contact Ginger Savely, DNP

Ginger Savely, DNP
450 Sutter St., Suite 1504
San Francisco, C.A. 94108
Email: gsavely@gmail.com

•CHAPTER 5•

W. Lee Cowden, M.D., M.D. (H)
PANAMA CITY, PANAMA

Biography

Dr. Cowden is a board-certified cardiologist and specialist in Internal Medicine. Internationally known and recognized for his proficiency in the Evaluative Kinesiology technique, Dr. Cowden has also refined treatment protocols for cancer, Lyme disease, autism, Parkinson's disease, fibromyalgia, chronic fatigue syndrome, as well as many other medical conditions, including the reversal of heart and vascular disease.

Dr. Cowden is the author or co-author of several publications and books including:

- *An Alternative Medicine Definitive Guide to Cancer*, 1997
- *Cancer Diagnosis; What to Do Next*, 2000
- *Longevity, An Alternative Medicine Definitive Guide*, 2001

In addition to these publications, Dr Cowden was also on the editorial board for: *Alternative Medicine, The Definitive Guide,*

(First Edition, 1993; Second Edition, 2002) and contributed to the *Alternative Medicine Guide to Heart Disease* in 1998, as well as to several other books. Dr. Cowden is the Chairman of the Scientific Advisory Board of IntegraMed Academy (2008). IntegraMed Academy produces Internet courses in integrative medicine for health professionals and lay public nationally and internationally. He is also an international integrative medicine health educator who has given presentations in the USA, Mexico, Brazil, Peru, Guatemala, Germany, the Czech Republic, Japan, China, Taiwan, England, the Netherlands, Curacao, the Dominican Republic, Singapore and Malaysia.

Note to the Reader

Dr. Cowden uses and recommends many products manufactured by a company called NutraMedix. Throughout this chapter, you will notice that many of the remedies described are not accompanied by manufacturer information. In most of these cases, the manufacturer is NutraMedix. Disclosure: Dr. Cowden is a paid consultant to NutraMedix.

Dr. Cowden's Healing Philosophy

In my opinion, Lyme disease is a condition that occurs because a person's total body load of toxins and other stressors has become conducive to the development of illness. As we go through life, we all accumulate a load of toxins from our environment. That load includes chemical toxins, electromagnetic pollution, geopathic stress, and heavy metals, as well as a variety of emotional traumas. The sum total of all of these stressors finally creates a situation that makes a person susceptible to illness, so if that person gets bitten by a tick or mosquito that's carrying Lyme-related microbes, then it becomes easy for him or her to succumb to illness. Evidence suggests that some people carry Lyme microbes around in their bodies for more than a decade before they finally have some type of trauma that causes the microbes to become active and cause illness. For instance, a motor vehicle accident or the death of a loved one can cause Lyme disease to "come out", if the bacteria and the toxic environment are there. So in my experience, I have found that if I reduce the load on patients' bodies, their symptoms of Lyme will improve, even if I don't specifically treat them for Lyme. One of my colleagues years ago said that the human body is like a swamp full of alligators; you can either fight the alligators one at a time, or you can drain the swamp.

For this reason, I can't say that Borrelia is the primary cause of Lyme illness because there are usually multiple causes. This idea ties in with the work of Antoine Bechamp, a contemporary of Louis Pasteur. Bechamp said that when it comes to healing the body, the microorganisms are nothing, and that the body's environment, or terrain, is everything. Pasteur, on the other hand, developed the germ theory, which is also called the pathogenic theory of medicine and which basically proposes that microorganisms are the cause of disease. Bechamp was a very brilliant microbiologist, whereas Pasteur was a flamboyant chemist. Even though Pasteur wasn't a microbiologist, he was more vocal and flamboyant, and his way of teaching practitioners at the time won out over Bechamp's. On Pasteur's deathbed, he acknowledged that Bechamp was right in his theory and that he was wrong; however, by then it was too late, because Pasteur's ideas were already being put into medical literature and journals of the time. Those ideas have been perpetuated in medicine to this day.

Treatment Approach

I take a naturopathic approach to healing my patients, using herbals and other natural therapies. The risk of harm to them is remote using this approach, but the chances of helping them are pretty high.

For this reason, I can justify doing empiric treatments on patients in my practice. Also, with the herbal therapies that I use most often for treating Lyme and co-infections, I find that I can get a very dramatic reduction in peoples' microbial loads without putting them at risk from the adverse effects of pharmaceutical medications.

I participated in a Lyme disease study in Dallas back in 2003, in which we performed darkfield microscopy tests every two weeks on a number of Lyme disease patients. In this study, we observed that those patients that were to be treated with a natural herbal protocol had massive swarming bacterial spirochetes in their first blood specimen that was taken, before any kind of herbals were started. Two weeks after starting the herbals, the number of spirochetes that were observed in these patients' specimens had been greatly reduced. And two weeks after that, very few spirochetes could be observed. Two weeks after that, none could be found unless we used a paper clip to press against the microscopic cover slip to crush the red blood cells so that the microbes could be released from inside the red blood cells. Two weeks after that, we were able to crush the red blood cells and not see any microbes at all! So we knew through this study and by our clinical observations that we were progressively lowering patients' microbial loads, as darkfield microscopy confirmed.

Fortunately, because of what I have witnessed through darkfield microscopy and because of the changes that I have seen in patients' symptomology as a result of herbal trials, I now know what remedies work for the treatment of Lyme disease. And I have observed that a large percentage of my patients can typically become symptom-free in ten to eighteen weeks with the herbal protocol used in the trials. It often takes at least this long for standard pharmaceutical antibiotics to have the same effect. Also, when patients use this herbal approach and stop treatments, they usually don't get a recurrence of symptoms, as is often the case with antibiotics. Relapses are less common with herbal therapy if patients are treated appropriately and for the right length of time, based on an energetic evaluation.

Testing For Lyme and Co-Infections

A lot of the conventional lab tests for Lyme disease and other Lyme-related microbes are not very good. We know that there are probably twenty to thirty common species of Borrelia besides Borrelia burgdorferi that cause Lyme, and most labs don't look for any of these. We also know that there are more than thirty-two species of Bartonella that are pathological in humans, but the average lab only looks for one or two of these. In addition, we know that there are more than fourteen species of Babesia that are pathological in humans and commonly found in Lyme patients, and that the average lab can detect only one or two, at best. So, one of the problems with diagnosis is that there can be all of these bugs in the body that the labs aren't even looking for. For this reason, I use energy testing on my patients to try to get a clue about what's going on in their bodies. Often, I find that the biggest problem for a patient isn't Borrelia burgdorferi, but some other Borrelia strain, or an unusual Babesia or Bartonella species.

For my patients' energetic evaluation, I primarily use the Zyto LSA Pro, because I find it to be the most precise device on the market. It's a fully automated, technician-independent, electrodermal screening device. That means that I can put it on auto-test mode, have my patients put one of their hands on the electrodes of the hand cradle, and then I can leave the room, while the machine analyzes them. Then, I can come back a few minutes later and get the results. The results come out the same, no matter which technician starts the process. So I like this aspect of the device—the fact that it is objective.

Further, the results of the Zyto seem to correlate well with clinical findings. One of the ways in which the machine functions is that it looks for things that distress the autonomic nervous system, using specific energetic frequencies. It's basically a very sophisticated lie detector test and is a galvanic skin response testing system that can test many "items", or potential stressors or energy-balancers in the body per second. This means that it can get through long checklists of items very quickly.

Treatment Protocol for Infections

For people with Lyme who want to try my protocol but who don't have access to an energy medicine practitioner to determine which remedies are most appropriate for them, my herbal Lyme protocol that's published on the Internet (www.bionatus.com/nutramedix) is a good place for them to start. One of the reasons why I allowed the protocol to be placed on the Internet was so that patients and other health care practitioners could learn about effective ways to treat Lyme and co-infections using herbal medicine. I decided to do this after receiving a phone call from Dr. Richard Horowitz in January, 2007. He told me that he had 10,000 patients in his practice, and that 500 were not doing well at all on pharmaceutical antibiotic therapy. He then asked if I had any suggestions for him. I asked him if he wanted to learn energy medicine, and he told me "No", because he could lose his license in New York for doing that, so I then developed an empiric herbal protocol for him to use on his 500 patients who had failed antibiotics. He started a large number of his patients on that protocol, and reported at the ILADS meeting in the fall of that year that 70% of the patients who had failed his antibiotic protocol had done well when they were given the herbal protocol. So when he called me, excited that 70% of his patients had greatly improved, I said to him, "Well, then, so what should we do about the other 30%?"

In April 2008, some of the Lyme patients who had failed to improve on the initial empiric integrative protocol were re-evaluated. The protocol was subsequently revised and condensed, to include reducing the total number of dosings per day to improve patient compliance and changing the types of some of the herbals that were being prescribed. For example, Dr. Horowitz had a large number of patients that had treatment-resistant Babesia species, so I recommended that they try a product called Enula, which then helped to get rid of some of the species that had not responded to other herbal or antibiotic treatments. Also, Dr. Horowitz had some patients with antibiotic-resistant Bartonella species and we found that by adding certain imprinted energetic frequencies to the herbal remedies that he was already using and by administering higher doses of those remedies, the Bartonella was effectively eradicated in these patients. So once he implemented these types of adjustments, approximately 90% of his patients got well using the new condensed herbal protocol. Also, greater than 90% of my own Lyme patients who had used this condensed protocol got well, whether they had previously been treated with pharmaceutical antibiotics or not. So now my question to practitioners is, "If 90% of your patients who have failed antibiotic therapy then heal using herbal medicine, why would you start patients on pharmaceutical antibiotic therapy in the first place?" It doesn't make sense to me.

Bartonella and Borrelia

I have found that Bartonella is a more difficult infection to eliminate than Borrelia; it often persists, even after Borrelia is gone, unless very high doses of herbals are administered. Dr. James Schaller, M.D., M.A.R., (a Lyme-literate physician) did an evaluation on a large number of herbs and essentially all of the pharmaceutical antibiotics on the U.S. market, and performed in-vitro testing with those herbs and drugs on patients with Bartonella. He found that there was no pharmaceutical drug that worked consistently to eliminate all species of Bartonella in these patients, and that only three types of herbal remedies could do the job. Those remedies were Cumanda, clove bud oil, and Houttuynia herb from China. He did not test Banderol, which I also find to be very effective for treating Bartonella when alternated with Cumanda.

It doesn't take long to get rid of Bartonella using the Cowden Condensed Protocol, just four to eight weeks, if high enough doses are used. Borrelia, however, is a different story, because it can change into different forms all of the time, which means that if patients don't treat cyclically for a long enough period of time, then they can relapse once treatments are stopped. In order to reduce the probability of relapsing, doing cyclical or rotational treatment for a sufficient period of time, as well as detoxifying the body, are necessary. The rotational protocol for Borrelia and other infections can be found on the Internet at:
www.bionatus.com/nutramedix.

Babesia

One of the herbal remedies that I use for treating my patients' Babesia is Enula. I sometimes have to prescribe fairly high doses of this remedy—as much as sixty drops, twice a day—in order to eliminate some species of the organism. I have seen some Babesia species that seem to be resistant to everything, so I often start patients who have these difficult strains at doses of thirty drops, twice a day, and increase their doses from there. That seems to do the trick most of the time. If not, I sometimes add artemisinin (3-5 capsules, 2-3 times per day, for 3-5 days each week, for 3-6 weeks) to the Enula therapy. The dosing of these herbs, however, depends upon which strain and species of the organism I am treating.

Babesia, like Bartonella, doesn't take long to eliminate from the body—usually eight weeks if patients do cyclical, or rotational, therapy. For Borrelia, I advocate cyclical therapy for anywhere from six to eight months. During that time, patients must also detoxify their bodies, so that their internal environment isn't favorable for stimulating the re-growth of organisms.

Dosing and Length of Treatment

A typical protocol might involve patients taking the two or three herbs that they test best for energetically, and administering these on a rotational basis so that they only take one herb at a time. Typically, they would take the first microbial defense herb for twelve and a half days, then take thirty-six hours off, during which time they don't take any herbs. Then they would take the second microbial defense herb for twelve and a half days, and then take another thirty-six hours off. They might then go on to take the third microbial defense herb for twelve and a half days, and then take another thirty-six hours off before going back to the first herb again. They would then continue with that rotational protocol for several months. The timetable of this protocol is especially useful when treating Borrelia, because I have observed in darkfield micro-scopy that spirochetes that have managed to hide from treatments come back out of hiding towards the end of the thirty-six hour period that patients aren't taking any microbial defense herbs. When the spirochetes come out again, patients can then hammer them with the herbs so that they can't form new offspring. In this manner, eventually all forms of the organism, whether spore, granule, L-form or cyst, come out of hiding at some point, and can be eliminated sequentially without creating new crops of organisms.

Patients and practitioners should bear in mind, however, that six to eight months of treatment is sufficient only if patients do an appropriate detoxification protocol. If not, then treatment may be required for a year or two. Dr. Horowitz, for example, does a little bit of detoxification in his practice, but not a lot, so some of his patients who do the herbal protocol must be on it for a year. Because I do a lot of detoxification in my practice, I find that most of my patients are well within six to eight months.

Specific and General Detoxification Strategies

I do specific as well as general detoxification strategies on my patients. One of the specific strategies that I do is called LED or Laser Energetic Detoxification. For this, I first do an energetic evaluation on the patient in order to discover which toxins appear to be causing problems for him or her. I then make up a clear liquid remedy in a clear glass vial, containing the homeopathic homaccord dilutions of the toxic substances that are represented in that particular patient's body. I then take that clear glass vial of homeopathic toxins and place it in front of a laser pointer, and shine the laser through the glass vial and onto the patient, which has the effect of carrying the energy of the homeopathic remedy into the patient's body.

If you shine a laser pointer on a wall, without any glass vial in front of the light, you will only see a red or green dot, depending upon whether you have a red or a green laser. If you put a vial in front of the light, however, you end up with a line of light on the wall, because the curvature of the glass vial causes a refraction of the light that is coming out of the laser. If you move that vial and laser pointer six to ten feet from the patient, then the line of light becomes long enough to cover the entire width of the patient. "Sweeping" is the name I give to the process of sequentially covering the body, from head to toe, and from front to back, with this refracted light. I also perform sweeping of light through the homeopathic vial on the ears, palms of the hands, and soles of the feet.

Through this process, I am able to cover enough of the body's surface so that sufficient energy enters in for the processing and release of physical toxins from cells. After doing the LED therapy, I then give my patients a combination of drainage/detoxification remedies. This is to ensure that the toxins which have been released from the cells move out from the space from in-between the cells, into the lymphatic system and veins, and from there, into the clearing organs—the kidneys, bladder, liver, gall bladder and bowels.

One thing that I have discovered about laser sweeping is that if I don't address the emotions that caused the body to hold onto the physical toxins in the first place, then patients will have a harsh detoxification reaction when we do the LED. The body often holds onto toxins when there is unresolved emotional trauma in people's lives. I deal with such traumas by giving patients homeopathic remedies containing the energetic imprint of certain flowers and colors, since these are known to positively affect mood and emotions. I put these remedies into a vial before the detoxification procedure, and shine the laser through them and onto the patient. Whenever I do this, the detoxification procedure that follows is smooth and effective.

With some patients, I will do just one session of LED; with others, I might do two or three. After that, I will teach them how to keep themselves from getting loaded up with toxins again, as well as how to keep heavy metals and other toxins flowing out of their bodies. When I do so, I find that after a few weeks or months, they are basically healthy again.

All of the above is what I call specific detoxification, because it is a protocol that is specifically tailored to each patient's problems.

My general detoxification protocol for patients involves therapies like far infrared sauna, clay plaster and oil pulling, among others. These target general toxicities that are common to many people.

Another therapy that I have found to be very important for aiding in detoxification is called Reverse Spin treatment. There is a quantum physical abnormality that occurs in tissues that get toxin overloaded, and when this happens, lymphatic drainage, venous outflow from tissues and capillary inflow into tissues all drop off dramatically. As a result, tissues become starved for oxygen and get overloaded with toxins very quickly. For treatment of this abnormality, I use Burbur and Parsley Detox drops because these herbals are imprinted with energetic frequencies that help the body to deal with this reverse spin. I also use a product called Right Spin Glutathione, by NatuRx, which is an energetically imprinted remedy that also works well for this purpose. This pale yellow powder, which is taken in 100 mg doses and held under the tongue for a couple of minutes, resolves reverse spin throughout the body fairly quickly. If those with Lyme take Burbur Detox plus Right Spin Glutathione, or Parsley Detox plus Right Spin Glutathione every ten minutes, their Herxheimer reactions generally last an hour or less, whereas if they don't take these combinations, their Herxes may last one to two days.

Also, I often use Pinella in conjunction with Burbur or Parsley, because it helps to move toxins out of the brain faster than the other two products. So if my patients have brain fog, I will recommend that they take Burbur Detox with Pinella, or Parsley Detox with Pinella.

Biotoxins from Borrelia, Bartonella and fungus are often patients' biggest problem because of the exacerbation in symptoms that they can cause. If patients have been on prescription pharmaceutical antibiotics, they will typically have a major fungal overgrowth in their gut and/or sinuses, and those fungi are producing mycotoxins that are far more toxic than any man-made toxin. For that reason, it's important to get rid of mold and fungi that are growing in the body (see section below on mold), and start binding up their myco-toxins, which poison enzyme systems. Dr. Ritchie Shoemaker, M.D., recommends using Cholestyramine to bind such toxins. I have found that some of the fibers, like rice mucil, slippery elm bark, marshmallow root, or psyllium husk, are better tolerated by patients than Cholestyramine. I also sometimes use a product called Nanotech Chitosan, which is a micro-chitosan from shellfish. Since some patients have shellfish allergies, however, not everyone can take this product.

Addressing Detoxification Defects

Laser Energetic Detox or LED therapy can correct problems of compromised detoxification to some degree. Some people have heterozygous genetic defects, which means that only one of the two strands of DNA which code for a protein is defective. When toxins are removed, then the impact of such toxins on the gene is reduced; the defective DNA strand stops coding for an abnormal protein, and the healthy one starts coding for a normal one. That's an epigenetic effect of detoxification, as well as a solution for some people that have trouble detoxifying.

If practitioners don't have access to LED therapy, they can make homeopathic dilutions of toxins in vials, and patients can rub drops of these on their skin, or take them orally. By doing this, a similar detoxification effect may be achieved, but the advantage of the laser detox is that results are achieved in days, instead of weeks or months.

Treating Hormonal Dysfunction

I prescribe bioidentical hormone replacement to some of my pa-tients, but I find that often, the body will make the hormones that it needs to make once its toxic load is reduced and it gets the nutri-tional building blocks that it needs. Some people have been sick so long that they develop adrenal exhaustion, and because of this, their thyroid malfunctions, and as a result, other systems start malfunctioning, too. I use adaptogenic herbs to stimulate their adrenals to recover, but don't treat their thyroid much until their adrenals are sufficiently healed. The adaptogenic herbal I use most often for this purpose is called Adrenal Support. Along with this herbal combination, I recommend moderately high doses (up to 1,000 mg daily) of Vitamin B-5, or pantothenic acid, and if tolerated, Vitamin C from a non-corn derived source. I find that when patients take a combination of Vitamin C, pantothenic acid and the Adrenal Support herbs, and perform stress reduction techniques several times daily, their adrenals can recover. At that point, I will then recommend that they take just a few drops of iodine per day to recover their thyroid. I often recommend a saturated solution of potassium iodide, which is rubbed into the forearms. Iodine also stimulates the immune system, since it's needed for the normal functioning of many white blood cells, and for stimulating the steroidal hormone receptors on cells.

Hormonal dysfunction can sometimes be the first consequence of Lyme disease and what causes patients' symptoms. It's also one reason why they accumulate toxins so easily. For such patients, supplementation with pregnenolone, low dose cortisol, estradiol, progesterone, testosterone, or DHEA may be necessary. These hormones are the ones that are most commonly out of balance in those with Lyme. Sometimes HGH, or human growth hormone, is also out of balance, but I don't typically give injections of HGH because patients can become quickly and irreversibly dependent upon this hormone, and I don't like for them to become dependent upon hormones. Instead, I use the Chinese solution, which is an extract of deer antler velvet; taken sublingually, it restores growth hormone pathways. HGH is also lowered when patients sleep in rooms with too many electromagnetic frequencies, too much light or geopathic stress, so reducing these influences can also be beneficial for restoring HGH levels.

William McJeffries, in his book, *Safe Uses of Cortisol*, suggests that short courses of cortisol can be helpful for restoring health. I don't advocate synthetic cortisol for my patients; however, I believe that a low dose of a true, bioidentical cortisol can give the body a bit of help. When cortisol levels are too low, the immune system is suppressed, just as when cortisol levels are too high, the immune system is also suppressed. The amount of cortisol in the body needs to be just right.

Treating Mold and Fungal Infections

Cumanda, Lakato and Banderol herbal remedies are superb for treating fungal infections, but it's sometimes necessary for patients to take fairly high doses of these. Also, some people make the mistake of taking these remedies while continuing to eat massive amounts of sugar. When they do that, it's as if there were two fire trucks with two different alarms going off in their bodies. The first fire truck comes along and starts squirting water (Cumanda, Lakato or Banderol) on the fire which represents the infection, and then the second fire truck goes around to the other side of the fire and starts squirting gasoline on it, (this gasoline is the sugar). As a result, the fire continues to burn. So I have to caution my patients to completely eliminate all sugars from their diets, including all fruit sugars, if they want to get rid of fungal infections. This means no fruit or fruit juice, except for lemons and limes, during the first six to eight weeks of fungal treatment. It also means dramatically reducing the amount of starches in the diet so that people are basically eating nuts, seeds, salads, meats, vegetables, lemons and limes. No grains, rice, dairy or beans, (including dried beans), as well as no potatoes or other starchy vegetables, are allowed.

Treatments for Symptomatic Relief

Anxiety and Depression

For symptoms of anxiety, I often recommend Amantilla to my patients. This is an herbal extract of valerian root that has been imprinted with a variety of energetic frequencies. It was evaluated on over one hundred patients with chronic insomnia at the University of Guayaquil in Ecuador, and was found to reduce insomnia in 82% of these. The herbal is therefore also useful for inducing sleep, and at lower doses, is effective for relaxation. I also use other herbal remedies, such as Babuna or kava kava for the treatment of anxiety.

In people with anxiety, the sympathetic nervous system is in overdrive, and when this happens, there is also too much vasoconstriction in the body, which creates oxygen deprivation in the tissues. The body then goes into a state of anaerobic metabolism, lactic acidosis develops, and the acid that builds up in the body binds to minerals, so that the minerals are no longer available to make enzymes work. The result is a metabolic breakdown inside of the body.

For the treatment of depression, I have found the NutraMedix product Avea to work well for patients, even though it's an herbal that one might not ordinarily consider for treatment of this symptom. Basically, Avea is a quantum energetic imprint of turmeric but I have seen it reverse suicidal depression in some, and in just a few hours when it's taken by mouth on an hourly basis.

Another product that I have found to be extremely helpful for treating the emotional aspects of illness is EZOV. It seems that when my patients take this at bedtime, a lot of their subconscious emotions come out in their dreams, because they start dreaming vividly and in color for the first time in their lives. Then they tend to wake up the following morning with a completely different (and better) feeling than what they had when they went to bed the night before. For example, one patient of mine, a guy who had suffered from symptoms of irritable bowel syndrome (IBS) for over ten years, took one dose of EZOV, went to bed and never had IBS symptoms again. So results can be dramatic with this product.

I rarely use pharmaceuticals for the treatment of my patients' depression. Instead, I try to get to the root cause of their depression. Usually, energetic tests reveal that their main problem is autoimmunity to one of the neurotransmitters that are necessary for normal mood, especially norepinephrine or serotonin, and I can use the Laser Energetic Detox treatment to resolve that. When I do, patients often go from being profoundly depressed to being cheery within twenty-four to forty-eight hours.

That said, sometimes patients have severe neurotransmitter deficiencies, and I have to make up for these deficiencies with nutrition. So if the deficiency is serotonin, I might give my patients 5-HTP or tryptophan plus tiny amounts of the co-factor B-6 so that the body can make its own serotonin. Often, serotonin production is shut down because of too much light in the bedroom at night, or because electromagnetic or geopathic fields are affecting sleep. So improving one's sleep environment can also help the body to make more serotonin. Other people have norepinephrine deficits as a result of a methylation defect. This problem can often be remedied by taking an appropriate form of folate—frequently 5-methyl-tetrahydro-folate, and/or the right form of B-12, either hydroxy or methyl B-12. When people with Lyme take these nutrients, they start producing better methylation, and start converting neurotransmitter precursors into the neurotransmitters that will prevent depression.

Finally, I will share another pearl on treating depression. If patients' depression is due to under-methylation, then a teaspoon of creatine monohydrate per day can significantly ameliorate that depression. The reason is because 70% of the S-adenosyl-methionine that is produced each day by the body is used up in producing creatine, which is then used to clear amino acid byproducts from the body. If S-adenosyl-methionine is spared through creatine supplementation, then there is frequently a lot more S-adenosyl- methionine available to increase neurotransmitters and their precursors. So practitioners can lift their patients pretty quickly out of depression this way.

If the above-mentioned measures aren't sufficient, then 5mg of Lithium (as the orotate form) three to four times daily, or one tablet of LiZyme-Forte (from Biotics), taken hourly, can sometimes be helpful for rapidly resolving depression.

Pain

One remedy that I recommend for the treatment of pain is Condura from NutraMedix, which can be taken as a dropperful under the tongue, or as several drops rubbed into the skin on the painful spot. The dose is repeated every ten minutes as needed. If that doesn't work, then I might recommend Bliss in a Bottle, a homeopathic remedy that can be sprayed into the mouth, and/or onto the skin.

I also teach my patients and their family members to do a pain reduction technique called Ki Therapy. This is a light touch, hands-on technique that can resolve a lot of conditions in body when the palm surface of the index, middle, and ring fingers of both of the practitioners' hands are simultaneously applied to certain points on the patient's body. The "practitioner" doing this might be a friend or loved one, and the technique is performed in the following manner:

First, the patient lies on his or her back in bed with his or her head placed at the foot of the bed, while that person's friend (or family member) sits in a chair at the foot of bed. The friend places his or her right hand fingers on the patient's forehead, above the patient's right eyebrow, and his or her left-hand fingers on the patient's forehead above the left eyebrow. The patient places his or her fingers on the rib margins below the breasts. Patient and friend should keep their hands in this position until strong pulsations are felt in all four hands, usually after about five minutes. Once the pulsations are felt, then they keep their respective hand positions for another minute, before releasing and going to a second hold position.

In the second hold position, the patient moves his or her hands to the pulses that are felt in the groin, (the point where the femoral pulses can be felt crossing each groin crease), and places the right hand on the right pulse, and the left hand on the left pulse. The "practitioner" friend then moves to the side of bed, and puts his or her hands together, and places them so that one sits above and the other below the patient's belly button. He or she then simultaneously slides both hands away from the patient's belly button until each hand hits a midline bony prominence on the patient's body. These prominences are the lower end of the patient's breastbone and the pelvic bone. Patient and "practitioner" then hold those hand positions for about five minutes, until strong pulsations are felt in all four hands. At that point, the patient should re-assess the pain level.

If the patient uses Condura or Bliss in a Bottle before performing this Ki technique, it will make it more effective. If, after doing these two hold positions, the patient's pain went from a level ten to a level five intensity, and he or she feels better but still can't sleep, then another Ki Therapy technique can be done. For this one, the patient lies on his or her back with his or her head at the head of the bed, while the "practitioner" friend goes to the foot of bed. The "practitioner" friend sits at the foot of the bed, with his or her palms beneath the calves of the patient, with the fingers together and with the tip of the middle finger behind the crease of the patient's knee. This is called "palming of the calves". The "practitioner's" left hand goes under the patient's right calf, and the "practitioner's" right hand goes under the patient's left calf. The "practitioner" holds that position for about ten minutes.

This calf palming technique helps to stimulate the patient's detoxification processes, thereby relieving the pain, because often, pain is the result of toxin build-up. For this reason, I will also give my patients Burbur and Parsley under the tongue or in ½ cup of water to take orally, as well as Pinella, if they have headaches or pain in their heads. I will also give them Right Spin Glutathione under the tongue for detoxification. If they keep repeating with these (Burbur or Parsley plus Pinella and Right Spin Glutathione) every ten minutes while doing the Ki Therapy, then their pain gets relieved much faster, so that they can go to sleep or do whatever it is that they need to do. This combination works for all kinds of pain, including head, muscle or joint pain. To learn more about Ki Therapy, visit the following website: www.KingInstitute.org.

Insomnia

For the treatment of insomnia, I recommend Amantilla to my patients. If that doesn't work, I recommend Babuna, which is an herbal extract of chamomile. This product was studied at the University of Guayaquil, in Guayaquil, Ecuador, and was found to induce sleep in sixty-eight of one hundred patients with insomnia.

Also, patients can take melatonin, but I don't recommend extended use of this supplement. Instead, I try to fix the cause of insomnia. Melatonin or serotonin deficiencies, for example, can result from an unclean sleeping environment, which may include the presence of too many electromagnetic frequencies or chemical odors, or too much geopathic stress or light in the bedroom. People need to create a sanctuary that is conducive to sleep.

When people wake up in the middle of the night, they shouldn't be able to see their hands in front of them. If they can, then the room in which they are sleeping is not dark enough. Studies have shown that even very low levels of light affect melatonin production. The only type of light that doesn't affect melatonin production is a pale red light, so if people have to get up in the middle of the night, then it's best that they use a red pin light or red laser pointer to guide them to the bathroom or to wherever they need to go.

To determine whether electromagnetic fields (EMF's) are affecting my patients' sleep environment, I tell them to take EMF readings over their beds with a low-frequency Gauss meter. The readings should be 0.2 milligauss or less; if they are above that, then they should turn off the master circuit breaker in the house, in order to determine where the source of the problem is. If the readings don't change as a result of doing this, then the EMF's are coming from outside of the house. If the readings go down but don't normalize, then the problem is inside, as well as outside of the house. If the readings normalize as a result of turning off the circuit breaker, then the problem is from inside the house only. In that case, I tell my patients to unplug all of the appliances in the bedroom, leaving the bedroom circuit breaker on, and repeat the Gauss readings.

In some cases, if there is an electrical wiring defect in the wall, unplugging appliances may not reduce the EMF's, in which case I advise my patients to either turn off the circuit breakers at night, or get an electrician to fix the defect. Unfortunately, many people live in cities and get bombarded with high-frequency EMF's from cell phone towers, radio stations, microwaves, and so forth, and obtaining an instrument to measure the effects of these in the home is much more expensive than purchasing a low-frequency Gauss meter. If people find that they have severely high levels of EMF's in their bedrooms, especially from sources that are coming from outside of the house, there is a material that has been fabricated in Germany that they can purchase and which will shield high frequency EMF's. This material is fashioned into a canopy that covers the bed, much like a mosquito net but instead of shielding the body from mosquitoes, it shields the body from high-frequency electromagnetic radiations (but not from the low-frequency radiation that is created by most home appliances or wall circuits).

Treating Gut Dysbiosis

If my patients use the herbals that I recommend to get rid of the pathogens in their guts, then their gut dysbiosis can be resolved to some degree. For example, Enula is quite effective against many parasites that cause dysbiosis, and Cumanda, Lakato and Banderol are effective for fungal infections and many pathologic bacteria.

To resolve gut dysbiosis, I also recommend that patients take sources of non-absorbable fiber, such as psyllium, slippery elm, marshmallow root and rice mucil along with a probiotic, to help get rid of toxins and replenish friendly bacteria in the gut. Typically, a probiotic should contain at least two species of bifidobacteria and two or three species of lactobacillus besides acidophilus, along with some other species of bacteria. A product containing all of the above will produce a hearty repopulation of bacteria in the gut. Some people rely on lactobacillus acidophilus alone, but this bacteria is really too weak and fragile; it won't kill unhealthy bacteria and can't stay implanted in the gut. When used alone (in the absence of other types of bacteria), it gets continually killed off by unfriendly bacteria.

Healing Emotional Trauma

I have observed that patients often develop inflammation due to microbial infestation in their bodies, but the microbes are there in large part because the internal body environment is right for them to grow (according to Bechamp and others). An internal body environment conducive to microbial growth can be created in part by unresolved "emotional toxins," and whenever these are present, microbes, as well as other physical toxins, will also be present. Thus, if patients want to go as far upstream as they can in their healing, it's important that they deal with the emotional toxins as well as the physical ones. These emotional toxins can be defined as stored traumas that they have experienced in the womb or some-time during the first few years of their life, and which the body can't get rid of. So sometimes, the things that are making people sick are the things that they can't even remember, which makes healing from chronic illness a bit more challenging.

To treat emotional toxins, I use the EVOX, which is voice analysis software from the Zyto Corporation. Patients speak into the micro-phone of the EVOX system and it records their voice, as they speak about a specific issue or person in their lives. Imbedded in the voice are energetic frequencies that correspond to the negative emotions that are being held in the body because of a particular issue or person. So if patients talk about themselves and say, for example, "My name is Jennie", as they say that simple phrase repeatedly, all of the information that is buried in their subconscious mind about themselves is being recorded. It is then possible to make an elec-tronic homeopathic-like dilution of those voice recordings and deliver them back out through a hand cradle to the patients. This then has the effect of "shifting" them energetically so that their emotional trauma gets released, even though they don't know what that hidden trauma is. And all of this is accomplished without having to go through a tear-jerking session with a therapist.

I also use numerous types of flowers for emotional healing as part of Laser Energetic Detoxification (see section on detoxification), including Bach, Bush, North American and Peruvian flowers. I use these in conjunction with the energetic imprint of colors. Every color in the color spectrum or rainbow has a vibrational frequency that can be stored in water or in water and alcohol, and which can also be used for healing trauma.

Homeopathy is a good starting point for healing emotional trauma, because it releases physical toxins that are there due to emotions. However, if patients are to fully heal from trauma, they need to go deeper and also do other things to get better.

Hence, there is another type of therapy that I recommend to my patients to deal with trauma, which is called Visualization Raging. Those in my office call it Emotional Release by Visualization—and only sometimes by raging! For this process, patients go someplace where they won't be disturbed and where they won't disturb anyone else. This is often a mountaintop, a park or hillside.

They start by visualizing a person not related to them who hurt them in the past and whom they still have anger or frustration towards. They visualize this person as he or she was at the time when he or she wounded them, not how they see that person now. Then they start shouting at that person. When I mention this exercise to patients, they will say things like, "I shouldn't shout at that person." But in order for the exercise to work, it's really important that they not judge themselves for what they are shouting— what matters is that they get their raw emotions out as they shout. As they do this, other emotions that are lying beneath the current one start to come up too, so they might need to stop and cry a little to fully release those. Or they might stop and tremble a little because the person who wounded them did something to make them fearful. After trembling or crying or releasing other emotions, then they can go back to shouting until all of the emotions related to the person they are visualizing are gone. When they shout, they must also shout directly at the person they are angry with, for having caused the hurt that they are experiencing. This is very important.

Then they move on to a second, third, fourth person and so on. After shouting at non-relatives, they shout at distant relatives, and finally, close relatives. It's important to work last on close family members including parents, siblings, grandparents, spouses, and finally, oneself. When patients get to themselves, they start by shouting at their bodies for not being perfect and healthy like they want them to be. Then they shout at their minds for doing or saying things that they regretted, or for failing to do or say things that they wish they had done or said. When they are finished shouting at themselves, if they believe in God and are angry with God, then they can shout at God.

After this, they go through a forgiveness process, whereby they forgive all those that they shouted at, including self and God. I find that if my patients do this in a certain way, then it is more effective. That process involves saying the name of the offending person aloud, and saying, "I forgive you both consciously and subconsciously, for all that you said or did, or failed to say or do and which has caused any anger or frustration in me or anyone else I care about." When they do it this way, there is usually a deeper release of unforgiveness than they have ever had before. Praying people often say a prayer at the end of this activity, such as, "Please forgive me for the anger I had. Please replace the roots of anger and frustration that were in me with unconditional love, joy and peace." Whatever a person's spiritual beliefs are helps to determine what the rest of the process needs to be.

Another powerful technique for healing emotional trauma is called Recall Healing, which has evolved from the work of several doctors in different countries. This work is based upon the idea that if practitioners know their patients' physical diagnoses, then they can also indirectly know the emotional conflicts that caused their patients' physical problems. If they then ask the right questions to resolve the emotional conflict that created the physical condition, then their patients' physical symptoms disappear. More information on this type of therapy can be found on the Internet at: www.IntegraMedAcademy.com. Also, I have produced a course on the IntegraMed website called Emotional Detox that describes a variety of emotional detoxification procedures that I have found to be very helpful.

IntegraMed Academy

The IntegraMed Academy site also contains courses on EMF pollution, bioenergetic medicine, and Art Therapy. The academy usually hosts a couple of new courses per month, so any doctor that wants to learn something about different areas of integrative medicine can go to that site and sign up for these courses. The information presented in the courses can be streamed off of the site, because the courses are mostly done via video with Power Point presentations and text information for practitioners to review. In the near future, once practitioners have reviewed the information, they will be able to take an exam if they wish, and get continuing education credits through the site. So they can learn and do all of this without having to pay for a hotel, rental car, airplane flight and meals away from home; travel expenses that they would typically incur in order to learn about new areas of medicine.

Profiling the Person Who Heals from Lyme Disease

The person that fully heals is the one who has the right attitude and support system, and who doesn't believe that he or she will always be ill. If people believe that there is a chance they will be well, then it is more likely that they will. A lot of patients have been told by well-intentioned practitioners that they will always be sick, and so if they believe what the practitioner says, then they won't get well.

Those with Lyme also need to ask themselves whether there are people in their lives who are sabotaging what they are trying to do. For instance, there are those who say things like, "Oh that therapy isn't going to work. How do you expect that kind of therapy to work? That's not studied in a peer-reviewed journal in an Ivy League institution in the United States." If they are getting that kind of talk all the time from the people in their lives, then it will be hard for them to get well. Or if they are speaking those kinds of words to themselves, they will also have a hard time healing.

On the other hand, if the people around them act loving, caring, giving and supportive towards them, then they will likely get well. If they say things like, "I can help you to get the foods that you need. I can help you to prepare those foods. I can help you to set up your nutrient protocol, and get it organized so that you can take your supplements at the right time," then their loved ones have a greater chance of healing.

There are other factors that come into play when it comes to healing, however. People with poor genetics, for example, will have a more difficult time healing, as will those who live in a terrible physical environment, with lots of EMF's or mold in their houses.

Strategies for Stress Reduction and Dealing with Life's Difficulties

One activity that I recommend that my patients do every night, which is extremely helpful and powerful for emotional healing and for dealing with the lifestyle difficulties of Lyme disease is called "good and bad" journaling. Patients take a piece of paper and write down all of the things that they don't want to ever think or worry about again. Once they are finished, they tear up that paper into tiny pieces or put it in a paper shredder or burn it. Then, after writing on this "negative" paper, they pull out their "good" diary, which is something that they will keep forever, and start writing down everything that was good, positive and a blessing on that particular day. They must come up with at least one thing that was good, in order for this exercise to work. And then a few days later, when they are having a really tough day, they can go back and find their good diary, open it up and read about all of the positive, good things that happened in previous days but which they forgot about. In this manner, their own writing uplifts them.

This exercise is very powerful. Studies have shown that the average child hears the word "no" one hundred times for every single time that they hear the word "yes." That means that most people arrive into adulthood with a deficiency of "yes's", and an excess of "no's", and as a result, are quite negative in their thinking. This process is a way of dumping the "no's" and filling the body and mind back up with "yes's".

Another stress reduction technique that I recommend for my patients takes just two minutes before each meal and before each bedtime. For this, they first close their eyes, and imagine themselves in a vacation spot where they once enjoyed themselves. They then breathe in and out deeply through their nose or mouth, as they visualize this place with all of their senses. So if they are walking on a beach, for instance, they will smell the ocean smells, see the clouds in the sky and the sun setting, feel the sand squishing between their toes, hear seagulls calling in the air, feel the warm breeze on their skin, and so on. Once they immerse themselves in the memory of that enjoyable place, it becomes hard for them to be negative, dwelling on stuff that is detrimental and harmful to their healing.

Exercise

For exercise, I recommend that my patients do whatever type of activity that they are able to handle. In general, I recommend that everyone do stretching and what I call self-adjustment techniques, which involve putting all of the body's major joints back into alignment. A lot of people with Lyme have "messed-up" organs, which are sending undesirable signals to the nerves, and then to the vertebrae in the back. The muscles around those vertebrae go into spasm, usually on one side and not the other, which causes the vertebrae to get pulled out of alignment. The vertebrae being out of alignment then causes the nerves leading back to the organs to be pinched, which keeps the vicious cycle going. For this reason, I teach my patients to do a series of stretches every morning and night, to align their major joints.

The first of the stretches that I teach them are called windmill twists, which align the mid-thoracic, lower thoracic and upper lumbar vertebrae. A second technique involves them laying down on their back near the edge of the bed and putting the leg that is furthest from the edge over the edge of the bed, while keeping both of their shoulders pressed against the bed. Using the other side of the bed, they can then stretch the other leg in a similar fashion. This exercise stretches the lumbar and sacral areas. To properly adjust the sacroiliac joint, it is important that the thigh be at a ninety-degree angle from the torso. They can also adjust the pubic bone joint at the lower end of their abdomen by putting a ball or pillow between their knees when their knees are flexed close to their chest, and then squeezing the ball as their legs are again fully extended. After doing an adjustment of the sacroiliac joints and symphysis pubis as described above, they can stand upright and reach simultaneously towards the ceiling with one hand and towards the floor with the other hand, then repeat the motions, but switching which hand is up and which is down. They can then reach simultaneously forward with one hand and backwards with the other, and then switch which hand is reaching forwards and backwards. This adjusts their upper thoracic vertebrae.

After asking patients to forgive everyone that they can think of, I show them how to turn their neck from side to side, to adjust the cervical spine. Sometimes, I even show them how to adjust their cranial bones as well. Just adjusting those major joints can help those with Lyme tremendously, because when they are out of alignment, especially in the lumbo-sacral spine, their bodies are sending signals to the sympathetic nervous system to pump out adrenaline. As a result, they can't sleep at night, when the body should be resting and recovering. So if they can stretch those muscles and adjust their major joints in the lumbo-sacral spine before bedtime, then the body's "sympathetic outpouring" and adrenaline levels diminish dramatically, and the body goes into parasympathetic dominance, which is conducive to sleep, healing and rest.

On Sunshine and the Marshall Protocol

People often read about the Marshall protocol on the Internet, and as a result, become fearful about sunlight. That is a mistake. I have found that all of my Lyme patients do well with sunlight exposure, as long as they don't stay in the sun so long that they get sunburned. Sunlight exposure programs the pineal gland to turn on melatonin production at night, as long as the person is sleeping in a dark room. Also, if those with Lyme get thirty to forty minutes of sunlight exposure per day in the late morning, while not wearing too many clothes, their bodies will produce Vitamin D, which is important for proper immune function. Vitamin D also aids in the functioning of several thousand genes in the body. Walking, deep breathing exercises and gardening are some examples of good outdoor activities that those with Lyme can do, and which are beneficial for health.

Final Words

There is hope for patients who suffer from Lyme disease, even if they have suffered for years, have become disabled and exhausted every pharmaceutical antibiotic therapy. A comprehensive protocol of all natural therapies has restored health to thousands of Lyme disease patients who were told by allopathic physicians that there was nothing else that could be done for their condition. If you suffer from Lyme disease, seek out an open-minded health care practitioner who will work with you using the approach described in this chapter. The empiric Cowden Condensed Protocol mentioned in this chapter is also described in some detail on the Internet site: www.bionatus.com/nutramedix.

How to Contact W. Lee Cowden, M.D., M.D. (H)

I am now involved in teaching integrative medicine full-time to healthcare practitioners in the USA and abroad and functioning as Chairman of the Scientific Advisory Board for IntegraMed Academy. Healthcare practitioners can reach me via email at: drc@integramedacademy.com. The information on the Academy's website can be accessed by the general public as well as by health-care practitioners. Not only should those with Lyme learn as much as they can from IntegraMed Academy's website and courses, but they should also encourage their health care practitioners, friends and family to access the valuable information at: www.integramedacademy.com.

• CHAPTER 6 •

Ingo D. E. Woitzel, M.D.
PFORZHEIM, GERMANY

Biography

Dr. Ingo Woitzel graduated from medical school in 1981 from the University of Heidelberg in Heidelberg, Germany. He is a medical doctor with training in naturopathic and environmental medicine. In addition, in 2004, he received a Master of Chiropractic certificate from the Ackermann College of Chiropractic, in Stockholm, Sweden. He is married with seven children and currently works in Pforzheim, Germany, where he treats Lyme disease (Borreliosis) and other conditions of illness.

Treatment Approach

I have been treating Lyme disease (Borreliosis) with photon therapy for about nine years. Over those nine years, I have observed a relapse rate of about 3% in my patients.

Biophoton Theory

One of the most important scientific contributions to our world today has been the discovery of biophotons, a type of electromagnetic light (quantum mechanics) that all living organisms emit and which cells use to communicate with one another.

First discovered in 1923 by Russian medical scientist Professor Alexander G. Gurvich (who called them "mitogenetic rays"), biophotons were widely researched in Europe and the USA in the 1930's. In the 1950's, Italian scientists developed the "photon multiplier technique" and proved that biophotons emit low levels of radiation. Subsequently, three Russian scientists, S. Stschurin, V.P. Kasnaschejew and L. Michailova performed over 5000 experiments and through these proved that all living cells transmit information via biophotons.

In 1974, German biophysicist Fritz-Albert Popp further established the existence of biophotons beyond any reasonable doubt, and proved that they originate in the DNA of the cell. He also developed and tested a number of hypotheses about their possible biological functions. He subsequently developed a number of applications for the use of biophoton measurements in microorganisms, plants, animals and humans.

From all these discoveries, French biophysicist Daniel Giron developed photon therapy, and is therefore called the 'father' of today's Bionic 880, a photon device that is used (mostly in Europe) to treat Borreliosis and other conditions. (Note: The Bionic 880 is also discussed in Chapter 11).

Dr. Woitzel uses photon therapy in his practice to treat Lyme disease and other illnesses. (*Note: Author Connie Strasheim traveled to Germany in April, 2009 to be treated by Dr. Woitzel. She received treatments with the Bionic 880 twice a week, for three weeks*).

How Disease Happens

Every cell of the human body has a nucleus with DNA. From this DNA, and as established by Popp, biophotons are emitted, which control the metabolism inside, as well as outside, the cell. A change in the balance of the cell's biophotons by toxins, bacteria, viruses or electromagnetic radiation brings about a disturbance in the cell and leads, over time, to disease in one or several organs.

Thus, any illness manifests itself first on an energetic level, and since energy is superior to matter (matter is comprised of energy), any change in the body's energy eventually leads to changes in the body's biochemistry, as well. The balance of the body's biophotons can be restored, however, by therapy that brings photonic light back into the cells.

Since disease manifests itself first on an energetic level, I always treat any disease with energetic methods first, if my patients are willing to collaborate. The most effective of these involves treatment with photons within the 880-nm (880 nanometer) infrared range. With this type of therapy, I can directly influence the biophotonic balance of my patients' cells and change or normalize the energetic information found therein. As a result of normalizing their energy, the biochemistry of their physical bodies normalizes, as well. In this way, they regain their health, but the process takes time.

How Bionic 880 Photons Are Transmitted Throughout the Body

Photons that are radiated by the Bionic 880 device are absorbed by the skin, then multiply in the body and spread everywhere. They reach all organs, even the brain, and pass through the branchings of the nervous system and spinal cord, where they harmonize (modify) the production of different hormones and neurotransmitters, such as endorphins and serotonin. The photon signals also reach other tissues and influence all systems of the body, including the immune.

The Cellular Effects of Photon Therapy

Life isn't possible without light. According to Popp, and as previously mentioned, photons radiate from every cell in the body. In cells affected by illness or toxins, the intensity of biophoton emissions is low. Regeneration of these darkened cells can be accomplished by administering photons from an external source, such as the Bionic 880.

Photons in the infrared wave band that are administered to the body can activate many metabolic processes. First, they increase the detoxification of all toxic matter, including pesticides, bacteria and viruses. They also increase the production of leukocytes and macrophages, CD-57 cells, and lymphocytes, as well as other immune cells, and normalize pathologic metabolism.

If macrophages are exposed to infrared light within the range of 880 nm, they release substances that are helpful for repairing damaged cells and which support the production of connective tissue.

Infrared light has proven to have positive effects not just upon leukocytes, but also upon several types of lymphocytes and enzymes. It can increase NK cell counts, but it can also decrease immune cell counts in those with autoimmune conditions.

Testing for Lyme Disease

Problems with Traditional Tests for Lyme (Borrelia)

Some patients with Lyme (Borreliosis) test negative for the disease on serologic tests; however, a tissue evaluation from their organs often reveals that in fact, they do have Lyme. Hence, I believe that it's important to diagnose Lyme disease using different energetic techniques, along with a clinical diagnosis. Such techniques produce accurate results, once mastered by the practitioner.

Testing in this manner is especially important because there are four categories of people with Lyme disease who don't meet the official criteria for a positive diagnosis under the traditional antibody system of testing, or who are difficult to diagnose for other reasons. These people may not present typical Lyme disease symptoms or have positive results on their lab tests. These categories (according to Henry Feder et.al. [N. Engl. Med. 2007; 357: 1422 – 1430]) include:

1. People who test negative on serologic tests, and live in non-endemic Lyme regions, but who have non-specific symptoms such as fatigue, insomnia, night sweats and myalgias.

2. People whose illnesses have been diagnosed as something else, such as MS, or who have not yet been diagnosed as having Lyme. Also those who have been diagnosed with Lyme but who have not accepted their diagnosis.

3. People who do not have clinical signs and symptoms of Lyme but who have antibodies to Borrelia.

4. People who get the classic erythema migrans rash and who have taken antibiotics for Borrelia but who are yet still suffering from symptoms. Such people have been labeled as having "post-Lyme syndrome".

Testing for Borrelia Using Homeopathy and Energy Medicine Modalities

When determining whether or not to treat patients for Borreliosis (as Lyme disease is called in Europe), I perform bioresonance tests on them using a variety of energetic devices, such as the Bicom, along with homeopathic nosodes containing original Borrelia bacteria. The Borrelia nosodes, in conjunction with the Bicom, are used to determine whether the energetic information contained within the nosodes resonates with the energetic information that is contained within the patient's cells and/or meridians. If it does, then that means that Borrelia is present in that patient's body.

When patients test negative for Borreliosis using this method, I do not treat them for the infection, even if their serologic or other lab tests are positive.

For the testing, I use homeopathic nosodes in dilutions of D 5 - D 200 (D 5, D 6, D 8, D 10, D 12, D 15, D 30, D 60, D 100, D 200, along with the original Borrelia organism). Usually, if Borrelia is present and causing problems in their bodies, then patients will test positive within this range of dilutions.

After administering five photon therapy sessions to my patients, I will then test the reaction of their cellular energy to the borrelia nosodes using the Bicom machine, using a range between 120 Hz and 152 KHz on the machine. If there is no positive reaction to the nosodes, then their borrelia is considered to be in remission. If there is a positive reaction, then I treat them once more, wait a month, and then test them again.

Once Borrelia is in remission, then patients must be tested on a monthly basis for the following three months. If test results continue to be negative after those three months, then they are considered to no longer have Borreliosis (Lyme disease). After the third test, they can choose to come into my office to continue to get checked on a yearly basis. Most decide to do this, but I have found that 97% of them remain symptom-free, even two or three years after the completion of their treatments.

It is important to note here that the lymphocytes destroy most of the body's Borrelia. Any Borrelia that remains in the body is inactivated and doesn't cause symptoms because the body's cells no longer resonate with the infection. Only in cases of extreme energetic stress can the organism re-emerge and cause symptoms again. Such cases are rare, but possible, and physicians who treat with the Bionic 880 should know this. Such stressors might include the problematic delivery of a child, a major accident, or the death of a close family member or loved one.

Clinical Procedure for Treating Patients with the Bionic 880

Photons have different frequencies, and using the proper frequency on the Bionic 880 device to treat a specific disorder is extremely important for success in healing that disorder. I establish the appropriate frequency for the treatment of Lyme and other conditions by testing patients using energetic methods, such as the

Biotensor, muscle testing, bioresonance, Vega device, and so on. The results of such tests enable me to determine which frequency is most appropriate for a particular condition and the individual patient.

For the treatment of Borreliosis (Lyme disease) I usually administer treatments with the Bionic for 320-340 seconds, at ten to twelve different points on the body, using 11.77 Hertz at 100% power on the machine.

For the process, I also use the Borrelia nosodes of different homeopathic dilutions, which I tape across the patient's solar plexus. Once the Borrelia nosodes are taped into place, treatment is then administered using the photon device.

The photons, along with the nosodes, normalize the body's own biophoton emissions and energy so that the cells are able to expel the Borrelia organism, along with other toxins. The photons basically enable the cells to eliminate all toxic things, the presence of which can be evidenced in the patient's blood after treatments.

The ten different treatment points

1 & 2: The inside of the right and left wrists, with the right wrist being treated first. (The points on the right side of the body are always treated first).

3 & 4: Over the right and left ears

5: Middle of the forehead

6: Top of the skull

7 & 8: Right and left thyroid gland (except in those with hyperthyroidism)

9: Upper third of the sternum, by the thymus

10: Above the navel, just below the homeopathic nosodes

(Warning: placing the head of the device over the nosodes themselves may break the nosodes).

Following the photon treatment, I administer a hyperbaric ozone
treatment to those patients who suffer from concentration disturbances (brain fog) or who have trouble with word finding. Ozone
increases the blood's oxygen level to 180 – 200 % (the normal
range is 96 – 100 %), thereby alleviating these symptoms.

Finally, all of my patients receive a detoxification treatment, which
includes an intravenous infusion of magnesium, zinc, Hepar comp
(a homeopathic liver decontaminant), Solidago comp (a homeopathic kidney support remedy), Lymphomyosot (a homeopathic
remedy to support the lymphatic system) and 100 ml of sodium
bicarbonate (NaHCO3 8.4 %).

Since photon therapy can reactivate dormant infections and diseases, it's important to get toxins from these out of the body, which is
why my patients always get a detoxification infusion after every
session. The infusions also help to partially alleviate any potentially
intense reactions to the photon therapy.

Five treatments, sometimes six, are usually required to eliminate
symptoms of Borrelia. I allow my patients at least two days of rest
in-between treatments in order not to interrupt or disturb the
activated regulation of cellular activity induced by the photons. If
these intervals are not maintained, patients may also experience
intense pathologic overdose reactions, and might be put at risk for
thyroid gland decompensation and subsequent Hashimoto's thyroiditis.

(Note: Anywhere from three to ten photon treatments are usually
required to treat other conditions of illness. Three is the minimum
required for any condition, even if the patient feels well before the
end of those three).

After administering five treatments for Borrelia, I test my patients. If my German patients test negative after the fifth treatment, then I tell them to come back to my office in a month to get tested again. If they still test positive after five treatments, then I administer just one more treatment and then tell them to come back again in four weeks, as they observe their symptoms during that time. After five or six treatments, it's very important to wait for four weeks before doing another treatment, because Borrelia is cyclical in its lifecycle, and dormant forms, which were not taken care of during the first round of treatments, may emerge during these four weeks. On average, however, I find that most people need only five or six treatments for Borrelia.

No other supplements (orthomolecular substances, such as chlorella or vitamins) are given during treatment, because the photons regulate the body's entire metabolism. I am convinced that the administration of additional substances (except vital medicines, such as heart or diabetic medications) negatively influences this regulation. So far, my experience seems to prove that I am right.

In order to increase the efficiency of photon therapy, I also give my patients a chiropractic adjustment. They welcome this additional treatment, which enables their energy to flow more freely from the top of their head to the bottom of their spine, as well as throughout their entire body. Any blocks in the body's flow of energy may lead to pain throughout the spinal column, particularly in the first vertebra/atlas/axis. After this adjustment, patients also feel more flexible and are able to move about more freely, which also means that the photons are able to work more effectively in their bodies. Some patients may occasionally require a second chiropractic adjustment, and may even have to learn to do certain exercises in order to maintain its effects.

Finally, I sometimes do SCENAR therapy on my patients, (Self-Controlled Energo Neuro Adaptive Regulation) which involves the use of a handheld, electro-stimulation therapeutic medical device to loosen ligaments and muscles, as it frees up movement within the body.

Using the Bionic 880 To Treat Other Health Conditions

Photon treatment can positively influence almost all diseases and medical conditions. In the realm of infections, this includes bacteria and viruses, fungus, mold, yeast, and just about any type of pathogen.

In addition, photon therapy can regulate hormones and neurotransmitters, reduce pain (of all kinds), treat allergies and gut dysbiosis, as well as other problems present in Lyme disease and other chronic illnesses.

Pain therapy is one of the main focuses of my practice. I have successfully treated, for example, cases of chronic recurrent lumbar spine pain and achillodynia after only six sessions. Some of these cases had previously been resistant to any type of therapy. One patient with acute lumbago, for instance, was free from discomfort after only two treatments. A superficial ulcer on the right foot of another patient, which had previously been resistant to all kinds of therapy, was healed after twelve treatments.

Other conditions that can be successfully treated with the Bionic 880

Psychosomatic illnesses

Somatic disorders

Other long-term and chronic illnesses

Dysfunction of the vegetative nervous system

Wounds

Depression

"Burn out" syndromes

Weight problems

Hyperactivity

Addictions (especially smoking)

Cancer aftercare

Brain fog

In addition, photons may do all of the following:

Improve lymphocyte differentiation

Improve pathological enzyme function

Regulate the immune system

Raise or lower lymphocytes, as necessary

Normalize and activate CD-57 cell production

Increase the amount of toxins that leave the body

Normalize serotonin and tryptophan metabolism

Have a positive influence upon the psyche

Normalize PSA (prostate) values

Reduce allergies

Positively impact insulin levels

Lower blood sugar (when necessary)

Increase the rate of wound healing

Decrease pain levels

Create an increased tolerance to cancer medications (for those receiving cancer treatments)

Positively impact immune markers - leukocytes, lymphocytes, IgG, IgM, CD-57, etc.

Reduce diabetic symptoms, even in those with Type One diabetes

Normalize immune system reactions

Increase the excretion of environmental toxins

Decrease bone necrosis

For those with high fever infections, bronchitis and pneumonia, photons create an increased CD-57 response to such infections

Since I am a general practitioner, I treat a wide range of ailments, not just Lyme disease. Recently, for example, I used the Bionic 880 to get rid of my daughter's oral Herpes infection, which I was able to eliminate with only three treatments.

Treating For Other Infections Using Homeopathic Nosodes and The Patient's Own Blood

After doing treatments for Lyme and co-infections, when patients are stronger and more stable, they may be treated for other infections or conditions, using their own blood as a homeopathic nosode, in conjunction with the Bionic 880.

This is a good way to treat any infections or issues for which a homeopathic nosode isn't available, or to mop up infections that could not be identified through energetic testing, since the blood contains the blueprint of all infections that are in the body.

If patients choose to receive biophoton treatments using their own blood, they should always get an intravenous detoxification cocktail afterwards, since the blood may contain multiple infections, which creates the potential for many toxins to be released. I don't advise practitioners to treat with their patients' own blood at first, because these patients might get a detoxification reaction that is too violent and which no intravenous infusion could fix. It's important to treat Borrelia first, using Borrelia nosodes, and then the patient's own blood may be used as a nosode to get rid of any remaining infections (and depending upon the results of energetic testing). Moreover, when using the blood as a nosode in conjunction with biophotons, I advise practitioners to initiate treatments at 25% power on the Bionic device, and gradually increase the intensity by 25% per week, until patients are able to complete two treatments at 100% power.

Troubleshooting Problems in Healing

Almost all of my patients can be successfully treated for Borreliosis. Those who already suffer from strong symptoms of paralysis and progressive muscular atrophy may have trouble healing, however, because cells that have died no longer emit biophotons, and so far, I have not yet discovered a method for re-activating these. So while I haven't yet found the right therapy for such conditions, I keep searching.

I am convinced that there is a key to healing all diseases, and we must simply find it. For the aforementioned, perhaps we just need new and different frequencies that are not found on this particular device.

Patients who are exposed to strong electromagnetic fields during therapy also have trouble healing, because such fields disturb the photon therapy and can weaken its effects or even make it ineffective. Whenever I suspect that my patients are being exposed to too much electromagnetic radiation, I recommend that they have their homes examined by specialists for electromagnetic "smog" and, if necessary, made "safe" again. This involves removing EMF sources, such as cellular radio, cordless phones, high-frequency and low-frequency radiation, military directional radios, and so on, from their environment. Cell phones can be especially problematic, as can computers, but if they put a diode (energetic protection device) on their computer or cell phone, this can minimize the possibility of the EMF's affecting their photon treatments. Whenever patients make the necessary changes to their living environment, I find that they respond better to the treatments. Those who become free from disease tend to have low EMF levels in their environments.

Patients with detoxification problems may also have trouble healing, but I do have techniques in my practice that can help them to detoxify better.

The Problem with Using Antibiotics for the Treatment of Lyme Disease

I consider the use of antibiotic medications for the treatment of Lyme disease and other infections to be highly questionable.

People with Lyme frequently observe positive changes in their symptoms as a result of antibiotic use, yet they are only that: a shift in symptoms. They may still have bacteria in their cells, but these may not be reflected in their lab results or symptoms—they may only be detected by some types of energetic testing. Most patients who have gone into remission from Lyme disease after antibiotic use have later suffered from other diseases, due to the immune suppression that the medications cause. Such diseases are seemingly unrelated to Lyme but were probably initially caused by Lyme. I have observed, for instance, that there is an increase in patients' risk of developing cancer after they have been on long-term antibiotics.

In any case, I believe that antibiotics prevent or hinder the defense system of the cell, and I haven't observed any cases of complete healing from Lyme disease as a result of antibiotic therapy. People take different antibiotics and try to heal Lyme but don't succeed, because the real cause of Lyme hasn't been dealt with. Only by using photon therapy have I been able to fully heal my patients of the symptoms caused by Lyme.

Also, organisms can develop resistance to antibiotics, and it can become increasingly difficult to find medications that will work well for treating different forms of the infection.

Adjunct Therapies during Photon Treatment

If patients test positive for Borreliosis, I will first treat them for this infection, since the symptoms that it causes can imitate more than 300 different diseases. By treating Borrelia first, I don't have to guess at the source of other symptoms, if any remain after the treatments. If patients still have symptoms after successful Borrelia treatments, then these symptoms are probably not caused by Borrelia, and they should keep in mind that not all disease symptoms are caused by Borrelia. Whenever this is the case, I then treat them for other issues, according to integral holistic principles.

For example, I might recommend intravenous detoxification therapy to help the body get rid of toxins, or treatments to heal the intestine such as colon hydrotherapy, dietary modification, and supplements such as Mutaflor and Symbioflor. I may also recommend vitamins and other supplements, depending upon what the patient's problems are. Removing dental amalgams and ridding the body of mercury and other toxins may also be important, and I have a number of remedies that I use for such problems.

Heal the Mind, Heal the Body

In addition to physical toxins, the cells release emotional toxins as a result of photon therapy. Whenever this happens, I do a type of mental training program with my patients to help them process the emotional toxins. The aim of the program is to give them the opportunity to heal themselves by using different mental techniques. I can only offer this type of therapy to patients who speak my language (German) well, however, and who are ready to change their way of thinking. One of the things that I always tell my patients is that I believe that any illness, including Lyme disease, originates on a spiritual level first and only manifests itself later in the body and soul. I also believe that illness is a prompting for patients to change something in their lives on a spiritual level, and often I am amazed at how successful they are at doing this.

The Use of Immune Markers to Measure Progress in Healing

I developed photon therapy for Lyme disease about nine years ago. I couldn't ask anybody about how to treat Lyme with photons so I relied on my own mental faculties and energetic tests to determine its effectiveness. The first patient that I treated was a four-year-old child. This patient's parents had refused a colleague's antibiotic therapy and asked me to do something different. The parents knew me well, so they knew that I wouldn't risk the child's health. Fortunately, after four treatments, the child was free from his troubles! Based on that success, I then performed a trial on 106 patients in which I used a LTT (lymphocyte-transformation test) to help determine the effectiveness of the photons. The positive change in lymphocyte activity in these patients after treatments was amazing.

Over the last years, I have performed several other types of immune tests, which have proven the positive effects that photons have upon Th1 and Th2 cells, as well as upon leukocytes and lymphocytes. To obtain such information, before and after every single photon treatment for Lyme, I took blood samples from my patients and analyzed these.

Currently, I am running trials to determine the effects of photon therapy upon the differentiation of lymphocytes. For this test, I use over thirty-four parameters before and after each treatment, and on one patient, I have even performed over 240 tests! Currently, I have received more than 1200 results from this test. These results, which are still being evaluated at the moment, so far show highly interesting reactions that will be important for further oncologic and immunologic scientific research.

It has also been demonstrated that photons have regulatory effects upon the cells, but more testing is still needed to conclusively confirm these phenomena.

190

I often lecture in Germany and my colleagues who have adopted my protocol have reported similar good results when using the Bionic 880 on their patients. Very often, I advise them on matters pertaining to the therapy.

The Difference between North American and European Patients

Treatment outcomes always depend upon the individual patient that I am working with. I have noticed that there can be slight changes in therapy outcomes according to the degree of each patient's disease. There are, as of yet, no significant differences between European and American patients when it comes to treatment outcomes, although other variations in these patients do exist.

North Americans tend to have more co-infections. Europeans have some, especially Chlamydia, Epstein-Barr and Rickettsia, but overall, North Americans have more and different infections, such as Bartonella, Babesia and Mycoplasma.

I have also noticed that North Americans tend to become too fixated on their diseases, which affects their healing. Europeans tend to get "free" from thoughts of disease more easily. North Americans must find mental exercises that will enable them to get free of their fixation on illness, if they want to heal fully.

Thinking too much about disease is a problem for our cells. We can influence our whole metabolism by our thoughts. So if those with Borreliosis are fixated on the idea that they are ill, they will get ill, and remain ill. The fact that I don't speak English as well as German means that it's difficult for me to fully explain this concept to my foreign patients, however, and offer them strategies for getting "unstuck."

It's important, though, that people with Borreliosis do some type of mental training to break their fixation on disease, or on whatever is disturbing their health. It's beneficial for them to not become too fixated on anything, and to live without fixations requires difficult mental training, but it can be done. We have powers within us that can be developed and cultivated, and if we are able to discover and develop these, then we have the ability to get rid of disease. For example, I just had a patient who got rid of Lyme by the power of her thought alone.

I teach my German-speaking patients four different mental techniques to enable them to discover more about themselves and to help them tap into their own healing power.

Relative Contraindications of Photon Treatment

Photon therapy is somewhat contraindicated in just a couple of situations.

First, in those with colitis, because the photons can increase bleeding and cramps.

Secondly, in those with depression who are being treated with medications, because the photons render ineffective the medications.

Also, it is critical that those with hyperthyreosis consult with a knowledgeable practitioner before using the Bionic 880 on the thyroid points.

Finally, those with pacemakers should make certain that the photons are not aimed directly at their pacemakers.

Sample Frequencies for Different Conditions

Below are some frequencies that are commonly used for treating other conditions that are often found in those with Lyme disease. These frequencies, however, should only be used as a guideline. Patients should be energetically tested before receiving treatment for any condition in order to determine what the best frequency for their particular condition is. This is because frequencies also depend upon the person being treated; each person has a different energy at the time that they are being treated, and a frequency other than the one listed below may be more appropriate for that person.

Also, when treating certain conditions, such as hormone and neuro-transmitter imbalances, using five points on the body instead of ten may be more appropriate. Again, patients should be energetically tested to determine which points would be most beneficial for their particular condition. For pain problems, treating locally on the area of pain is often best.

Finally, it is generally best to treat patients for only one issue at a time, and no more than twice a week (except for pain or other local issues, which can be treated 4-5 times per week). Over-treating with photons can cause problems in the body, and when treating for multiple infections, a break should be given in-between treatments for each infection, so that the body has time to fully process the effects of a particular treatment.

Recommended frequencies for conditions often found in those with Lyme disease

Psychological problems	7.83 and 80 Hz
Pain	Between 2.7 Hz and 9.88 Hz
Wounds	9.88 Hz
Hormonal Imbalances	Between 7.83 Hz and 80 Hz
Infections	Between 9.88 Hz and 28 Hz
Detoxification Problems	9.88 Hz and 11.77 Hz
Immune system imbalances	9.88 Hz and 11.77 Hz

Allergies: It's very important to accurately test for allergies, in order to avoid strong reactions to treatment. Different frequencies can be used for allergies, depending upon the allergy and the person.

Finally, when energetically testing patients for specific conditions, it's important for practitioners to place the nosode or the matter that will be used for treatment directly on their patients' epigastria for most accurate test results.

Final Words

This newly developed energy medicine technique should be more widely used for the treatment of Lyme disease (Borreliosis). Research in the field of biophotons should also be intensified and other physicians encouraged to learn about this method, so that the number of positive treatment outcomes may be increased. Fortunately, many of my German colleagues in medicine are already going in this direction.

Technical Data for the Bionic 880

Description of the device

Bionic 880 with Cluster Probe (Applicator). Frequency, power level and duration of treatment may be programmed into the device. Operator guidance is included.

Dimensions:	L 27 cm x W 17 cm x H 8 cm
Weight:	2.3 Kg
Radiation source:	84 (LED) diodes 880 Nm
Wavelength:	880 Nm, pulsed
IMF:	2.471 Hz, 4.942 Hz, 7.833 Hz, 9.88 Hz, 11.77 Hz, 28 Hz, 80 Hz
Density of EFM energy:	ca. 3.000 mw on the surface of the treated tissue or ca. 150 mW/cm2

Additional Information on Photons

Their effect upon the body is dependent upon their wavelength. The shorter the wavelength, the stronger they are.

How to Contact Ingo D. E. Woitzel, M.D.

75172 Pforzheim, Luisenstr. 54 – 56, Germany
Tel: 0049 (0) 7231-313533 Fax: 0049 (0)7231-357268
e-mail: praxisdrwoitzel@t-online.de
Website: www.drwoitzel.de

Author's note:

Dr. Woitzel recommends that patients who live outside of Germany stay at Gästehaus Klein in Dobel while undergoing treatments in his clinic. This friendly, welcoming guesthouse is located in a small town where electromagnetic levels of pollution are low. For more information, contact:

Karin Klein
Neuenbürger Str.59
75335 Dobel, Germany
Tel.: 0049 (0)7083/3665
Fax.: 0049 (0)7083/3665
email: info@gaestehausklein-dobel.de

Translation Note

This chapter is based on an interview that was conducted in German and translated into English. While we made every effort to ensure that the translation was accurate, the reader should be aware that translation errors may have occurred.

• C H A P T E R   7 •

Ronald Whitmont, M.D.
RHINEBECK, NY

Biography

Ronald D. Whitmont, M.D. is a second-generation classical homeopath. He graduated from the State University of New York Health Sciences Center at Brooklyn, completed a transitional (rotating) internship at St. Vincent's Hospital and Medical Center in New York City and an Internal Medicine residency program at the Reading Hospital Medical Center in Reading, Pennsylvania.

He became board certified in Internal Medicine in 1995 and in Holistic Medicine in 2000. He currently maintains offices in Rhinebeck and Manhattan, New York.

Healing Philosophy

My healing philosophy for Lyme disease is not substantially or significantly different from my philosophy for other conditions of illness. I utilize the classical homeopathic technique, which involves (a) using only one medicine at a time, (b) using this medicine at the lowest possible dose, and (c) basing the prescription upon the psychosomatic totality of all the symptoms involved in the case: mental, emotional and physical.

Homeopathic medicine isn't based on theory. It's an empiric science. Each of the homeopathic medicines in the United States Homeopathic Pharmacopoeia (HPCUS) was first tested by administering them to healthy subjects. This process, known as "drug proving," forms the basis of homeopathic prescribing. Every substance that is proven in this manner demonstrates an ability to disturb the state (whether mental, emotional or physical) of healthy subjects in a specific, reproducible manner. When these patterns of disturbance are recorded, both objectively and subjectively, then the full picture (or proving) of the substances becomes known.

The key element of homeopathy involves the recognition that extremely small amounts of a substance that are capable of creating a disturbance in health can also lead to the resolution of a similar pattern when the treated disturbance is part of an illness. The closest concept to this conventionally is immunization. However, with an immunization, an actual material dose of a substance is administered which can actually cause harm to the person. In the homeopathic model, only an energetic imprint (an infinitesimal dilution) of the substance is administered to the patient, not the material substance itself. Homeopathic medicines are made from many substances, both toxic and non-toxic, but in homeopathic (infinitesimal) dilution they are all safe.

Homeopathic science bases the prescription of medicine for the sick upon the symptoms that develop in a healthy person during the drug proving, and involves administering a substance that acts in the most similar manner to the actual illness. In other words, a homeopath would administer a non-material dose of a medicine to a person who is ill, by utilizing the medicine that most closely mimics the actual symptoms of the illness based upon the patterns evoked during the homeopathic drug proving. Many homeopaths believe that this prescription actually acts as a type of "feedback", providing information for the energetic body to utilize when formulating a healing response to illness. It's as if the body was receiving a blueprint of instructions, or a computer program of pure information to help it solve the riddle of illness. The substance used (the homeopathic medicine) might make a person ill if it were administered in large material doses, but in infinitesimal doses, it stimu-stimulates, paradoxically, a healing response.

After the symptoms of the healthy person taking the substance in the drug proving are fully catalogued, this information is integrated into an encyclopedic reference text known as the "Materia Medica" of homeopathic prescribing. The job of the homeopathic physician is to then determine which medicine most closely matches proving symptoms to those of actual illness. This principle is known as "the Law of Similars", or "Let likes be cured by likes". The process of prescribing the homeopathic remedy is a lot like matching a sick person to an abstract painting of himself or herself. It is both a science and an art.

When choosing a homeopathic medicine, besides symptoms, knowing patients' medical history and understanding their individual constitution are also important. For example, if a patient has a strong family history of cancer, tuberculosis or other medical maladies, then this might influence the practitioner's remedy selection for that patient. Similarly, knowing that a patient has previously reacted strongly to an immunization, for example, might also influence remedy selection. In a drug proving, however, only the symptomatic results at the moment of testing are included in the database, not the personal histories of the subjects.

In actual practice, the homeopathic practitioner takes a three-dimensional approach to treatment, which includes looking at a patient's history, as well as which treatments have been effective and which have been suppressive for him or her in the past. When working with patients that have Lyme disease, this is all beneficial information, because one of the things that Lyme disease challenges is how well the immune system functions. There are many people with the Borrelia infection that have never developed symptoms and who have never been sick with Lyme, because their immune systems have been able to adapt to and address this infection. Then there are others, with chronic, unremitting, waxing and waning symptoms whose immune systems have been unable to cope with the infection. These people can't seem to get over their illness, because their immune systems aren't able to come to grips with it. Others might be somewhere in-between these two extremes—that is, Lyme may be playing a role in their illness, but it may not be the principal cause of their symptoms.

Lyme disease is a particularly challenging condition for many reasons. Getting an accurate diagnosis can be extremely difficult and can lead to tremendous confusion, in part because there is no perfect test for Lyme. Also, there are different varieties of spiro-chetes that cause the illness and patients often have multiple co-infections along with Borrelia, which complicates their symptom picture and diagnosis. Under-treated cases may also present diagnostic dilemmas since immune response to treatments in such cases may be either incomplete or partial. For instance, it may be difficult to discern when someone is actually responding to an infection with a healthy immune response, or overreacting with an autoimmune inflammatory response in the absence of an actual infection. Diagnosis can be treacherous since most tests only meas-ure the immune system's (antibody) response to illness.

Treatment Approach

My treatment approach to Lyme involves obtaining a very detailed and accurate understanding of my patients. I review their lab tests and medical history and frequently perform a focused physical exam. From all this, I make a selection of the best homeopathic medical solution for their entire condition using the classical ap-proach. This means that patients are treated on the basis of their symptoms and history, as well as other factors that influence their current state of being. They are not treated on the basis of a Lyme disease diagnosis, but instead upon the basis of their own situation in extremely specific terms. It makes no difference whether they test positive or negative to Lyme disease. The approach is based upon their actual state of being, not their presumed diagnosis, which can include an entire spectrum of different states, and false positives as well as false negatives on lab tests.

Hence, in classical homeopathy, the prescription of medicine is based upon patients' individual constitution and symptom picture— it has nothing to do with the diagnostic nomenclature of Lyme or other tick-borne infections, whose definitions are incredibly broad and non-specific. Confirming that a patient has a diagnosis of Lyme disease is purely an academic exercise, and irrelevant to the homeopathic treatment. While it can be reassuring for many people to know what their diagnosis is, in classical homeopathy, the diagnosis has no bearing upon the actual treatment protocol. As mentioned above, the classical homeopathic approach is not diagnosis-driven; it is determined solely by an individual patient's set of symptoms, history and characteristics. That person's symptoms may be static or they may change and evolve over time. When the practitioner is able to capture, describe and elucidate these symptoms at a given point in time, or over a period of time, however, he or she learns what that person is experiencing on a physical, emotional, cognitive and whole body level. When this discovery process is handled with meticulous care, and the homeopathic Materia Medica is utilized appropriately, the most accurate homeopathic medicine can be selected.

The classical homeopathic approach is not only highly specific, but extremely practical, as well. In Lyme disease and other chronic illnesses, it's often very difficult to determine exactly what's causing patients' symptoms. Are they related to the Lyme bacteria, to an associated infection, to an immune inflammatory reaction, or to the interaction of all three? Invariably, and in the end, it is probably a combination of many factors. That there can be many factors involved poses significant challenges to the conventional antibiotic-based system of therapeutics, but not to homeopathy. Since homeopathy doesn't offer one standard protocol for all those with Lyme, therapy is based upon the individual patient.

And because patients are all unique, genetically, environmentally and with regard to their treatment history, by focusing on their symptoms and constitution, the most specific, individual form of treatment can be rendered. Categorizing infections is more important from a pedagogic perspective, and is more relevant when a practitioner needs to select the right antibiotics for treatment. Since many of those with positive Lyme tests don't necessarily have Lyme disease ("false positives"), their symptoms may be more relevant to their treatment plan than the actual laboratory tests. Antibodies to Borrelia can be present for many years following the resolution of the infection. Practitioners that are intent upon proving the presence or absence of active infection can become bogged down in an expensive and time-consuming morass of incomplete and inadequate data. An active infection may be indistinguishable from an inflammatory immune response that has gone off on a tangent of its own, (even though the Lyme may not be active anymore). Frequently, symptoms of the immune reaction and those of the actual infection are confused with one another. The signs of a functioning immune response can be suppressed when antibiotic medications are given, which can further complicate the picture.

Knowing when the body is simply overreacting to something can be extremely beneficial. Augmenting the immune system to help it deal with such problems is essentially what homeopathy is all about. Since patients are invariably at different stages of illness, treatment is usually different for each patient. It's not based on imperfect diagnoses, but on actual symptoms of illness that are affecting the patient in the present moment.

I must emphasize that the treatment approach that I advocate is based upon the classical model of homeopathy. There are other uses of homeopathy that don't follow the same guidelines as those found in the classical model. Homeopathy can be prescribed as a form of allopathic medicine, but this method forgoes the highly specific and sensitive nature of classical prescribing. Practitioners that use this form of homeopathy frequently administer homeopathic medicines according to diagnosis, not on the basis of individual symptoms. An example of this would be a practitioner routinely prescribing Lyme Nosode or Ledum for a diagnosis of Lyme. But by ignoring the highly specific nature of the individual patient and focusing on the epidemic nature of the disease, such practitioners trade the potential for deeper curative responses for rapid symptom alleviation and crisis management. They are following a formula that has very little to do with classical homeopathy, although it may be helpful in certain uncomplicated cases of illness and even prophylaxis.

There are certainly homeopathic medicines that I have used repeatedly in cases of Lyme disease, but any of the (roughly thirty-five hundred) homeopathic medicines currently regulated by the U.S. FDA could potentially be used in cases of Lyme. Of course, the determination of the most appropriate remedy for a particular patient is based upon that patient and his or her unique situation. Because of the highly specific and individual nature of classical homeopathic prescribing, it's nonsense to name, or outline, a particular group of remedies that should be used or considered for the treatment of Lyme. Choosing remedies in such a manner doesn't allow the practitioner to take advantage of the true potential and strength of classical homeopathic prescribing, and would be applying an allopathic framework to a homeopathic methodology. The results from such an approach, though sometimes beneficial, are limited. Also, this approach should be used cautiously, since it may suppress patients' symptoms. Whenever this is the case, then the effectiveness of homeopathy might be extremely limited. Remedies are only as targeted as the practitioner makes them.

How Many Remedies Are Required To Bring About A Cure?

This depends on the case. Sometimes one remedy is enough to do the whole job, but I have also seen extremely complex cases that have required multiple remedies used in succession. These cases often involved patients who had been mismanaged for many years with suppressive antibiotic therapies. Unfortunately, this is a common scenario. For such cases, a series of different remedies may be required to achieve a resolution of symptoms. Homeopathy is a science, but not an exact science, since no two people are exactly alike. Instead, it involves some trial and error, since the homeopathic tools rely on human judgment and individual human responses.

How Long Does the Healing Process Take With Homeopathy?

The healing process can be extremely fast. In cases of uncomplicated, early illness and prophylaxis, the results of remedies can be seen within days. In more chronic cases, one may first observe responses such as increased energy and the return of old symptoms (before such symptoms resolve) within a short period of time following treatment. It's not uncommon to see a progressive, stepwise increase in these people's overall functionality over time on a cognitive, emotional and physical level, and the process can start very quickly when the right homeopathic medication is administered. Improvements can take place over a period of weeks, but the healing process also depends upon how long patients have been ill. If they have been sick for a short period of time, in general, their recovery will be faster. If they have been ill for many months or years, it generally takes longer for improvement to occur. Healing may stretch over several years if the case is very complicated or if patients received a lot of suppressive treatments prior to undergoing homeopathic care.

The other goal of homeopathic treatment, beyond immediate recovery, is helping patients to achieve a healthier state of being so that they are less likely to become ill after a potential re-exposure to Lyme disease in the future. In many cases, Borrelia acts as an opportunistic infection, and causes symptoms only because a person's health and immunity was already inadequate due to a myriad of other causes. In such cases, simply treating the infection and eradicating it with antibiotics does nothing to prevent recurrence or relapse in the future. The antibiotics do nothing to improve health, they only deal with a crisis. A carefully selected homeopathic medicine can not only help to eradicate the infection, but can also strengthen the immune system so that a serious relapse of symptoms becomes less likely in the future.

One of the most common causes of immune deficiency is the prior use of antibiotics. Frequent antibiotic use has been associated with many health complications, including immune dysfunction, treatment-resistant infections, symptom suppression and even cancer. Even the short-term use of antibiotics weakens the immune reaction, which, paradoxically, makes one more susceptible to Borrelia and/or other Lyme-related infections. It's a bit like an undefended ship being attacked by pirates. The pirates (bacteria) are able to easily take over the ship (the body) when it is less strongly defended, whereas those with stronger immune systems are able to offer more resistance to invasion (infection).

In the end, and over a lifetime, homeopathy can be extremely effective for a variety of health concerns and issues. Patients can become very frustrated by the failure of different therapies to give them symptomatic relief, but because of this, if a particular strategy isn't working for them, I am one of the first to say: "If this isn't helping you, we need to try something different". There is no single approach that works for everyone.

More Thoughts on Using Antibiotics for the Treatment of Lyme Disease

There has been a lot of debate, even amongst homeopaths and other health care practitioners, about whether antibiotics should be used in the treatment of Lyme disease, and if so, then at what stage? As health care practitioners, we don't have all of the answers. My opinion has certainly evolved over time.

Currently, one of my concerns about the use of antibiotics is that we might not be effectively and thoroughly treating the infections, but through the use of a "chemical warfare" approach are instead making a smokescreen that muddies the water and which forces the infection into deeper areas. There is good data in the medical literature to suggest that antibiotic overuse is associated with drug resistance and more aggressive infections. The use of antibiotics in such circumstances could be considered "suppressive"; an ineffective treatment. Suppression is a bad word in homeopathy because we have seen that whenever illnesses are suppressed, they tend to show up again at a later date and often in a more serious form.

We also know from experience (and research) that antibiotics are frequently anti-inflammatory. The implication of this is that they may provide symptom relief, and help patients to feel better, while actually allowing their illness to become worse. Because they act as anti-inflammatories, suppressing the immune system, they may mask symptoms of the infection as it continues to thrive, undetected. Antibiotics also turn off parts of the immune system and thus prevent the body from mounting a complete immune reaction to the infection. Hence, patients on antibiotics may experience improvements in their symptoms, but no real improvement in their underlying condition. Medical data suggests that overall health frequently suffers from antibiotic treatment.

There may be a role for short courses of antibiotics during the early stages of Lyme disease, and this has been debated, but so far, there is no clear consensus of data on the matter. In my experience, it is generally advantageous to postpone the use of antibiotics for as long as practically possible, if they are to be used at all.

There are also many unfortunate side effects and complications associated with antibiotic use. Yeast infections are among these, but are only part of the problem. Antibiotics change the whole body's bacterial flora, most obviously in the gastrointestinal tract, but also on the skin, as well as in the respiratory and urinary tracts. The entire body is altered by these medications and when the bacterial balance of the body is significantly changed, then a host of other changes tends to follow. It's not a benign process to give people antibiotics. By altering bacterial flora, the body's nutrition and defenses are altered. The short-term effects of this may be minor and insignificant, but the long-term effects of prolonged antibiotic treatment can play a role in the development of many conditions including allergies and recurrent respiratory, skin and urinary tract infections. Susceptibility to fungal, viral and other bacterial infections also increases. Candida is the most common example of the infections that typically occur with antibiotic use, but it's really just the tip of the iceberg.

Another problem with antibiotics is that they don't deal with the core of the problem, which is a weak immune system and consequent susceptibility to illness. The role of the practitioner should be, first and foremost, to assure that no harm is done to patients as a result of their treatment. Antibiotics are toxic to many organs of the body and can damage the kidneys, ears, gastrointestinal tract, and liver. Their use comes at a high cost.

I don't forbid the use of antibiotics in my practice, but I am careful to recommend them only when necessary. Such medicines should be used in a rational, careful manner. They should never be used to quell a state of fear or panic. They should be used sparingly and for limited periods of time. Their use should be based upon the science of their indications and the data on their effectiveness. One of my jobs as a practitioner is to support the immune system in the healing process. If I'm not able to do that, then I must examine other approaches to treatment, including antibiotics. I do not believe they should be utilized as a first line of defense in most cases of Lyme disease.

Are Adjunct Remedies Necessary in Homeopathy?

No single medical specialty contains all the healing methods that are sufficient for the complete attainment of health in all possible scenarios. Homeopathic treatment, for instance, works best when combined with a proper diet and lifestyle changes that support and augment physical and emotional well being. Hahnemann, the founder of homeopathy, strongly believed that patients should remove toxic elements from their diets and environments, lest these factors become "obstacles to cure." People heal at different rates because they are different. One of the reasons why homeopaths spend so much time with their patients is so that they can learn about the many factors that influence their patients' health. Many patients benefit from lifestyle and nutritional counseling, while others benefit from emotional counseling that enables them to deal with socially toxic and personally traumatic situations.

Dietary Recommendations

I don't recommend the same diet to all of my patients. Like all things in homeopathy, I take a very individualized approach to diet. First, I want to hear about what kind of diet my patients are already on and if any foods have been a challenge for them. People frequently have sensitivities to different foods, so it would be crazy for me to recommend the same type of diet to everyone. I generally advocate whole foods, fruits and vegetables. I frequently recommend a Mediterranean-based diet that is high in fruits, whole grains and vegetables and low in processed foods and refined carbohydrates. I also believe that it's important to keep the diet as organic as possible. Sometimes, I recommend vegetarian diets to my patients, but it depends upon the person and his or her other health needs. In any case, a proper diet is very important for recovery and healing. One can work against health with the wrong diet.

What about Treating Patients for Environmental Toxins?

When treating my patients, I don't address environmental toxins directly. I believe that an effective homeopathic treatment will frequently take care of the problem of toxins. One of the amazing things about symptoms is that if you listen to them, they will tell you precisely what is affecting the body. Even if a particular toxin can't be identified, a health-promoting homeopathic treatment will facilitate the body's elimination and disposal process so that many toxins can be more easily released. When taking a patient's history and doing an exam, certain toxic exposures may become apparent to the practitioner. Toxic living environments, dental amalgams, mold and chemical exposures, (including pesticides), may be a problem. It may be important for patients to mitigate these factors.

Important toxic exposures frequently show up in symptoms, because the body expresses its need for the right medicine through these symptoms.

Lifestyle Recommendations for Healing

Consuming refined sugar, tobacco, alcohol and other drugs can compromise and slow recovery. One common problem that I run into with my patients is that as they start feeling good again, they tend to overdo things. They want to jump right back into their old lives as though they had never left them. It's a very important thing to get people to listen to, and honor their bodies. They often need to re-learn which activities they can tolerate and which ones they can't. Treating their bodies appropriately also means exercising and eating moderately.

Emotional problems also frequently need to be addressed, including those that involve the patient's family, partner and job. Getting adequate sleep is also important. Dealing with whatever other lifestyle factors that might be causing stress is also essential for healing.

The Role of Emotional Trauma in Healing

Emotional trauma can delay or obstruct healing, and this is probably one of the most important aspects of chronic illness that has been ignored by conventional medicine. When it isn't ignored, it's generally relegated to a psychopharmacologist for "symptom management". Unfortunately, conventional medicine draws a pretty sharp line between emotional and physical ailments (ever since Descartes). It doesn't recognize that emotional factors directly affect and may even precipitate physical ailments. From my perspective, emotional and physical problems are two manifestations of same thing; the emotional details are just another expression of what is happening physically (and vice-versa). These two expressions of illness mirror and closely interact with one another. When you look at them together, you see two sides of the same coin. And it's more or less the rule that chronic illness is always connected to some history of emotional trauma. At the same time, the circumstances of chronic illness cause emotional problems. Either way, emotional and physical health need to be addressed simultaneously.

One of the nice things about homeopathy is that it's truly a psychosomatic discipline. Every homeopathic medicine embodies, and therefore addresses, physical, as well as emotional, states. This is one reason why homeopathy is considered a truly holistic discipline. Also, taking advantage of the breadth of each homeopathic medicine allows for incredible individualization in treatment.

During office visits, I review my patients' family history, as well as their parent, sibling and other important relationships. I am also curious about their relationship to the world and society. Self-image, confidence and goals play important roles in health. All of this information helps me to determine the most appropriate remedy for them.

At times, the patient-practitioner visit might even resemble an actual counseling session. It's important to remain open to, and address the emotional and behavioral contributions that patients make to their illness. This can even include emotional reactions that manifest as a result of their failure to progress on a regimen. For example, they may be experiencing a particular emotional state as a result of being physically ill. The specific pattern of that state may be connected on an unconscious level to previous life experiences that have shaped their outlook and sense of self. Examination of this reaction can frequently help reveal the connection to their current dilemma. Such understanding can "unlock" an impasse in healing so that they can move on to the next level of recovery.

Our emotions are not just "byproducts" of chemical synapses in our brains. Substantial evidence suggests that our emotions are the precursors of our physical state as often as they are the result. To subject these feelings to psychopharmacological suppression is one

210

of the most egregious errors that can be made in healthcare. It's important to identify patients' emotional state and take that into account in their healing process, along with their physical condition. Healing isn't just about treating the individual parts of the body or mind separately. These parts are always working together, and their interaction and interplay is one of the most amazing things that homeopathy addresses.

I frequently recommend that my patients seek outside assistance for their emotional concerns, depending upon their level of insight into the emotional issues at hand. I believe that most people can benefit from additional emotional support. I sometimes recommend hypnosis, counseling, visualization, psychotherapy or another form of psychological assistance. At other times, patients just need clarification; for someone to reflect back to them what they are experiencing. A "reality check" into their lives can be helpful. Addressing these issues in addition to physical symptoms can be empowering and encouraging in the healing process.

The Practitioner-Patient Relationship

Success in healing has a lot to do with the encounter that takes place between the practitioner and patient. When these two meet within the context of illness and the healer sees the patient in a thorough, non-judgmental fashion, then healing can take place. When either the patient isn't living in the present or the healer doesn't "get" what the patient is experiencing, then they "miss" each other and healing becomes more difficult. When a patient isn't aware, or isn't able to pay attention to his or her experience, then that can also be a problem.

As a healer, I am there to witness. Each patient is a completely new phenomenon and learning experience for me. I'm not there to make a "diagnosis". I'm there to validate and help explore the phenomenon of illness that's taking place in the person that's in front of me. This exploration leads to a gestalt of the illness that allows for the appropriate homeopathic prescription. This gestalt is a whole process that happens during the patient-healer interaction, and which enables the practitioner to understand what the patient is going through, not just intellectually, but also emotionally. That experience in itself can catalyze a change in both the patient and the healer. The practitioner is not immune to the effects of this interaction, and if he or she tries to insulate, or remain distant from it, then he or she risks "missing" the case.

Two of my most sensitive barometers in practice are intuition and emotion. Hearing what is said beyond words, non-verbally, is extremely important. Sensing and interpreting what is said is just as important as hearing what is being spoken. Patients who aren't aware of their symptoms and who can't effectively verbalize what is going on in their minds or bodies are more difficult to treat.

One way that this can occur is by taking pain relievers and anti-inflammatory medications that mask symptoms. Several studies in the homeopathic literature suggest that patients who are unable to describe their symptoms in adequate detail, and who can't clearly articulate what's going on in their bodies, tend to fare worse with homeopathic treatments than those who can. Homeopathy is definitely advantageous for those who are willing (and able) to listen to their bodies, explore their symptoms and pay attention to their present emotional and physical state. If patients aren't willing (or are unable) to do this, then I find it more difficult to effectively treat them. If someone were to come into my office and say to me, "I have Lyme disease, but I can't tell you what my symptoms are", then I have a very poor chance of helping them. There's very little that I can do homeopathically if I can't individualize their symptoms and if I don't know how the person in front of me is unique and different from others. If close relatives or family members can provide this information, then we may proceed, but if there is a paucity of subjective experiential information, then patients may need a medical intuitive, not a homeopath!

Are There Herxheimer Reactions in Homeopathy?

There are no Herxheimer reactions (that I am aware of) in homeopathy! I haven't seen any Herxheimer reactions, anyway.

Homeopathy does pose a risk for a curious reaction called a "homeopathic aggravation", however. This has been shown to occur in about half of all cases, and not just in those with Lyme disease.

When this happens, whether the patient's problem is rheumatoid arthritis or irritable bowel syndrome, there is initially a worsening of symptoms or a return of old symptoms that takes place following the administration of a remedy. What determines whether patients are experiencing an aggravation or not is how they feel after this return of symptoms: If there is a subsequent improvement accompanied by a return of energy, then a homeopathic aggravation is presumed to have taken place. This is generally a good indication that the remedy is doing what it should and is working. Symptom aggravation is sometimes part of the healing process, though not always. Homeopathic aggravations are distinct and different from Herxheimer reactions. Patients don't get an aggravation every time they take a homeopathic remedy, but it's not unusual after the first prescription.

Why are there are no Herxheimer reactions with homeopathy? Since there has been a paucity of funding for homeopathic research, it's impossible to know. We (in the medical community) understand the theory behind the Herxheimer reaction to be a "die off" of infectious organisms following the application of an antibiotic, (as if you had sprayed napalm on a rainforest, and as a result, got a huge organic die-off reaction from the dissolution of all the wildlife). Homeopathic treatment doesn't seem to act in this manner at all. It doesn't poison the ground, and it doesn't act like chemical warfare. It's not toxic, either to the body or to the infecting organism. This much we know. Homeopathy seems to alter resistance so that the body no longer remains a hospitable place for the infectious organism, but it doesn't do so by sudden chemical annihilation. Thus, we don't expect a Herxheimer, or massive die-off reaction.

Curiously, the fields of microbiology and infectious disease were initially based upon the assumption that bugs are bad and unnecessary for the body. Lately, however, many in the medical community have changed their opinion on this, and science now accepts that bacteria are overwhelmingly good and necessary for the body to remain healthy. In fact, bacteria are so important that we can't live without them. Apparently, the mass of bacteria naturally occurring in and on our bodies even weighs more than we do. We are only beginning to learn about the ecosystem that exists in and on our bodies, and it's changing the way that we view infectious disease. It now appears that the most optimal health scenario involves having a diversity of organisms that co-exist together in the body.

I don't think that homeopathy kills bugs, but it does change the environment in and around the body so that the bugs cease to be as aggressive as before and cease to be a problem for the person. These organisms seem to become integrated into the ecology of the body as non-aggressors, peacefully co-existing with their human host. The use of homeopathy encourages them to reduce their numbers, act less aggressively and assume a balanced niche in the system. They fade into the background because they establish a role in the body that is not parasitic in nature, but rather, commensal. This is a theory that is backed by science and research.

We know that there is even an evolutionary role or an advantage to becoming infected with certain organisms. After all, the science behind the use of probiotics is based upon this premise. Certain theories of evolution suggest that bacterial and viral infections may have been responsible for the development and inclusion of mito-chondria and other organelles into our cells. Mitochondria reproduce independently from the rest of our cellular machinery and contain their own genome. Something similar happens with viral infections since they routinely incorporate their genomes into our own. If you aren't aggressively killing bugs with antibiotics, but are instead creating an environment where the bacteria can co-exist with their human host (without causing infection), then these bugs might sometimes end up providing an advantage to their host. This exact scenario has occurred with gastrointestinal parasites. Some varieties of hookworm parasites, for example, protect against the development of allergies and inflammatory bowel disease when they are allowed to co-exist with their host.

True immunity is actually based upon the concept of exposure (to an organism) with subsequent acclimation and accommodation by the host to this organism. Both the organism and the host change and adapt to this new relationship. It doesn't happen when one member of this relationship is bent upon annihilating the other. Developing immunity requires the presence of two different organisms, so that the immune system can adjust to the organism and the organism can adjust to the immune system. Molecular biology has shown that organisms adjust to the human body, becoming tamer and less virulent with time when they aren't treated with antibiotics.

These complex relationships suggest that the antibiotic approach to infectious disease and, in particular to Lyme disease may not be advantageous. Antibiotics may trigger a more aggressive, adversarial and invasive form of illness, which is antithetical to the concept of accommodation and commensalism. Therefore, getting the bacteria to adjust so that they live in harmony with the immune system, and adjusting the immune system to the bacteria, may be just the trick to establishing an effective healing response.

On a cultural level though, we may not be ready to accept this approach. We want our food supply to be sterile and to wash with antibiotic soap. We may even have backed ourselves into such a corner where we can't live without antibiotics anymore. More and more scientists and biologists are recognizing that this super-hygienic approach to better health is not beneficial, neither ecologically nor environmentally. Health-wise, we are seeing increases in allergies, autoimmune disease and infections as a result of immune systems that have no experience in dealing with foreign organisms. We have a whole society that is unaccustomed to bacteria. Sterilizing the food supply and overusing antibiotics may limit the ability of the immune system to mature properly. These medications eliminate key developmental factors in the formation of the immune system. Over the long run this is a dangerous thing.

Finally, herbs, like antibiotics, may also make bacterial infections more aggressive and harder to treat. These agents are precursors to, and grandparents of, antibiotics, the only difference being that they are a little weaker and a bit more heterogeneous. They may be more "natural", but they function in the same manner as antibiotics and can also relieve symptoms, even while allowing the infections to proliferate.

The Process of Administering Remedies

My initial evaluation for new adult patients is two hours long. This visit allows me to take a fairly extensive and detailed history of the patient and perform a focused physical exam, if needed. After that, I generally suggest a follow-up within four to six weeks, to make sure that the patient and I are on the right track. If we wait too long, and the medication isn't working, then we have lost time. If we don't wait long enough, then we don't have sufficient opportunity to see if the treatment is working. After the second visit, if things are going well, I will generally recommend a follow-up in two or three months. I will keep pushing the time back after every visit, as long as the patient continues to improve. After a few visits, I might recommend a return visit in another six months, and if things are going really well, then I might suggest another visit in a year. The frequency of visits is based upon progress; sometimes, more contact is necessary, and at other times, less.

Several different treatment strategies are available using homeopathic medicines. Depending upon the complexity of the case, a single dose of the homeopathic medicine may be all that is administered in the first month of treatment. At other times, and in more complex cases, a daily or weekly dose of medicine might be recommended. Dosage might be repeated up to three times daily in severe cases or as little as once for less severe cases.

The selection of the homeopathic medicine's potency is based entirely upon the individual case at hand. If I expect patients to have a sluggish response, then the potency of their remedy will be adjusted accordingly, as will their dosing schedule.

Advantages of Homeopathy over Other Types of Treatment

Homeopathy is safe. It doesn't produce toxic or allergic reactions. It doesn't cause noxious side effects or peripheral damage to the body. It doesn't interact with other medications or herbs. It's also extremely well tolerated by those who have a history of drug sensitivity and adverse reactions to conventional medications.

Homeopathy treats each person individually. It can adjust to nearly all contingencies and levels of severity and complexity. It can be adapted to each individual case and address the most prominent areas of disease.

Homeopathy doesn't cause Herxheimer reactions, and if there is a homeopathic aggravation, then it's generally brief, mild and transient, posing no risk to the patient's health.

Homeopathy is inexpensive, easy to administer and holistic. It fosters a more intimate knowledge of and closer relationship with oneself and one's health. Homeopathic medicines are well tolerated; kids love the taste of them and don't mind taking them.

Homeopathy promotes long-term health, not just short-term symptom alleviation and crisis management.

Homeopathy is ecologically and environmentally sustainable. The use and manufacture of homeopathic medicines doesn't pollute or damage the environment or ecosystem, or produce a large carbon footprint. The development of homeopathic medicines doesn't exploit the environment, injure animal species or cost tremendous sums of money.

Comparing Homeopathy to Other Types of Energy Medicine

I am not aware of any significant differences between homeopathy and other types of energy medicine, but I have not studied other systems extensively. Classical homeopathy follows a very definite protocol of analysis and prescription. Laws of prescribing and healing are observed. It is not a matter of "anything goes". It doesn't follow whim or fancy. Classical homeopathic prescribing can't be accomplished by using a biomeridian machine or through Applied Kinesiology. It is based upon a definite and reproducible science of history-taking, repertorization and prescription. Its effectiveness has been confirmed by repeated observation of phenomena over more than two centuries in the Western hemisphere. Today, it is practiced on a worldwide basis.

Why Homeopathy Isn't Used More Widely for the Treatment of Lyme Disease

Ah, now we come to the interesting question! As I mentioned above, it may be that our society is just not ready to use homeopathy extensively. Our mainstream form of medicine, as well as our culture, supports an approach to health that is relatively paternalistic and non-interactive. Conventional wisdom fosters a "quick fix" mentality that demands very little from the patient. One doesn't even need to take responsibility for one's own behavior in the conventional system because there always seems to be a drug that can be taken to alleviate symptoms or a surgery that can be performed if the drug approach fails.

Homeopathy thrives in an environment where cooperation and communication between the physician and patient is strong. Our society fundamentally believes in antibiotics and a "chemical warfare" approach to health and the environment. "Slash and burn" is a slogan of surgeons. Homeopathy advocates a gentler, safer and more ecologically sustainable approach to health and the body, but many are unwilling to entertain a fundamental shift of thinking in this direction.

The history of medicine in our society is based upon "following the money". There is a huge amount of money invested in the current biomedical model of illness. Altering this pattern means large shifts in the way that our medical-pharmacological and academic institutions do business. The allopathic medical profession strongly influences the path that people choose for their health, and what drives the medical system is money. Insurance companies, pharmaceutical companies and physicians are deeply entrenched in a mode of treatment and in a relationship that they are reluctant to see change, even if it is towards a system of safer, less costly and more holistic care.

Even though science is advocated as forming the basis for most of modern medicine, it is actually only evident in a small percentage of the therapeutic interventions. Medical research is not free of conflicts of interest and profit-driven motives. Scientific research is funded heavily by pharmaceutical for-profit interests, while many CAM (Complementary and Alternative Medicine) investigations go unsupported and unfunded. The field of medicine has never been free of ideological constraints, so why should it be any different today? The history of medicine is rife with examples of suppression and ostracism of ideas whose time had simply not come. The science of medicine is a highly politicized arena and largely dependent upon the free-thinking tendencies and biases within a society. Bias and prejudice are strong factors working against truly objective scientific research in homeopathy and other areas of CAM.

If medical researchers were truly objective, then we would be using homeopathy and many more CAM practices today (as the rest of the world is already doing) not only in the treatment of Lyme disease, but in a great many other conditions as well.

Last Words

I strongly advocate a scientific approach for the treatment of conditions like Lyme disease. I also support a holistic, integrative approach to health care. A long-term view of health and the environment should be part of any sustainable therapeutic regimen.

There are many unanswered questions in health care today and even the concepts of health and healing are poorly understood. There is widespread disagreement regarding what even constitutes good health. The issue of healing is a far more complex issue than most people assume. I do not believe that "healing" resides in a little white chemical pill, but in a relationship and in an energetic balance between a person and the physical and emotional elements of his or her life. Health care isn't something that is done to us, but something that we actively participate in on a day-to-day basis with awareness and creativity.

For this reason, the practice of classical homeopathy can add a much-needed support to the person suffering from Lyme disease and other related medical disorders. Not all cases can be cured, but many can. Others can be helped tremendously by this process, which supports and augments autonomy and truly holistic healing.

How to Contact Ronald Whitmont, M.D.

Ronald D. Whitmont, M.D.
6250 Route 9
Rhinebeck, NY 12572
(845) 876-6323
www.homeopathicmd.com

• CHAPTER 8 •

Deborah Metzger, Ph.D., M.D.
LOS ALTOS, CA

Biography

Dr. Metzger is the medical director of Harmony Women's Health in Los Altos, California. She is also a gynecologist, reproductive endocrinologist, and integrative medicine practitioner devoted to the treatment of men and women with challenging medical problems. After graduating from college (SUNY at Buffalo, 1973), she obtained a PhD in molecular endocrinology from Baylor College of Medicine in Houston, Texas (1979). She graduated from the University of Texas Medical School at Houston (1982), completed her residency in both Obstetrics and Gynecology (1986) and a fellowship in Reproductive Endocrinology and Infertility (1988) at Duke University in North Carolina. After spending six years on the faculty of the University of Connecticut Health Center (where she was an associate professor) she went into private practice in Hartford, CT, specializing in chronic pelvic pain, endometriosis, infertility and advanced laparoscopic surgery.

In 1998, Dr. Metzger moved to the San Francisco Bay Area and joined Dr. Arnold Kresch in creating Helena Women's Health. After

Dr. Kresch's untimely death in 1999, Dr. Metzger continued to expand the breadth and depth of the practice's services. In January 2004, she decided to give up her surgical practice in favor of an integrative medical practice and then opened Harmony Women's Health, which is dedicated to the treatment of the whole person, using integrative and holistic care in a nurturing environment.

Dr. Metzger is recognized as one of the leading authorities in the integrative and holistic treatment of endometriosis and chronic pelvic pain. By necessity, she is also an expert in chronic fatigue syndrome, fibromyalgia and Lyme disease since these problems often accompany pain issues. She has lectured extensively throughout the world, and has published widely in peer-reviewed journals and textbooks. Dr. Metzger is one of the editors of *Chronic Pelvic Pain: An Integrated Approach*, the first book on the subject of pelvic pain. She is also one of the authors of the first edition of, *Operative Gynecologic Laparoscopy: Principles and Techniques*, a groundbreaking overview of modern laparoscopic surgery. More information on her other published works can be found on the Internet at: www.harmonywomenshealth.com.

Healing Philosophy

Everyone carries microbes in their bodies that could potentially cause infections, but people with healthy immune systems live in peaceful co-existence with lots of bacteria, viruses, yeasts, and parasites. When the immune system gets overloaded and/or distracted, these infections can no longer be controlled and they then cause problems. Therefore, treatment for Lyme disease and chronic illness can't just be aimed at getting rid of infections. If practitioners and patients aren't doing anything to improve the immune system, then patients may not improve or may relapse on a treatment regimen.

Also, I believe that the "chronic fatigue" or "fibromyalgia" labels that are often given to the chronically ill (with Lyme) are often the only diagnoses that conventional medicine has to offer them. Sadly, these diagnoses are typically based only on the most cursory of test results, i.e. CBC and TSH levels. In reality, both chronic fatigue and fibromyalgia are inflammatory disorders, which are caused primarily by allergies and infections. Therefore, Lyme may be just one of many causes of inflammation for those who have this disease as part of their inflammatory disorder. Regardless of the cause of inflammation, however, in order to reduce it, it's important for practitioners to improve their patients' immune systems, beat back the "critters" in their bodies and get them back into a state of peaceful harmony and co-existence with their bacteria, viruses, yeasts, and parasites.

All of the following must be addressed in order to heal the body of inflammation and Lyme disease:

1. Disordered sleep

2. Digestion

3. Diet and nutrition

4. Allergies

5. Stealth infections

6. Hormonal problems

7. Exercise

8. Detoxification

9. The Mind/Body Connection

Let's take a more in-depth look at each of these areas.

Sleep

First, sleep is essential, and is the most important component of any treatment plan. If my patients aren't sleeping, then none of my treatments are going to work for them. Often, those with Lyme disease have a completely disordered sleep/wake cycle. I address this problem by prescribing my patients three milligrams of melatonin two to three hours before bedtime, then at bedtime, they take two to four grams of the amino acid glycine. If they wake up during the night, they take additional glycine. Since using this protocol, I have had to write far fewer prescriptions for sleep medications. In any case, it's necessary that people with Lyme get eight to nine hours of sleep at night, and this may require them taking two or three different prescription medications at the same time.

The other problem that I commonly see in my patients with Lyme disease and sleep disorders is sleep apnea. This is often found in those who consistently require at least ten hours of sleep per night and who snore. Sleep apnea can be easily diagnosed through a sleep study. Patients shouldn't overlook the possibility of their partners having sleep apnea either, since their partners' snoring may wake them frequently during the night and disrupt their sleep, which then compromises their healing.

Intestinal Dysbiosis

Cleaning up the intestine is an essential component to healing. Disordered digestion contributes to overall inflammation and interferes with the body's ability to absorb nutrients. Fifty percent of the immune system is associated with the intestine, so problems in the intestine affect immune function. The most common problems that I find in my patients are H. pylori infections, hypochlorhydria (low stomach acid secretion), inadequate release of digestive enzymes, small intestine bacterial overgrowth, candidiasis, bacterial dysbiosis, inadequate levels of beneficial bacteria, food allergies, and gluten sensitivity. These problems can be easily identified by simple testing and treated with supplements, herbs, antifungal remedies and probiotics.

Diet & Nutrition

The root of all evil is not the love of money, but the love of sugar. In general, I recommend that my patients follow a low glycemic diet called "Sugar Busters", which disallows the consumption of 'white foods' such as table sugar, white bread, processed flour, white potatoes, white rice, white pasta, etc. Also, consuming caffeine is akin to drinking a cup of sugar and should also be avoided because it causes the liver the release large amounts of sugar. Finally, if my patients have gluten sensitivity (which is about 90% of them) and food allergies (100% of them), then I further personalize and refine their diets.

When I put my patients on the "Sugar Busters" diet, they start getting better, and not only because the diet lowers their inflammation, but also because chemicals and other toxins get automatically removed from their bodies. Boxed cereals, canned and other processed foods are loaded with chemicals and toxins, so I encourage my patients to eat organic fruits, vegetables, and protein instead.

I also like to be conservative when recommending nutrients, and rather than taking a 'one-size-fits-all' approach, I do blood and urine testing to determine my patients' specific nutrient needs. NutrEval by Genova Diagnostics is the lab that I use for this.

Allergies & the Immune System

Allergies are not commonly taken into account in Lyme disease, but Lyme makes allergies worse and allergies make Lyme worse. In addition, allergies to inhalants, foods, hormones, and neurotransmitters can cause many of the same symptoms as Lyme disease. And when patients' immune systems are fighting mold and pollen like they would a virus or bacteria, they easily become distracted and the resulting immune response creates inflammation. Treating their allergies with antihistamines may improve some of the their symptoms, but their inflammation, fatigue, brain fog, and achiness will continue until their practitioners attempt to re-focus the attention of their immune systems, by desensitizing them to their allergies.

Most of my patients have hyper-alert immune systems. If they get a common bacteria or virus, their immune systems take care of it right away, and this is a positive thing. Having a hyper-alert immune system can also be detrimental, however, because it tends to focus on minor insults from the environment, including mold, pollens, foods, and so on. This means that it gets distracted from other, more important problems, at the same time that it becomes overloaded from having to focus on a multitude of less important ones.

I do intradermal allergy testing for environmental and hormone allergies, as well as for fourteen foods that patients are typically allergic to. Because the results of IgG blood tests for allergens does not correlate well with those of skin tests, and because I have had good results with skin testing, I don't use blood tests to test for allergies. Allergists do a 'prick test' which is also not as sensitive as an intradermal test.

I find that 100% of my patients have allergies of some type, and not just to food, but to pollens and other environmental allergens, so I test them for things like allergies to mold, trees, grass, and dust. I even test their hormones, because some develop auto-immunity to their own hormones. If patients have PMS, for example, then I know that they probably have allergies to progesterone or serotonin. If they have weird responses to supplemental thyroid hormone, then it is likely that they have allergies to T3/T4 hormones. If they have symptoms of adrenal fatigue, but feel worse on cortisol replacement, they are usually allergic to cortisol. Patients with depression and anxiety (and who are barely hanging on by a fingernail), tend to have neurotransmitter allergies. I can pick out the hormonal and neurotransmitter allergies that my patients are likely to have, based on their symptoms.

To treat their environmental allergies, such as to trees, molds and grass, it's not enough for me to give them an antihistamine, because this type of medication doesn't address their inflammation, which is the source of their symptoms. Therefore, desensitizing them to these allergies is essential. To accomplish this, and rather than administering injections, I give them sublingual drops containing the allergenic substance, which they self -administer. Symptomatic improvement is often seen within one to three months with this type of treatment.

To treat my patients' food allergies, I first desensitize them to allergenic foods by taking them off of the suspected foods for six weeks. Then, I add foods back into their diet, one at a time, to see which ones they respond negatively to. I try to determine not only the foods that they are allergic to, but also the ones that they are sensitive to, because some foods can be eaten, but only in moderation, while others need to be eliminated completely.

I also treat hormone allergies using the same sublingual desensitization technique mentioned earlier, after which time patients are able to take hormones, if necessary, to correct any imbalances. I also treat allergies to neurotransmitters using this method.

Supplements that I use to improve my patients' immune system function include andrographis, (which is useful not only for the treatment of infections, but also for increasing natural killer cell counts), as well as colostrum, transfer factor and arabinogalactan. When I give them any of these, however, it has to be for a good reason. Not just because they *might* work for them, but because testing indicates that they have a high probability of working. Guessing on treatments just becomes too expensive for them otherwise.

I refer my patients with lymphatic drainage problems to a physical therapist for lymphatic massage and myofascial release. This therapy is essential for some people. If they can't afford massage, I may recommend that they take homeopathic remedies that aid in lymphatic drainage, since these are inexpensive.

Sometimes, the treatments that I use for other problems (certain herbs, for instance) are also effective for the lymphatic system. So before prescribing a new treatment to patients, I first consider how much of a difference that the new treatment will make for them. Why add another treatment to their regimen if the problem is being taken care of through some other means?

Stealth Infections

When the immune system becomes overloaded or distracted, infectious critters that are ordinarily kept under its control become problematic. Many infections are effectively treated with Lyme protocols, but others may require a different approach. There is no way to determine at the onset of treatment which, if any, of these infections are causing the majority of patients' symptoms, though. Therefore, a coordinated approach to treatment is important.

I routinely test my patients for Mycoplasma, reactivated viruses (EBV [Epstein-Barr], CMV [Cytomegalovirus], HHV-6 [human Herpes virus six], and parvo virus), toxoplasmosis, chronic strep, Rocky Mountain spotted fever, parasites, Candida, and Chlamydia pneumoniae. To treat these infections, I often use herbs, because they have a wide spectrum of activity against bacteria, viruses, yeasts and parasites; however, I also sometimes use antibiotics and antiviral medications. Treatment is individualized to the patient's diagnoses and personal preferences.

Hormonal Dysfunction

I have found that women who have been well for most of their lives can crash around the time of perimenopause. During this time, estrogen and progesterone levels start to get out of whack, and both of these hormones are involved in regulating the immune system. About half of the men that I see are deficient in testosterone. Once people crash as a result of hormone imbalances, they can't just pick themselves back up again by fixing their hormone levels. Their infections, diet, allergies and sleep must all be separately and simultaneously addressed.

I don't rely solely upon blood or saliva hormone tests to determine what hormone deficiencies and excesses my patients have, because hormone levels fluctuate all of the time. Also, there is no way of knowing what an individual patient's "normal" levels are, since these differ from person to person and do not necessarily correlate with what the labs consider to be "normal". And because it's so difficult to determine beforehand exactly what type of hormone replacement and the dose that patients need, I tend to prescribe them the form of hormone that they choose, through the route that works best for them. Some women don't want to take replacement hormones, however, because the popular press has made it impossible for them to feel comfortable with this type of therapy, when, in fact, there is so much medical literature that supports the safe use of it.

Personally, I prefer that my patients take either prescription bioidentical or compounded hormones. Prescription bioidentical hormones are often cheaper than compounded hormones, so I only use compounded hormones for patients that request it or who need it because of sensitivities. There is such a wide range of products available for hormone replacement: patches; transdermal creams; vaginal tablets, creams, and rings; injections; subcutaneous pellets —there is something for everyone. In the end though, I prescribe the type and dose of whatever product makes my patients feel right, rather than relying solely upon their blood test results.

In addition to estrogen and progesterone, I also test my patients' DHEA-S (DHEA-Sulphate) levels and testosterone, and do a complete thyroid panel that includes TSH, free T3, free T4, reverse T3, and anti-thyroid antibodies. I treat the thyroid gland with whatever works for my patients (somewhat like my approach to progesterone, estrogen and testosterone). Many of my patients prefer dessicated porcine thyroid hormone (Armour thyroid or Naturethroid). If they have Hashimoto's thyroiditis (an autoimmune thyroid condition), I use Levoxyl, Cytomel or sustained release T3.

I also test my patients' adrenal gland function by performing an a.m. and p.m. blood cortisol test. I prefer blood cortisol tests over saliva because I have found that there is a poor correlation between saliva and blood test results due to the presence of cortisol allergies in many of my patients. The antibodies that bind to cortisol prevent the cortisol from appearing in the saliva. Cortisol allergies produce all the signs and symptoms of adrenal insufficiency, but often, adrenal function in people who have these allergies is normal. Many patients with cortisol allergies cannot tolerate cortisol replacement until they are desensitized to these allergies.

Other hormonal problems that I frequently encounter in my patients are insulin resistance (which can be diagnosed with a two hour glucose tolerance test that measures glucose and insulin levels) and growth hormone deficiencies. Insulin resistance is treated with a low glycemic diet, herbs to control sugar cravings (my favorite is cinnamon—five capsules a day) and sometimes Metformin, which is a diabetic medication.

Growth hormone deficiency occurs in about 5-10% of my patients. A five-hour growth hormone stimulation test can confirm whether this deficiency is present. If so, and if patients have health care insurance, then most companies will generally pay for them to get growth hormone injections to correct for this deficiency.

Exercise

People with Lyme disease find most physical activity exhausting, often requiring several days of rest to recover. At the same time, they feel compelled to continue their usual exercise program to stay in shape. Many of my patients insist on going to the gym every day of the week, and I must tell them that they are not allowed to do this! Even though they feel awful after their workouts (this is not always a good thing), they think that they are doing something positive for themselves. In order to recover, they must carefully budget their energy expenditure, and make sure that they leave themselves as much energy as possible after their workouts, so that they may properly recover from the exercise. Physical activity that leaves them exhausted will complicate their recovery.

I tell my patients that it's better to walk instead of going to the gym, but only as far as they are comfortable with and only if it improves how they feel. If they feel poorly afterwards, then it means that they are doing too much.

Detoxification

We live in a chemical soup that we cannot avoid. Some people are genetically equipped to handle it better than others. Those with Lyme disease often have genetic deficiencies that compromise their body's ability to detoxify. For this reason, their detoxification system needs to be supported as much as possible during healing.

I test all of my patients for heavy metal toxicity. I have found that at least sixty percent of them have high levels of lead and mercury. If they have dental amalgams, I recommend that they get these removed. I also do oral chelation therapy. I don't like intravenous therapy, because I believe that the oral therapy gets the job done just as efficiently as an IV, but is less costly. I have heavy duty, as well as light, heavy metal chelation protocols for my patients. Some want to get started right away on a heavy metal chelation protocol, but discover that they aren't strong enough to do the "heavy duty" protocol, so for such patients I prescribe one capsule of DMSA, every 3rd night, as well as chlorella every day. The heavy-duty protocol consists of 400mg of DMSA, three times per day for three days, followed by eleven days off DMSA and mineral support.

I also perform a urine chemical screen on those patients who have a strong history of chemical exposure. If their test results reveal that they have high levels of chemicals in their bodies, then I recom-mend that they do saunas to remove these (There is a controversy over whether infrared or moist heat is better). Some of my patients feel awful after spending just five minutes in the sauna, because they are releasing so many toxins. Most chemical toxins are re-leased through the skin, but some are released through the intestines, as well, which is why taking toxin binders is also important for getting rid of chemicals.

So many of my patients are chemically sensitive, too, whether to things in the environment or to medications (often the fillers). Trying to address all of their chemical problems is a challenge, but I believe that environmental toxins are a major reason why so many people are getting chronically ill, and why more and more are getting symptoms of chronic fatigue and fibromyalgia. Toxins interfere with the functioning of the immune system.

A lot of people with Lyme disease also have mold toxicity. Often, they move into houses, and start to feel bad shortly after their move. One of the questions that I ask my mold patients is whether they have water damage in their house, because that is an indication that the house probably has mold, even if the water damage is in the crawl space under the house. It's difficult to get people to move, though, because nobody wants to believe that their house is toxic.

When testing patients for mold, I look for serum antibodies (IgE, IgG, and IgA) to stachybotrys and aspergillus, two common, but dangerous, household molds. I also have them do mold plates to help ascertain whether there is a problem. If there is, then it's vital that they move out of their house! I also encourage people with mold problems to call a mold remediator and have a proper inspection performed on their house, so that whatever mold is present can be removed. Sometimes, mold exposure comes from people's workplaces (particularly schools!), and uncovering the source can require persistence and a lot of detective work.

Mold allergies are quite common though and are associated with symptoms such as fatigue, fibromyalgia, and brain fog (sound familiar?). If I discover that my patients have mold toxins in their bodies, then I use sublingual mold drops to desensitize them. However, unless they get away from the source of their mold toxins, their recovery will be precarious. I treat some of my patients with mold biotoxin binders such as Cholestyramine or Actos, but I believe that a mold diet may be more effective for them. Such a diet would involve avoiding the consumption of fermented products, such as wine, beer, vinegar, mushrooms or yeast-containing breads. As with other issues in chronic illness, however, it's important for practitioners to not focus solely on their patients' mold problems, because it's just one piece of their healing puzzle.

For detoxification, I also give my patients IV Myers' cocktails and glutathione. These treatments can be miraculous for some, especially when performed once or twice per week.

Mind-Body and Spiritual Strategies for Healing

> *"God grant me the serenity*
> *to accept the things I cannot change;*
> *the courage to change the things I can;*
> *and the wisdom to know the difference."*

This serenity prayer alludes to the complexities of life and might describe those with chronic Lyme disease who are looking for a way to be able to enjoy life the way that they used to, rather than how they might be at the present time. Since nobody can foresee what it will take to get better, much less when it will happen, people with Lyme should incorporate some type of spiritual practice into their healing regimen, but I think that everyone needs to find their own outlet and way of recharging spiritually. While dealing with chronic Lyme disease closes some doors, it often opens windows that the sick person never saw before. This can be a time of intense personal growth.

Sometimes I will suggest practices for my patients, such as yoga, and they will say things like, "I used to do yoga and really enjoyed it!" And it's as if a light bulb has gone off in their heads, and they are reminded of a great practice that they can do and which will help them to heal. In any case, I tell them to listen to their inner voice, because it doesn't matter what type of activity they do, as long as it's meaningful and not just an exercise in going through the motions.

I have patients who are workaholics and who will say things like, "I really need to work", even though they are exhausted. These people are totally ignorant about their bodies and will have difficulty healing if they don't slow down. Yoga, acupuncture, and other mind-body strategies found in energy medicine can help them to re-connect with their bodies and spirits that have been overshadowed by constant activity. I advocate energy medicine strategies because I believe that it's important to take the energetic body (not just the biochemical) into account when healing. If patients have blocked energy fields, for example, they may not get better by just taking an antibiotic or changing their diet. They need someone to re-channel their energy for them. Also, energy medicine strategies address areas of healing that biochemical treatments can't.

I also have patients who don't want to deal with their emotional issues. For these people, illness has become their way of expressing their feelings of anger or betrayal towards their loved ones. They may need to assess their marriages, unrealized goals, or unresolved childhood trauma, because any suppressed feelings that have been caused by such things are being expressed in their bodies. They often aren't ready to face their trauma though, and are often reluctant to see therapists, but their progress in healing can be hindered because of this. Once they start to understand and face their emotional problems, however, then true healing can begin.

About twenty to thirty percent of my patients have been sexually abused, but interestingly enough, in the general population, about thirty percent of people have suffered this type of abuse, so the statistics of those in my practice are lower than I would expect. The medical literature states that those with sexual abuse trauma have more difficulty healing than those who have never been abused, but (in my experience) they do as well as anyone else. Many of my patients have physical and emotional trauma, but I find that those who have the most trouble healing have post-traumatic stress as a result of invasive and impersonal medical care.

Treating Lyme (Borrelia)

When asked what I use to treat Lyme disease infections, I often answer, "whatever works". It is important for practitioners to keep an open mind and not continue to follow a protocol if patient response indicates that it isn't working. In general, I start off by treating my patients for Borrelia with doxycycline, Biaxin (clarithromycin), or herbs such as Samento or andrographis. If it's spring through fall, I don't use doxycycline, because people want to be outside during this time of year, and doxycycline causes sun sensitivity. A good summer antibiotic is Biaxin. If I find it necessary for my patients to be on a tetracycline drug, then I prescribe minocycline, which causes less sun sensitivity. I should also add that I do an inventory of their overall health problems during their initial consultation with me and make recommendations for testing and treatment based on what I learn from this consultation.

I request that my patients set up an appointment with me six weeks after their initial consultation so that I can evaluate how well they are responding to the antibiotic that I have prescribed them. I want to know if they have had any kind of healing crisis, or Herxheimer reaction. At six weeks, I expect them to have had at least an hour, or a day, where they have felt great. If I don't see any change at this stage, then I start adding other antibiotics or herbs to their regimens. If they have been taking Biaxin, for example, I may then add hydroxychloroquine. Then I evaluate their symptoms again after another six to eight weeks, at which time I may add ciprofloxacin, another antibiotic, or an herb to the mix.

Basically, I will keep adding remedies to their regimens until they say, "Wow, now I know that this stuff is working!" Sometimes I use herbs, sometimes antibiotics, and I often use a combination of both. Some of my patients prefer to use herbs only, though, and have good results with just these, while others need the pharmaceutical medications.

Also, when dosing antibiotics and herbs, I allow my patients to decide whether or not they want to hit the infections hard with high doses of remedies right away, or start low and gradually ramp up on the dosing. Some patients just want to "dive in", while others don't want to, or even shouldn't, deal with unbearable Herxheimer reactions.

Also, when treating Borrelia, I don't necessarily differentiate between the different forms of the organism when deciding upon which antibiotics to give a patient. I know that a lot of doctors use Flagyl (metronidazole) or Tindamax (tinidazole) for the cyst and L-forms of the organism, but most of my patients find the side effects of these medications to be intolerable. So to treat these resistant forms of the organism, I commonly use pulse therapy, which involves taking antibiotics on a days-on, days-off schedule.

I have found that I need to use intravenous antibiotics in only about five percent of my patients, mostly because I do a lot of intramuscular Bicillin injections before considering IV antibiotics. Many patients think that they will get better faster with IV antibiotics but I find that if we take a comprehensive approach to treating their infections and immune system, then this isn't the case.

The bodies of those with Lyme disease are completely discombobulated, so I can't just get rid of my patients' infections. I must treat their whole body, taking into account all of the factors that were mentioned in the first part of this chapter. When I do, I find that I don't have to be as aggressive in treating them with antibiotics.

Treating Co-Infections

I tend to not extensively test my patients for co-infections. From the onset, I try to formulate a treatment plan that will at least begin to address whatever co-infections I suspect that they have, based on a clinical diagnosis, particularly if their symptoms indicate a specific one. Also, if I treat them for Borrelia and they don't seem to be getting better, this can be another indication to me that they need to be treated for co-infections. Not everyone has Babesia, Bartonella, and Ehrlichia along with Borrelia, but most people have at least one co-infection.

If my patients have neck pain, fatigue and night sweats then this often means that they have a Babesia infection. For treatment of this infection, I may prescribe five capsules of artemisinin, twice a day, on a rotating basis of twelve days on, two days off. If artemisinin doesn't work, I may then prescribe a combination of Mepron (atovaquone) and Biaxin (clarithromycin), but unfortunately, there are Babesia strains that are also resistant to these medications.

For Bartonella, I also typically use a combination of antibiotics and herbs, although in some cases, it can be either/or, but I usually try to exploit the full breadth of what is available in medicine. If I'm going to prescribe just antibiotics, I usually combine a macrolide drug with ciprofloxacin or Septra, along with another drug. Some doctors prescribe Levaquin (levofloxacin) for the treatment of Bartonella, but all of my patients who have used this medication have developed tendonitis afterwards. For that reason, I don't prescribe it anymore.

I try to put together the broadest treatment protocol possible for my sickest patients, since they tend to have the most co-infections. If I suspect that they have Ehrlichia, Bartonella and Borrelia, for example, I will prescribe doxycycline or Biaxin, along with Zithromax, in order to cover all of the infections. If I am suspicious that they have Babesia, then I will also start with artemisinin, too.

For the herbal treatment of Borrelia, I often use Samento (cat's claw) and andrographis. I have been really impressed with the results of these herbs. I also use a product called Spiro Kete, which is a five-herb combination product containing stinging nettle, yerba santa, goldenrod, monolaurin, and organic tobacco. More information on this product can be found at: www.kroegerherb.com. While these herbs are generally targeted towards Borrelia, other herbal combination products exist which are effective against the other infections.

In addition to Lyme co-infections, many of my patients also have opportunistic infections; that is, infections that were once dormant but which have been reactivated by their compromised immune systems. Such infections include Chlamydia, Epstein-Barr, HHV-6 (human Herpes virus 6), Mycoplasma, helicobacter pylori and tuberculosis, as well as others. I treat some of these infections, but I tend to find that by addressing immunity and the major infections, some of the other infections will go away on their own. Awhile back, I used the drug Valcyte for the treatment of viruses, but I wasn't very impressed with its results. Since then, I have used Lomatium to treat re-activated viruses and have witnessed better results in my patients with this medication.

It's Not All About Borrelia

It's not always easy for me to discern the most important causes of my patients' symptoms. The major player in their symptom game may not be Borrelia, but rather Mycoplasma or a re-activated virus. The major player could also be food allergies, gluten sensitivities, or a lack of sleep. For most patients, there is no one single major player, though, and multiple problems are causing their symptoms. Occasionally, I get patients with only one major problem, such as gluten sensitivity, and when I take them off of certain foods, they feel like a million bucks. This is why it's important for practitioners to address multiple healing components when treating their patients, because they can end up treating them endlessly for Lyme disease, when in fact, Lyme disease is a relatively minor player in their overall symptom picture.

Doing detective work is important. I have been treating patients for so long that I know that it's important to assess up front all factors that could be causing their disease, instead of waiting until I have treated their Lyme for six months or a year and then realizing that another issue is primary.

My initial patient evaluation involves doing tests such as the ANA (anti-nuclear antibody) and rheumatoid factor. Such tests help me to determine the source of my patients' problems, because again, it's not good to assume that everyone's symptoms are all due to Lyme disease. It might be that they have multiple sclerosis. Then again, is there any difference between MS and Lyme? Are they just different manifestations of the same disease, or are they two different diseases entirely? It's controversial, but since all Lyme practitioners are being closely scrutinized these days, we need to make sure that we haven't just jumped in and assumed that a patient has Lyme until all of the pertinent tests have been performed and assessed.

Also, by doing tests such as the rheumatoid factor, as well as others, practitioners can sometimes make interesting discoveries. For instance, I once had a patient whom I had treated with intravenous antibiotics of all kinds. She improved a little, but not proportionate to the amount of stuff that I had shoveled into her! She had a lot of joint pain and her rheumatoid factor test was negative, so I checked her ASO titers. They came back really high, which demonstrated to me that she had a strep infection, not Lyme disease. I gave her clindamycin, and within a day or two, she was a new person. Now, if my patients have a lot of joint pain, I perform an ASO titer along with a Borrelia test, and am finding that there are other people with chronic strep infections and which are causing them symptoms. So this is another major player that practitioners treating Lyme disease might overlook.

As another example, I once treated a patient for Lyme disease who felt great after her treatments but then subsequently crashed. However, her symptoms after the crash were different than those she had experienced when she had Lyme disease. So I cast out a wider net, figuratively speaking, and tested her for some other infections besides Lyme, including valley fever and histoplasmosis, and it turned out that she had the latter infection. So I prescribed her an anti-fungal medication, and within a week or two, she had recovered completely.

Treating chronic illness is an art. It's making decisions based on intuition (patients' as well as practitioners') and a lot of experience.

Patients read a lot and might suggest, for example, that I treat them for a certain infection based on a suspected past exposure to that infection. Take the patient with histoplasmosis, for instance. I mean, where in the heck did she get the idea that she might have this infection? Well, it turns out that she had been working for the government, cleaning up ammunition dumps where there had been an infestation of bats.

Again, it's important to look into a lot of areas, and check under a lot of rocks in order to discern what patients' issues are. As practitioners, we can't just stay in the same testing rut, especially when we treat the usual suspects (infections) and don't get the expected results. We must stop and ask ourselves whether we are missing something.

Other Treatments for Symptomatic Relief

Depression/Anxiety

Depression and anxiety are a problem for people with Lyme disease. Most of my patients have been to psychiatrists, and have tried the whole spectrum of medications, but nothing works for them. Food and neurotransmitter allergies, as well as Lyme disease, can cause anxiety. By treating these problems, patients can beat back their anxiety a little, but sometimes, there are deeper causes for this symptom, and it requires a lot of detective work by both patient and practitioner to discover what these are. For example, I once had a patient who had anxiety and neurotransmitter allergies, and after I gave her some neurotransmitter desensitization drops, her anxiety was gone within two weeks. It was incredible. Not everyone is healed in such a straightforward manner, however, and multiple strategies, such as working on eliminating allergies and improving the diet, are necessary for most, but then the pieces of the puzzle eventually all come together and people feel better. For some, treating B-6 and zinc deficiencies (pyroluria) with high doses of both nutrients can be helpful to varying degrees, depending upon how much of a factor these deficiencies are in their anxiety.

240

It's often difficult to distinguish fatigue from depression and patients are reluctant to take anti-depressants. My first line of treatment for depression is nutritional (based on testing), and also involves eliminating food allergies and gluten from my patients' diets, as well as treating their intestinal dysbiosis. If these approaches don't work, I may then prescribe them an anti-depressant. I find Wellbutrin to be a good anti-depressant, because not only does it relieve the depression, but also helps them to focus and stay alert.

Pain

Pain can be a difficult symptom to treat, especially when patients have generalized pain. Sometimes, it seems that nothing relieves this symptom. In general, I recommend high dose omega-3 oils, but I believe that medical marijuana works the best, especially if patients have bad fibromyalgia. Taking medical marijuana isn't feasible for everyone since there are only a few states where its use is legal.

Another treatment that I recommend for pain is an anti-inflammatory medical food called Limbrel, which contains flavocoxid, a proprietary blend of natural ingredients from phytochemical food source materials. Flavocoxid is comprised primarily of flavonoids such as baicalin and catechin. I also recommend the herbs boswellia and curcumin. Some products combine boswellia, white willow bark, and sour cherry for pain, and these can be effective. Like all things, however, these treatments work great for some, but not others. Everyone is different, so I give my patients samples of different products to try.

Patient and Practitioner Challenges and Roadblocks to Healing

The biggest challenge for patients and practitioners treating Lyme disease is ignorance. It is all too common for patients to be told that they do not have Lyme disease by ignorant practitioners, which then creates a delay in their diagnosis and treatment and prolongs their pain and suffering.

The two biggest mistakes that patients make in their healing journey are that 1) they give up on their treatments too easily or, 2) they fail to follow through on a treatment plan. Patients must be involved in their own healthcare and have faith that they will get better. Where there is a will, there is a way. They must be advocates for themselves.

Not fixing dental problems creates another significant roadblock to healing, because some patients that I have treated didn't respond well to antibiotics until they addressed their dental problems. Patients who have conditions such as osteomyelitis of the jaw, or root canals and dental amalgams, must treat these conditions or problems if they are to fully heal.

Finally, it's almost impossible for patients to get better unless they significantly decrease their normal physical and emotional demands of life. This often requires them taking a medical leave of absence from their jobs. Taking time off from the "rat race" is one of the most important things that they can do, because it's so hard to do treatments, keep a good sleep regimen going, stay on a good diet and work, all at the same time. Also, patients learn so much about themselves (and their conditions) when they can take time off from work. While it may be difficult for them to do this, it's necessary.

Mistakes in the Treatment of Lyme Disease

I think that it's a mistake when practitioners treat their patients with only antibiotics, while doing nothing else to improve their patients' immune systems. Fortunately, most Lyme-literate doctors now include some sort of physical therapy, dietary recommendations, and other holistic practices into their protocols.

It's also a mistake to assume that all of a patient's symptoms are due to Lyme disease and co-infections. Practitioners must do a comprehensive health evaluation and address any problems that interfere with the normal functioning of their patients' immune systems.

Labs support diagnoses, but they can't be used to diagnose. Lyme is a clinical diagnosis, and when I see someone with muscle aches, brain fog, chronic fatigue, and crazy neurological symptoms, Lyme disease is at the top of my list of suspects. If I see a woman with vulvodynia, I consider the possibility that she might have Lyme disease, even though she many not have any other symptoms. Bad nerve pain going down the arm can alone be indicative of Lyme. I even had one patient who only had hormonal issues, but when we treated her for Lyme, she got better. Funny thing, though, even the Lyme-literate doctor who had treated her previously thought that she only had hormonal problems!

How Finances Affect Healing

Money is not the only factor that determines whether patients will recover, but having it helps a lot. If they don't have a lot of money to spend on treatments, however, then I try to find low-cost resources and treatments for them. For example, if they have food allergies, rather than paying for a skin test, I will recommend that they do the food elimination test, which doesn't cost anything. I also belong to a co-op organization where patients can get blood tests for about 25% of the regular lab cost. Herbs can be cheaper than antibiotics, and I often recommend these to my patients. I also tell them about the $4.00 generic drug plan that is available through Wal-Mart and Target. If they can't afford stool tests, I treat them empirically, based upon what I know about the most common abnormalities found in those with certain gut symptoms. I have patients who don't have a lot of money but who will do anything that it takes to get better. I have other patients who have money, but who won't do things because (they believe) that it just costs too much.

The most important thing when it comes to being able to afford treatments is that patients need to feel that they are worth it. That they are worth spending money on and that they are worth being well. That sometimes means going out and asking for money. Some of my patients have asked family members to help out, and it's very hard for them to do this, but most of them get better when they are able to receive such help.

How Friends and Family Can Help the Sick

Family and friends of Lyme disease sufferers should learn everything that they can about the disease. They should learn about the treatment controversies and believe what those with Lyme tell them about their symptoms and disability. Some people don't believe in Lyme disease, or they think that it's their loved ones' fault that they are ill. They think that they aren't getting on with their lives, or aren't doing enough to be well. It is very hard for those who have never had illness or pain to understand what their loved ones are going through, but these people need to open their minds. Their loved ones may look totally normal, but are in reality, totally disabled. The same thing happens from the physician's perspective. Many doctors tell patients that their illness is all in their head, or that they just need to learn to live with their disease.

I put a lot of faith in my patients' ability to assess things. I am amazed at how much they know, and at how much they can sense. The patient is always right. When someone tells me, "There's something not right here," I say, "Okay, let's track it down." One of the most difficult aspects of my job is hearing about what patients have to go through with other health care practitioners. Being told, "Well you're just getting older, deal with it!" or "Go to a shrink!" makes patients feel betrayed when they finally find out what is causing their symptoms.

Final Words

I believe in my patients. I believe in their ability to make intelligent decisions for themselves. And I believe in being non-judgmental and available to them. I communicate with them via e-mail, which is a great way of being available 24-7 when they have concerns or questions about their treatments. It makes a huge difference for them, because practitioners are such an important part of their patients' treatment.

How to Contact Deborah Metzger, Ph.D., M.D.

Deborah A. Metzger, Ph.D., M.D.
851 Fremont Ave, Suite 104
Los Altos, CA 94024
(650) 229-1010
www.harmonywomenshealth.com
Email: drdebmetz@pol.net

• CHAPTER 9 •

Peter J. Muran, M.D., M.B.A.
SAN LUIS OBISPO, CA

Biography

Peter J. Muran, M.D., M.B.A. entered medical practice as an emergency room physician. Throughout his eight years in emergency medicine caring for the most critical conditions, he never lost his desire to provide care that effectively considered all aspects of the patient's well being.

Following his experience as an ER physician, he began to practice in what were two of the most innovative areas of health care at that time; in-home geriatric and hospice care. His experiences in these areas cemented his belief that optimal health care can only be achieved through consideration of the physical, emotional and spiritual facets of the patient. Dr. Muran is one of the world's leading experts in holistic, alternative and functional integrative medicine. He is a founding member of the American Board of Holistic and Integrative Medicine. In addition, he is a licensed medical physician with over twenty years of experience.

Dr. Muran specializes in Lyme disease and the related conditions that complicate recovery. He is a member of the International Lyme and Associated Diseases Society (ILADS). Raphael Stricker, M.D.,

247

Richard Horowitz, M.D. and Charles Ray Jones, M.D. were his preceptor supervisors.

Since his training in Western medicine doesn't enable him to address all aspects of his patients' health, he has also developed expertise in complementary healing techniques that draw upon the innovations and experiences of conventional and natural medicine.

In addition, he has become a recognized expert in the treatment of candidiasis and natural hormone replacement therapy, and in the use of chelation therapy for cardiac disease and heavy metal detoxification. He integrates traditional primary care, alternative and complementary medicine into his practice and his goal is to seek out the most effective and natural, as well as the least invasive means of promoting optimal health for his patients.

Dr. Muran currently practices functional medicine in partnership with his wife, Sandy Muran, PhD Clinical Nutritionist, at Longevity Healthcare for New Medicine in San Luis Obispo, CA. More information on Dr. Muran's work can be found on his website: www.longevityhealthcare.com.

(Note: The below article was reproduced with permission. Following the article, this chapter will resume with the presentation of information from Connie Strasheim's interview with Dr. Muran.)

Lyme Disease: A Functional Medicine Approach

By Peter J. Muran, M.D., ABIHM / Copyright © 2008

"Lyme disease is the latest great imitator and should be considered in the differential diagnosis of MS, ALS, seizure and other neurological conditions, as well as arthritis, CFS, Gulf War Syndrome, ADHD, hypochondriasis, fibromyalgia, somatization disorder and in patients with various difficult-to-diagnose multi-system syndromes." [1]

As Lyme disease spans the entire body, affecting all systems, an equally encompassing and individualized treatment approach is required to recover health. Functional Medicine [2, 3] is a comprehensive, individualized approach that focuses on the interrelated physiologic functions of the whole person, instead of on the disease itself. In my practice, Functional Medicine provides the context within which I can fully address the needs of my chronically ill patients. Their bodies are encouraged to heal when I relieve their systems of excessive stress and dysfunction at a cellular level.

The following diagram, Functional Medicine Matrix, identifies the components of my treatment approach and emphasizes the recovery of body function as the most effective means of combating disease. When treating Lyme disease, it is important to recognize that all bodily systems are interconnected. What appears to be an overwhelming treatment task, however, can be sorted out and points of dysfunction addressed, according to the Functional Medicine Matrix described below. Whenever this is effectively done, then the body is able to heal.

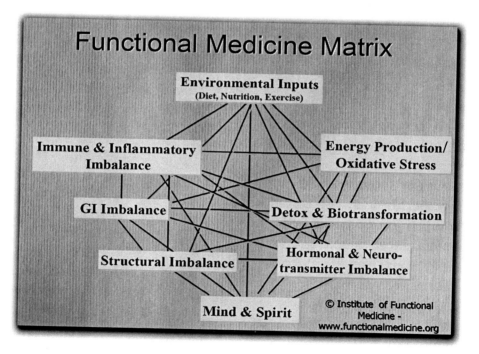

The following sections in this chapter illustrate the application of each component of the Functional Medicine Matrix, beginning at the top of the Matrix and proceeding clockwise. Emphasis is placed on how each area influences the treatment of Lyme disease and on how understanding the integration of the Matrix influences healing outcomes.

Environmental Inputs

This first point on the Matrix includes balanced nutrition coupled with regular exercise. Moderate exercise impacts the disease process by influencing gene expression, which leads to changes in the body's internal terrain. Exercise increases circulation and lymphatic flow throughout the body, thereby decreasing the collection of toxins that can further damage cells. Similarly, a lack of exercise results in gene expression that may trigger disease and increase toxicity, as well as render ineffective the body's overall functioning. Moderate exercise can be defined as the body in motion, and may include exercises such as daily walks, swimming or rebounding to tolerance.

Hippocrates' famous injunction to "let food be thy medicine" is conversely evident today as we see how industrialized food invokes disease. Simply, we are what we eat. Industrialized foods comprise the Standard American Diet (SAD diet), which consists of processed simple carbohydrates (white flour and sugar) that are stripped of nutrients, and which contain added artificial flavors, dyes, hormones and chemical preservatives. In the same manner that genetically modified and hormone- and/or antibiotic-laced feed grain increases fat deposition in animals, so too, the consumption of refined grains laden with chemicals increases fat deposition in humans. Most people are unaware that a cup of pasta, which is quickly converted to glucose, provides the same insulin impact upon the body as a Snickers® candy bar.

In recent decades, we had no choice about the source of our food. Supermarket shelves offered only industrialized or chemically treated foods, and proclaimed the scientific benefits of enriched, synthesized nutrients. After all, Tang® must be better than oranges, since it's the drink of astronauts, right?

Gratefully, today we have recovered the means to obtain foods that can be our medicine. Farmers' markets are ubiquitous and super-markets have organic food sections. People are increasingly interested in healthier, nutrient-rich, whole food diets that balance complex carbohydrates (fresh vegetables and fruits) and whole grains with proteins derived from hormone, antibiotic and preservative-free sources. Examples of these include the UltraMetabolism, Mediterranean, Zone, and South Beach diets. The benefits of eliminating attractively packaged, bleached white, unnatural foods have been documented to contribute to the proper management of cancer, obesity, diabetes, cardiovascular and autoimmune disease.

A proper diet is important for achieving health because food communicates a biological response to the body through the genes' signaling system, by sending it either dysfunctional or health-promoting messages. Healthy messages calm inflammation, strengthen the detoxification process, provide nutrients for effective metabolism, increase usable energy and influence the proper secretion of hormones. Laboratory tests can be performed which determine the body's nutritional balances and imbalances, as well as its cellular incorporation of nutrients, not just their concentration in the blood. Also, some clinicians successfully use other means of identifying nutritional stresses, such as Applied Kinesiology or Electro Dermal Screening (EDS).

A proper diet can be far-reaching in its effects; for preventing DNA damage, remedying genetic metabolic errors caused by enzyme deficiencies, providing the building materials for rejuvenation of the body, and decreasing cellular decay caused by oxidative stress.

Although it is impossible to recover and maintain health without nutritional balance, my patients, including those with Lyme disease, tend to resist dietary and lifestyle changes more than any other component of their treatment. They may take their nutritional supplements, but the use of these plays only a small role in achieving nutritional balance.

As reflected in the Matrix, there is an interconnection between diet, nutrition, and all of the body's organ systems and their biochemical and physiological processes. Conversely, all of the organ systems have a direct impact upon the body's ability to achieve proper nutrition. For example, an imbalance of the gastrointestinal (GI) tract can render useless nutrients that might otherwise make a positive contribution to the health of the body.

Further complicating the care of Lyme patients is the fact that they have high levels of food and environmental sensitivities, due largely to disruptions in their immune systems. These acquired sensitivities cause inflammation of their GI tracts, which then decreases the amount of nutrients that are available to their bodies. This increase in inflammation also produces an increase in antibodies, which affects the immunological system as large protein molecules leak through the walls of the intestine into the gut-associated lymphoid tissue (GALT). This causes the adrenal glands to become over-stimulated, as they produce more cortisol to overcome the inflammation, which subsequently starts a cascade of hormonal responses resulting in psychological changes and an increase in patients' struggle to get better. This explanation thus provides a panoramic view of how illness can affect the functioning of the whole body.

Energy Production and Oxidative Stress

The second point on the Functional Medicine Matrix involves addressing problems with energy and oxidative stress.

Many of my Lyme disease patients often say, "I'm so discouraged because I'm so tired all of the time. I can hardly find the energy to do the simplest things." Fortunately, managing the byproducts of energy production, oxidative stress, antioxidant defense and repair of oxidative damage, can restore energy and promote healing.

The conversion of nutrients into energy is accomplished by oxidation. The cells of the body can be likened to a mini-nuclear reactor that produces energy via oxidation. Like a nuclear reactor, the body needs to contain its energy production and byproducts in order to prevent harm to itself and so that it's able to repair the cells wherever containment of the energy reaction failed. Lethargy and fatigue are expressions of decreased energy production, as well as of a decrease in the containment of oxidative byproducts, which causes increased oxidative stress.

Fatigue is the most noticeable symptom of low energy production and high levels of oxidative stress. Insufficient detoxification and immunological response also contribute to the manifestation of this symptom.

Returning to the discussion of nutritional habits, oxidative stress is increased and immunological response decreased by an abundance of glucose, (which is created when people consume simple carbohydrates). The consumption of simple carbohydrates can also lead to insulin resistance, which, at some point, can become Syndrome X (also known as metabolic syndrome). Those with Syndrome X have a combination of elevated cholesterol and blood pressure, as well as a pronounced waistline and diabetes. Improper glycemic control is also a contributing factor to polycystic ovarian disease (PCOS) and adolescent obesity. These syndromes cause more inflammation in those with Lyme disease, which leads to increased infection and greater debilitation.

Laboratory tests can measure levels of oxidative stress in the body, as well as show the resultant DNA damage and toxicities that this stress causes. (Toxicities are stored chemicals in the body that decrease the efficiency of energy production). These values can then be used as markers to evaluate the improvement of patients' condition based on their physicians' interventions to reduce oxidative stress and improve immunological response.

Detoxification and Biotransformation

The next component of the Functional Medicine Matrix demonstrates how energy can be increased by freeing up resources in the body that are needed to make energy, balancing hormones, including the thyroid, and enhancing the body's overall metabolism.

Finally, it addresses the proper use of antioxidants, either from food or supplemental sources, which reduce oxidative damage and increase energy.

Detoxification is the metabolic process whereby toxins, facilitated by enzymes, are changed into less toxic or more readily removable substances that can be eliminated by the body. Biotransformation is the body's use of enzymes to cause a series of chemical alterations to a compound, especially when that compound is a drug, so that a different chemical than the original is formed for the body to use. The body's processing of medications is similar to its processing of toxins. The key to successful detoxification and biotransformation is the presence of specific enzymes in sufficient quantities to permit the chemical change.

If there are insufficient enzymes for proper detoxification, the result is increased toxicity, which increases cellular damage. This is best illustrated in cases of Parkinson's disease, which have increased 70% as a result of the increased use of pesticides and herbicides. Such chemical agents, when introduced into the body, are either improperly detoxified by the body or turned into more harmful products through improper biotransformation. This produces nerve cell dysfunction and possibly cellular death, and subsequently, diseases such as Parkinson's.

Enzyme production and variation is seated in the genetic structure of the DNA. Extensive work on genetic coding has provided insight into the duality of genetic expression. The body's DNA acquires its genetic expression and phenotype by means of the body's internal terrain, which is influenced by its exterior environment. The DNA switches on and off to form different messengers which then convey information throughout the body. Patients can have a balanced and healthy internal environment, or they may be nutritionally deficient and have an inflamed internal environment, which in turn affects their DNA expression. In any case, they control their internal environment by means of their lifestyle and dietary choices.

A good illustration of this is when women take folic acid prior to conception, because taking this B vitamin greatly reduces the possibility that their babies will develop a birth defect called spina bifida. This is an abnormality in which the spine is malformed and lacks its usual protective skeletal and soft tissue coverings. Folic acid deficiencies do not affect all pregnant women in the same way, however, which further illustrates how individualized genetic expression can be.

Knowing that:

1. Specific enzymes are the key to detoxification,

2. These enzymes are turned off and on by the genetic coding of the DNA,

3. DNA expression may be altered by external inputs to the internal environment ...

... then it follows that the effectiveness of the detoxification process is greatly dependent upon how we manage our internal environment.

Toxic load, by definition, is the sum total of the accumulation of chemicals or molecules that are foreign to our biological systems. Toxins may originate externally from toxic chemicals in the environment, and/or they may originate internally from foods that we eat or medications or supplements that we take.

Doing a laboratory evaluation of Phases I and II of the liver detoxification process is the first step in determining what needs to be done to invigorate the body's detoxification pathways. This information, when coupled with the patient's genetic coding for detoxification and biotransformation, provides the road map, or instructions, that are needed for reducing the body's toxic load and improving the detoxification process.

As demonstrated in the Functional Medicine Matrix, detoxification and oxidative stress are closely related. The improvement of one usually leads to improvement of the other. The management of one's internal environment through proper diet and nutrition greatly and positively influences the body's DNA signaling processes. Yet, the integration of the Matrix's other components plays a role, too. For instance, when there is an imbalance of intestinal flora (which causes bloating, Candida overgrowth or Leaky Gut syndrome), then the GI tract absorbs toxins from other living organisms throughout the body, thereby increasing the body's overall toxic load. This then changes the body's expression of DNA, and leads to the production of inflammatory proteins.

Hormonal and Neurotransmitter Imbalances

The endocrine system is a control system that maintains a stable internal environment in the body through the production of chemical regulatory substances called hormones and neurotransmitters (which are involved in brain chemistry). The endocrine system responds either through sensory inputs via the brain or through direct environmental and food exposures, the former of which are mediated by the immune and digestive systems. The dynamic interplay of all the factors included in the Functional Medicine Matrix gives rise to a balance or imbalance of the endocrine system, which then affects the synthesis and secretion of messenger chemicals to cells throughout the body.

It's important to note here that balance and imbalance are relative terms for positive and negative sensory information. A positive sensory response promotes growth and reproduction, along with energy, a vibrant immune system and vitality. Positive sensory response is associated with balanced levels of the hormone insulin, which has an anabolic, or building, effect upon the body when it interacts with other minor anabolic hormones such as growth hormone, thyroid, estrogen, testosterone and DHEA. A negative sensory response leads to the body avoiding the toxins found within its cells and a contractual response, which results in the body shutting down as it decreases its growth and reproduction. Depression and immune suppression also result from this type of response. Two major stress response hormones, cortisol and adrenaline, are implicated in negative sensory responses, as a chronic, excessive response of these two hormones is found in many neurological and cardiovascular maladies.

The body's hormonal signaling system affects all of its functions, from glucose metabolism to inflammation and cognitive capacity. All of the hormones work together to create a symphony of health, and whenever there is disharmony between any of them, a thorough investigation must be done to determine the reasons why this is happening. Simply replacing hormones without such an investigation can result in imbalances that create new clinical risks and complications for patients. Hence, a laboratory and clinical understanding of their individual situation is important for establishing a proper treatment protocol. Determining individual hormonal interactions, investigating cellular sensitivity to hormone messages and availability of transport binding proteins, as well as detoxification capacity at cellular receptor sites, are factors that practitioners should consider when attempting to safely restore hormonal harmony to their patients. A follow-up evaluation on patients is also required so that any changes that develop over time can be appropriately addressed.

A balanced endocrine symphony supports the function of every bodily system. Of particular concern for those with Lyme disease is the interplay between the adrenal and thyroid glands, although all endocrine instruments must be considered. If one is out of tune, then all are affected.

Mind and Spirit

Both the mind and spirit play an integral role in physical health.

> *"Even the greatest skeptic must now admit that a wealth of evidence exists to prove, in the most stringent scientific terms, that the functions of the mind influence the health of the body, and that sickness in the body can affect our moods and emotions through molecules and nerve pathways"* [4]

Healing the mind and spirit is of utmost importance for overcoming Lyme disease, and Functional Medicine recognizes the influence of emotional and spiritual health on all other components of the Matrix.

Groundbreaking work published in 1993 by neuroscientist Candace Pert, M.D., identified the physical and molecular expression of these intangible aspects of health:

> *"We must take responsibility for the way we feel. The notion that others can make us feel good or bad is untrue...Why we feel the way we do is the result of the symphony and harmony of our own molecules of emotion that affect every aspect of our physiology."* [5]

Our mind and spirit affect our emotions, which in turn directly impact stress mediators of functional health. Problems in these areas, for example, can manifest in immune system suppression, elevated levels of cortisol, central obesity, an increase in inflammatory cytokines within the brain, and in symptoms of brain aging, such as memory impairment.

A popular artist, Sally Hass, conveys this idea in one of her works. "Attitude is everything, pick a good one." How one achieves a balance of mind and spirit is as unique to each individual as his/her DNA. Recovery and the maintenance of health are dependent upon those with Lyme recognizing and attending to this aspect of their healing, along with all others found in the Matrix.

Structural Imbalance

Addressing and treating structural problems is crucial for the proper treatment of Lyme disease, since Lyme (Borrelia) destroys the musculoskeletal system. Migratory musculoskeletal pain is usually one of the first heralding symptoms of Lyme disease. Sometimes this is further complicated by an autoimmune presentation that is often diagnosed as rheumatoid arthritis (RA). Rheumatoid arthritis is one of the common look-alike diagnoses of Lyme disease. When the Lyme disease is properly treated, however, some of those with a rheumatoid arthritis diagnosis will undergo a degree of remission, dependent on the degree of joint destruction in their bodies.

In keeping with the confusion and complexity of Lyme yet others with RA may experience a continuation of their symptoms, even following treatment for Lyme disease, and this has been demonstrated both clinically and in laboratory testing. Such "dual diagnoses" individuals must monitor and decrease as many inflammatory factors as possible that are contributing to their symptoms. A medication-only route to reducing inflammation can suppress the immune system and complicate the body's healing. My Functional Medicine approach addresses treating inflammation via non-pharmaceutical means, which reduces the possibility of patients needing to take anti-inflammatory medications for RA symptoms.

Also, it's important to note that any increase in joint and muscle discomfort in Lyme patients leads to increased structural compensations and improper use of muscle groups, which further contributes to destabilization of the spine and increases the risk for injury. The accompanying chronic pain also creates neurogenic inflammation, which sets the stage for the development of chronic fatigue or fibromyalgia syndromes.

Substantial evidence exists to suggest that inflammatory joint disease is also directly related to inflammatory bowel disease, as suggested by these quotations from journals of rheumatology:

> "In ankylosing spondylitis the incidence of gut inflammation was significantly higher … These findings provide further arguments … joints disease is triggered through the gut." [6]

> "The arthritis also resolved promptly, suggesting that it was associated with the bowel disorder." [7]

Conversely, resolution of bowel inflammation leads to a resolution of joint inflammation.

Gastrointestinal Imbalance

The next component of the Functional Medicine Matrix addresses gastrointestinal imbalances. Such imbalances are evidenced by defects in the body's absorptive and digestive functions and are based primarily on an imbalance of the intestinal flora and a break-down in its mucosal integrity.

A breakdown in the intestine's mucosal integrity results in de-creased nutrient uptake and activation of the gut-associated lymphoid tissue (GALT) and mucosa-associated lymphoid tissue (MALT), which represent 70% of the immune system. There is significant documentation in the medical literature to demonstrate that gut, liver and immune function are all interrelated. For exam-ple, the following quote hints at how a problem with the gut can affect the immune system:

> *"An elevated prevalence of clinical and sub-clinical thyroid autoimmunity was found in Sardinian celiac patients"* [8]

The Functional Medicine approach to strengthening the gut is called the "4R Program," and involves:

- REMOVING any causative agents of intestinal distress, including food allergies and sensitivities, antigens, pathogens and parasites

- REPLACING the enzymes necessary for digestion, and

- RE-INOCULATING the bowel with friendly intestinal prebiotics and probiotics

These are then followed by:

- REPAIR of the gut mucosal integrity nutrients.

Dr. Jeffery Bland comments,

> *"Basic science and clinical observation indicate that significant signals that control (metabolic) function are being sent from the gut as it is*

exposed to the products of food and microbiological activity. The gut translates the message it receives and sends it on to the rest of the body through the release of various mediators that influence receptor sites on tissues very distant from the gut. The influence can be associated with diseases ranging from dementia to cardiovascular disease, liver disease and behavioral disorders in childhood, potentially even autism." [9]

One of the cornerstones of Lyme disease treatment is aggressive antibiotic therapy, which further disrupts the balance of the GI tract and results in an overgrowth of Candida. Candidiasis can become a chronic condition, making its own destructive contribution to systemic health. Dietary changes to discourage Candida growth, along with the 4R program, can re-balance the gastrointestinal tract.

Restoring GI balance increases the effectiveness of nutritional therapy and the immune system. Increased immunological response and the reduction of other inflammatory factors, in turn, improves patients' chances of overcoming Lyme disease.

Immune and Inflammatory Imbalance

Inflammation and immune imbalance are among the foremost characteristics of Lyme disease. By comprehensively addressing the preceding aspects of the Matrix, an automatic support of immune system function at the cellular level results.

Usually, when people think of allergies or immune system activation, an antigen-antibody response (which is determined by blood testing), or the classical immunological pathway, comes to mind. The problem is that there are several immunological pathways other then the classical one through which an immunological response can occur, and which can cause a cascading inflammatory reaction. Hence, identifying the primary causative agent of inflammation and the symptoms that are caused thereby is important, in order to reduce or modulate the proper inflammatory immunological pathways.

The immune system can intensify its response to toxins via complement activation, which means that one of its actions creates an amplified cascade of reactions throughout the body. This is very similar to the "Butterfly Effect", whereby a minuscule action can lead to a large overwhelming effect. The immune system may also function in an opposite manner, with a single response creating a calming, balancing effect throughout the body. Hence, optimizing diet, nutrition and exercise, increasing energy production and reducing oxidative stress, using detoxification protocols, re-balancing hormones and neurotransmitters, attending to the mind and spirit, implementing structural therapies and optimizing the GI environment, all contribute to a healing response along all immune system pathways and to a subsequent strengthening of the system. A strong immune system can then respond better to Lyme disease infections.

Conclusion

In closing, there is not and never will be a medication that can surpass the ability of the body to overcome disease and promote health. The key to health lies in the body's ability to efficiently express its DNA code, and in our ability to redirect any imbalances that cause illness, by enhancing the functionality of our internal environment.

When we consider all of the factors that contribute to illness, the task of recovering health appears insurmountable at first. However, the Functional Medicine Matrix provides a practical road map to recovery. By working clockwise from the top of the Matrix and addressing the components to healing contained therein, those with Lyme disease can rediscover health, and especially when they work in partnership with a Functional Medicine practitioner.

(End reproduced article)

Note: The following information is based on Connie Strasheim's interview with Dr. Muran, which focused on Lyme disease treatment guidelines and their application to the principles found in the Functional Medicine Matrix.

Treatment Approach for Borrelia and Lyme-Related Infections

I follow the antibiotic regimen used by the ILADS physicians,[10] but antibiotics are just a part of my treatment approach for Lyme-related infections.

My protocol for patients depends upon many factors, including the severity of their symptoms and how they present those symptoms. Lyme disease is best managed symptomatically; in other words, by the symptoms that patients present, rather than by laboratory evidence. Laboratory tests can present too many false negatives and practitioners might miss important aspects of their patients' diagnoses if they rely exclusively upon labs. Symptoms provide a better indication of the infections that patients have.

Symptomatic indicators also provide me with an understanding of the severity of my patients' disease. I introduce antibiotics into my patients' regimens in a stepwise, or incremental fashion, which decreases the possibility of them having any unwanted reactions. I will usually start by prescribing two antibiotics that disrupt the replication of the bacteria, (which are called bacteriostatic, or intracellular drugs), and follow those with an antibiotic that attacks the cell wall form of Borrelia, (such antibiotics are called bactericidal or extracellular drugs). If no adverse symptoms or laboratory changes result from these antibiotics then I will subsequently treat their Borrelia cysts using a pulsed antibiotic regimen.

If I'm working with patients who are exhibiting strong neurological symptoms, then I will usually initiate their treatment with some form of parenteral therapy, which involves the administration of an intramuscular or IV cell-wall inhibiting drug, such as Bicillin or Rocephin. If they tolerate this, then I will slowly introduce an intracellular drug, such as minocycline or azithromycin, into their regimen. Going slow with these medications is important, because

I've learned that the worst thing that I can do is to increase my patients' inflammation by adding too many drugs, too fast, to their regimens. A lot of people think that it's good to have a Herxheimer reaction, but I don't necessarily believe this to be true. "Herxing" sets the body back in its healing, by creating an inflammatory reaction that the body now has to deal with, along with the infections.

The threshold on treatment, however, should be determined by patients' level of improvement on a particular regimen. If they aren't improving, then I know that their regimen needs to be changed. The rate at which improvement should occur depends also upon the severity of their symptoms and where those symptoms reside.

Laboratory evidence has demonstrated that the borrelia organism exists in three forms: as a spirochete with a cell membrane, as a spirochete without a cell membrane and as a cystic or biofilm-encapsulated form. The cell membrane form, which is the most active form, responds quickly to penicillins and cephalosporins. Treatments for this form, however, tend to increase the presence of the cell-wall deficient (also known as L-form) of the bacteria. This L-form is resistant to penicillins and cephalosporins, as is the cystic form. When treating patients with neurological Lyme, it is important for practitioners to quickly reduce the most active form of the organism (that which has a cell-wall) using Bicillin, long acting penicillin, or Rocephin. At the same time, it's important that they slowly introduce an intracellular antibiotic, such as minocycline, azithromycin or Bactrim DS into their patients' regimens. Slowly introducing these medications avoids the potential for creating too much inflammation in the body or a Herxheimer reaction that is too strong for patients to manage.

If my patients have symptoms that more closely resemble those found in CFS (Chronic Fatigue Syndrome), then I view such symptoms as being caused by an imbalance in the endocrine system that was created by Lyme and co-infections. I perform a saliva cortisol test on such patients, and look for a drop in the phasing of their diurnal cortisol cycle. Any abnormal hormonal response (i.e., low cortisol in the morning hours) reflects an inability of their bodies to manage chronic stress, which means that symptoms in those with CFS-like symptoms are not necessarily reflective of just Lyme disease, but of problems in their endocrine system, as well. Such patients require not only antibiotics, but also a protocol to balance their hormones, if they are to fully heal.

The number of antibiotics that patients require also depends upon their response to treatments. For example, if they get diarrhea, or other problematic symptoms as a result of medications, then I have to change the course of their treatment. There is an ongoing type of treatment "positioning" that occurs by practitioners when treating chronically ill patients. Like playing chess, they have to constantly revise their moves.

For instance, when my patients get migratory arthralgia or joint pain, this indicates to me that they have an active Borrelia infection. At the same time, however, I must consider the possibility that Borrelia is activating an autoimmune response in them, which can cause rheumatoid symptoms and joint degeneration. Whenever this is the case, then I know that I am dealing with a specific type of antibody response, not just strictly Lyme disease. So when formulating a treatment plan, I must take into account all possible reasons for my patients' symptoms.

Diagnosis and treatment is further complicated by the practitioner having to determine which major immunological pathway that the disease is following. Paul Cheney, M.D., best describes the Th1 and Th2 immune pathways in his paper on balancing the Th1/Th2 immune system.[11] In short, he writes that the Th1 response cells generally combat intracellular bacteria, cancer, yeast and viruses. Normal (extracellular) bacteria, parasites, toxins and allergens usually trigger a Th2 response. Viruses and Lyme have a tendency to divert the immunological system from the Th1 mode that fights intracellular Lyme to the Th2 mode that does not. This tends to be similar to the shifts that are seen in other diseases like multiple sclerosis, where patients shift between a Th1 and Th2 response. An excessive Th2 response hinders the immune system's ability to effectively combat Lyme, and for that reason, imbalances in these responses must be corrected.

Other Common Infections Found in Those with Lyme Disease

Besides the common Lyme disease co-infections, I find that Mycoplasma fermentans, Mycoplasma pneumoniae and Chlamydia pneumoniae are prevalent infections in my patients, as well as Candida albicans or other forms of yeast. While C. albicans is the most common fungal infection, patients can also have other forms, which, like other Lyme co-infections, cause night sweats. Fungi are opportunistic and proliferate as immune function declines.

I use lab tests to help me determine whether my patients have opportunistic infections and co-infections, as well as what treatments are most appropriate for these. Once I have established a protocol for treating such infections, I watch for symptomatic changes in my patients over time to determine the effectiveness of their particular protocol.

Babesia and Bartonella

If patients have Lyme disease that isn't responding to treatment or if their symptoms are protracted, then they are probably also dealing with a co-infection, such as Babesia. Babesia mimics the malaria organism in the timing of its life cycle, which is shorter than that of Borrelia's. Borrelia cycles every three to four weeks, and patient symptom flares coincide with the timing of this cycle, but with Babesia, the life cycle is shorter, about every two to three weeks.

My standard antibiotic protocol for Babesia and Bartonella is similar to that of ILADS, but as I mentioned previously, I take a functional approach to medicine, which doesn't solely involve the administration of a standard, systematic antibiotic protocol.

Dietary Recommendations

My approach to diet for those with Lyme disease follows the model advocated by the Institute of Functional Medicine (an organization that equips and trains physicians to treat the underlying clinical imbalances of chronic disease). This diet focuses on restoring gastrointestinal tract function, and on avoiding foods that are inflammatory.

When determining patient sensitivities or allergies to food, it's important for practitioners to look not only at their patients' anti-body test results, (such as to gluten), because it's possible for the body to have a negative cellular response to a food without actually creating antibodies to it.

Fortunately, Sandy Muran, a Ph.D. nutritionist, works in partner practice with me and is able to determine the food allergies and sensitivities that patients have, beyond their usual antibody responses, using the Zyto Limbic Stress Assessment (LSA) system. The Zyto is a device that functions according a principle similar to that first developed by Dr. Voll, whose work dates back to the early 1940's. Basically, Dr. Voll demonstrated that if a person is sensitive to something (in this case, a food), then he or she will have a built-up resistance in the body to electrical conductivity when exposed to that food. The concept of the Zyto, LSA is based upon this principle, as is Applied Kinesiology. Dr. Muran also uses NAET, which is a technique used to desensitize patients to foods and other allergens. Eliminating food allergies helps to lower the body's total stress load and improves its immune response.

The Problem of Getting Patients to Change Their Diets

One of my biggest challenges as a practitioner is getting my patients to change their diets. I can't tell you how difficult this is. If I had a nickel for every time that I get a patient with a whopping gluten or yeast problem and who doesn't understand the importance of this issue, I would be rich! For example, whenever I tell patients that they can't eat wheat products, refined carbohydrates or gluten, they say things like, "Well, can I still have my ice-cream?" So it's really a problem, but to get to the next level of healing, they must understand that food is information for the metabolic function of the body and the quality of their choices determines at a very basic level the quality of their metabolic function.

Also, I have found that the question of dietary compliance is subject to broad interpretation by patients. Sometimes they say, for instance, "I've done everything that you told me to, and I'm still not getting better." Or, "I'm not losing weight." I will then ask them to keep a log of what they are eating, and when they do, I find that they are eating foods that are contraindicated for their healing. When I can get them to make the appropriate changes, they then start losing weight and feeling better. It's a constant challenge, though.

Finally, weight reduction is actually a big indicator of whether or not people with Lyme disease are getting rid of toxins. When they don't lose weight, then it means that they aren't getting rid of toxins.

One thing that I do to help my patients modify their diets is give them amino acids, which modify neurotransmitters. By prescribing amino acids, such as L-tyrosine, L-tryptophan, 5-HTP, and GABA, I am able to cause a shift in their craving for caffeine and other unhealthy foods. Patients self-medicate with certain foods in order to manage their symptoms. Unfortunately, it becomes a psycho-physiological problem, and sometimes, I end up with patients with food addictions that need to be managed both psychologically and physiologically. I can't get them to stop medicating themselves, however, without first explaining to them why the process is happening and then helping them to do something about that. If patients have caffeine addictions, for instance, I will look at their diurnal cortisol pattern and neurotransmitter levels and provide support to both their hormones and neurotransmitters, to bring these up to an optimum level, which in turn reduces their cravings for caffeine.

Other Uses for Amino Acids

All proteins are made from different combinations of amino acids. Amino acids that must be obtained from the diet are called "essential amino acids", while amino acids that the body can manufacture on its own from other sources are called "non-essential" amino acids. Sometimes, the body can't properly produce sufficient amounts of the non-essential amino acids and for such cases, supplementation is required.

The body utilizes proteins to determine biological function and to control most processes at the cellular level. Therefore, it is reasonable to conclude that a deficiency or over-utilization of certain amino acids can negatively impact the body and lead eventually to symptoms. Laboratories can measure patients' amino acid levels by taking urine samples from them. They can also compound amino acid supplements, which are then prescribed to patients to correct for any nutritional deficiencies. For instance, amino acids that interact with opiate receptors can be prescribed to decrease pain. Such amino acids include the essential amino acid phenylalanine, which is used by the brain to produce norepinephrine, a chemical that transmits signals between nerve cells in the brain, promotes alertness and vitality, elevates mood, decreases pain, and aids in memory and learning. In addition, this amino acid is used to treat arthritis, depression, menstrual cramps, migraines, obesity, Parkinson's disease, and schizophrenia. When used in conjunction with enzymes that are needed to promote its conversion to the appropriate protein, phenylalanine can heal the above-mentioned conditions and/or symptoms.

The Usefulness of Metabolic Testing

When formulating a protocol for my patients, I also perform lab tests to determine what metabolites their bodies are processing. Usually, I will use urine labs for these, but blood and serum tests can be useful, too. Blood tests are useful because technicians are able to remove and process cells to determine intracellular deficiencies. An analogy is important here. The blood is composed of many elements that can mostly be categorized as cells and fluid, or serum. Testing serum doesn't accurately reflect the overall composition of the body at a cellular level. It's like the ocean and the fish. The fish have a constitution that's different than the water in which they are swimming, yet the constitution of the fish is influenced by the water in which they live. So it's important to discover what the body is actually using inside of the cells in order to obtain an accurate evaluation of its overall metabolism, which is why it's important to be able to examine the cells, not just the serum.

The Role of Emotional Trauma in Illness

Emotional health significantly impacts the healing process. People with Lyme disease, just like those in the general population, possess varying degrees of emotional health and resilience. Whatever their level of emotional health, I encourage my patients to integrate some form of emotional and spiritual practice into their treatment regimen which will support their efforts to heal on all levels.

One resource that we in my practice provide is a free meditation group that meets at our office. Both patients and community members are welcome to attend free of charge.

Detoxification

Energy Medicine Strategies for Detoxification

In my practice, we work with ONDAMED, a device that's effective for detoxification and balancing the body's energy, both of which are important components to healing. In Chinese medicine, it's believed that there are blockages that occur within the body's energy meridians, or channels. By opening up the meridians and balancing the body's energy chakras or healing centers, healing can be accomplished, and the ONDAMED is a device that many of my patients have found to be useful for this purpose.

We also use homeopathy for treating certain conditions, as well as for liver detoxification and for supporting the other organs of excretion. Additionally, we use it to bolster our patients' immune systems.

There are two types of homeopathy that I see my patients benefiting from. In the first, which is classical homeopathy, remedies are developed based upon the individual patient's characteristics and symptom presentation. In the second, which is mixed homeopathy, remedies are more cookbook-like and standardized for certain conditions. The type of approach that I use is based upon patient response and the condition being treated. Lyme-literate physician Dr. Richard Horowitz, M.D., is doing exceptional work with homeopathy, in conjunction with Dr. Lee Cowden, M.D.

Other Detoxification Strategies

Another component of detoxification involves getting rid of biotoxins. Genetics factors into people's ability to detoxify. If they have the genetic capability for recognizing toxins and getting rid of them, then this is one less problem that needs to be addressed in the healing process. The problem of compromised detoxification due to genetic variation is illustrated well by Dr. Ritchie Shoemaker in his book, *Mold Warriors*.[12] Dr. Shoemaker describes his experiences with patients whose genes interfere with their bodies' ability to recognize and remove biotoxins. Biotoxin levels must be reduced in order to reduce the overall toxic burden placed on the immune and hormonal systems.

In order to effectively do this, however, the source of biotoxins must be discovered, and an effective protocol formulated for their removal. When dealing with patients who have neurological Lyme disease symptoms, for example, it's important for practitioners to first determine whether their patients' symptoms are a result of their genetic immunological constitution, and whether this constitution prevents mold and other biotoxins from clearing from their bodies. It's also important to determine whether their symptoms result strictly from the Borrelia organism, or from a combination of the above and other factors. That symptoms can have multiple causes, and that tests are fallible, creates treatment challenges for practitioners.

A large amount of detoxification occurs in the liver, and is usually managed in two phases. Jeffrey Bland, one of the founders of The Institute for Functional Medicine, eloquently describes how these phases affect healing. Basically, he states that in Phase 1, the toxin is prepared to be "packaged" for easier excretion by the body. In Phase 2, it's packaged for removal by the body. If there is an error in the Phase 1 or 2 processes, due either to genetics or vitamin or enzyme deficiencies, then this will cause a build-up of toxins in both the liver and bloodstream, which then increases the burden on the immune and hormonal systems.

If patients are able to detoxify and remove substances from their bodies, then healing may just be a matter of increasing their immune function, decreasing their bodily stress caused by infections, and adopting a healthy diet and emotional attitude.

One thing that I do in my practice and which is different than some other Lyme doctors is to administer intravenous forms of Vitamin C and other nutrients to my patients. The IV's stop night sweats and other aspects of Herxheimer reactions, and I have had great responses using this therapy.

Healing the Gut

To heal the gut, and as described in the Functional Medicine Matrix section of this chapter, it's essential to get rid of the pathogens that are found there. Parasites, as well as pathogenic bacterial and fungal flora must be addressed. When treating patients, I also look for other problems in their GI tracts such as gluten sensitivity, poor absorption of long-chain fatty acids, and poor creation of short-chain fatty acids. Many practitioners, when they test their patients for gluten sensitivities or allergies, only look at patient antibody response to gluten. However, if the surface of the intestinal tract has a very low capability for producing an antibody response, then patients may test negative on a gluten sensitivity test, yet may still react to gluten, as evidenced by their inflamed gastrointestinal tracts. I see this happen often.

Treatment for gastrointestinal problems, like all areas of healing, is highly individualized. It's unfortunate, because readers might want to know specific details about my treatment protocol, but because every patient has different needs, I can't say that there is a standard protocol that I use for everyone. Also, determining treatment regimens is like playing in a labyrinth. Every time I go down a corridor of treatment for a particular patient, it's as if the labyrinth opens up and becomes more complicated and I find that there are yet more issues that I must contend with in that patient. So I go down another corridor where the patient has a positive response to treatment, and as soon as I go down that corridor, the same thing happens, revealing yet more issues or problems that must be dealt with. That's why treatment must be individualized; it's why I need to have the patient in front of me, so that I know which corridors to go down and so that I can see which doors are going to open up for me and the patient.

In general, to treat gut infections, I prescribe both pharmaceutical drugs and herbs, along with digestive support aids. These include various types of anti-parasitic medications, from oil of oregano all the way down to black walnut, digestive enzymes, and betaine HCL with pepsin. So I work with a large repertoire of remedies, taking into account factors such as patient sensitivity to different remedies. Because if I give my patients a remedy to get rid of their fungus or parasites, and they are sensitive to that remedy, then it can increase their gut inflammation, which in turn causes them to improperly absorb their food. This then leads to leakage of large food proteins into their GALT (gut-associated lymphoid tissue) and creates what is called Leaky Gut Syndrome. As mentioned in the Functional Medicine Matrix section, this syndrome creates a drop in immune system function, which means that the expression of the inflammatory response in the gut ends up affecting the whole body. This is another reason why treatment needs to be individualized and personalized, and why I can't write a cookbook for this type of medicine.

Treating Hormonal Dysfunction

Practitioners must take into account many hormones when balancing their patients' hormonal profiles. For the purposes of this book, it is best to only briefly mention a few of the most common imbalances here, which involve thyroid, cortisol, estrogen, progesterone, testosterone and DHEA hormones. The three most common ways to measure hormone levels is through blood, urine and saliva tests. A blood test is convenient and easy to do but is not always indicative of active hormone levels because it doesn't take into account binding proteins, which are sometimes present and which bind up or reduce the bio-availability of hormones. Accurate measurement of a hormone's availability is better accomplished with a 24-hour urine test, which is especially useful when paired with serum test results. Salivary tests can also be useful, and the results from this type of test usually reflect the amount of hormone that is available to the body, but there have been problems with establishing an appropriate "normal" range of results for patients. For this reason, I only use salivary testing for two things: to look at my patients' cortisol cycling or if I want to see how a woman's estrogen and progesterone levels change throughout her monthly cycle.

When determining thyroid function, many practitioners will look only at TSH and free T4 hormones in their patients' blood test results. In doing so, they miss the next layer of the profile, which involves testing for T3 (the principal active form of thyroid hormone) as well as reverse T3, which is a less active form of thyroid hormone that indirectly competes with the formation of active T3. The body creates an increase in reverse T3 under conditions of inflammation, pregnancy, famine and illness, which in turn decreases the body's metabolic rate and creates symptoms that are very similar to those of hypothyroidism, including constipation, hair loss, fatigue, weight gain and dry skin, just to name a few. If practitioners only test TSH, free T3 and freeT4 in patients whose symptoms appear to reflect hypothyroidism, then these patients might not be considered to have hypothyroidism, because their test results may turn out to be normal, even though their levels of available T3 are in reality, low.

I generally use bioidentical hormones to correct my patients' hormonal deficiencies. Use of bioidentical hormones is especially important for supplementing estrogen deficiencies in women. Conjugated equine estrogen (Provera) is commonly prescribed to women, and has been construed in the medical community as being a "normal" form of estrogen replacement, but there is a big difference between the natural estrogen that women produce, and the estrogen that a horse produces. Equine estrogen causes inflammation, but there are political and economic reasons why this medication is so widely prescribed. Yet, it has been scientifically documented in the medical literature that such estrogen causes inflammation and alters hormonal balance.

It's the ingestion or production of inflammatory estrogen that causes breast cancer in women and prostate cancer in men. The medical community must consider a very important fact when linking breast cancer with estrogen. If all estrogens were the cause of breast cancer, then the prevalence of this disease would be high in women who are in their twenties and thirties, but it's not. Only certain types of inflammatory estrogen, the levels of which tend to be elevated in those with unhealthy bodies, or which result from taking certain pharmaceutical medications, cause breast cancer. Also, as women age, the risk of them producing inflammatory estrogen increases, as does their risk for cancer. They may start to produce more estrone from fat cells, which can be easily converted to an inflammatory estrogen. This inflammatory estrogen, which is a pre-carcinogenic form of estrogen, attaches to cells at estrogen receptor sites, where it can produce cancerous cells. Hence, supplementing with bioidentical estrogen is most appropriate for women with estrogen deficiencies.

Women with progesterone deficiencies also benefit from bioidentical progesterone, which is better than the synthetic progestin that is so commonly prescribed. Using bioidentical estrogen and progesterone in combination is beneficial, and many women have used both throughout all of their healthy reproductive years.

When men's bodies are stressed by inflammation or illness, including Lyme disease, then their total and bio-available levels of testosterone usually drop. It has become almost too common for practitioners to treat low testosterone with supplemental testosterone, but such liberal use of testosterone may lead to testicular atrophy, a condition whereby the testicles stop producing testosterone and shrink. In many cases of premature testosterone replacement, the testicles are unable to recover from the use of pharmaceutical testosterone and the men who use it become dependent upon the pharmaceutical medication to maintain their vigor. Testosterone, however, is very important for men's health and mental well being, and properly addressing deficiencies is important, so that they can eventually build up their own production of this hormone.

When stress or inflammation is present in the body, the hormones, of which cortisol is a major player, are set off balance. When people are exposed to increased chronic stress or inflammation, they then begin to develop a profile of adrenal fatigue. Cortisol is one of many hormones produced by the adrenal glands and a chronic stress environment will lead to a higher demand for this hormone than the adrenal glands are able to produce and maintain.

When determining my patients' adrenal function, I have them do a diurnal saliva cortisol test, in order to establish what their cortisol levels are at different times during the day. This information is then charted on a graph. I have found that treating them with low dose bioidentical hydrocortisone can be beneficial when given during the time of day that their chart, or graph, shows a "dip" in their cortisol levels. In any case, the goal should always be to bring the body's cortisol levels up to normal, during the times of day when they are low. Doing so helps to balance the body's overall cortisol pattern.

The bioidentical hydrocortisone that I use in my practice contains a compounded base of Vitamin C. I don't prescribe pharmaceutical cortisol because it's made with other compounds that can be harmful to patients. Also and as previously mentioned, I use only low dose, physiological levels of cortisol, as described in William McK Jefferies' book, *Safe Uses of Cortisol*. Also, the cortisol that I use is very short acting with a half-life of four hours. Using this type of cortisol prevents accumulation of the medication in the body as well as any unwanted side effects.

To treat adrenal fatigue, I may also give my patients cortisol precursors, such as pregnenolone and/or DHEA, along with adrenal-supporting nutrients, so that the body can eventually make enough of its own cortisol. Licorice root, bioflavonoids and B-vitamins are among such nutrients. In the end, however, to adequately treat adrenal fatigue, I must look at its underlying cause, which includes all of the factors that I describe in the Functional Medicine Matrix. The underlying cause isn't always Lyme disease.

Finally, many people with Lyme disease have some degree of insulin resistance, and I believe that diet and exercise are mainstay solutions for solving this problem. Unfortunately, exercise can be a problem for those who are really fatigued, so I may also recommend that my patients take alpha-lipoic acid, which helps to lower insulin resistance, as well as L-carnitine, which helps the body to utilize the glucose that it has available to it to make energy.

Bacterial Behavior, Inflammation, and Hypercoagulation

In the Functional Medicine Matrix section of this chapter, I discuss the reasons why it's important to reduce inflammation in order to heal the body from Lyme disease. Here, I will discuss a couple of other reasons why reducing excessive inflammation is important, apart from what I already mentioned in the preceding sections.

First, borrelia is in some regard, opportunistic. It's a stealth bug that waits until the immune system is weakened before fully unleashing its devastating effects upon the body. In the meantime, it remains dormant inside the cells, waiting for an opportune moment to attack. It has a genetic code, and the only thing that it's meant to do is propagate. It doesn't really care if it's flourishing, so if it's put into a hostile environment, it will simply shut down into cystic form. When conditions become more favorable for its propagation, then it will grow, so it's important to keep the body's levels of inflammation down, so that the immune system will be ready and effective against it.

Also, excessive inflammation causes hypercoagulation, a condition in which the blood becomes more viscous and syrupy. Whenever this happens, blood can't flow into capillaries properly. Borrelia happens to be a low oxygen pressure organism, unlike tuberculosis or Mycoplasma, which are high oxygen pressure organisms. The latter infections rest in the apices of lungs, where the highest concentrations of oxygen in the body are found, whereas borrelia hides in tissues where the lowest concentrations of oxygen are found. For this reason, addressing hypercoagulation is important, so that blood (and oxygen) can get to the cracks, crevices and crannies of the body, where borrelia resides.

When treating my patients for this condition, I first establish a coagulation profile for them based on test results. Then I use enzymes, as well as sublingual heparin, to break down blood fibrin products that occur as a result of hypercoagulation. Hypercoagulation also leads to endothelial dysfunction. (The term "endothelial" refers to the lining of the inside of the arteries). If this lining is coated with blood fibrin products, then the arteries will become and stay constricted, which then results in hypertension. Using serrapeptase or a proteolytic enzyme diminishes the endothelial fibrin coating and normalizes blood pressure.

Treatments for Symptomatic Relief

For Insomnia

Several factors must be taken into account when treating patients' insomnia. First of all, pharmaceutical drugs are not always the best solution for this symptom, because inflammation is often an underlying cause of insomnia, and if I can reduce my patients' inflammation, then I can resolve their insomnia, too. High night-time cortisol levels are one indication that inflammation is present in the body, so if I can decrease that inflammatory response, then I notice that my patients' cortisol levels will also drop and that they will then sleep better.

For Fatigue

To increase my patients' energy, I sometimes recommend that they take nutraceutical supplements such as D-ribose, which is a great sugar that aids in heart function. One great combination of nutrients that creates healthier mitochondria, (which is the energy source of every cell), is alpha lipoic acid, resveratrol and arginine. Many other strategies increase energy as well, but the greatest improvements in energy occur when practitioners take their patients' entire profile into account. For example, there might be a food that they are eating that's causing their adrenals to be stressed and which is in turn decreasing their energy. It's usually not just one thing, however. Multiple factors integrate to cause fatigue, which is why it's important for practitioners to look at their patients' entire profile. One error in medical investigation lies in all of the experimentation that we do to determine, for example, whether Vitamin C or E does this or that in the body. We can't generalize and isolate the effects of a particular substance upon the body, because all of the substances work together in a synergistic fashion. To try to do this is akin to isolating your eyeball from your brain, and saying, "I can't see." You need the brain in order for the eyeball to deliver sight.

For Pain

For the treatment of pain, I use a device that delivers frequency-specific micro-currents to the body. This therapy is a spin-off of Carolyn McMacklin's work. McMacklin is a chiropractor who often uses micro-currents to treat joint and muscle pain. She has demonstrated in animal models that this type of therapy can immediately decrease inflammatory cytokines. Treatments with this device can be done in the practitioner's office or at the patient's home and doing them decreases the need for pain medication.

Other Factors That Affect Healing

When people overextend themselves and do not properly rest or have restless sleep patterns, then these situations compromise the body's ability to heal. Rest is very important for the body to heal itself and a lack thereof will reduce the hormonal and immune response that it needs to manage infections.

Philosophy on Pharmaceutical Medications

I use pharmaceutical medications throughout my practice, but not as my mainstay. I try to use them as safety nets, and only for limited periods of time. I use them to bring patients back to as normal a state of functioning as possible. When that happens, I start to taper the medications off, so that their bodies can take over the function of the medication. And in reality, my whole practice of medicine is designed with this goal in mind.

Less than Beneficial Approaches to Treating Lyme Disease

As practitioners, I anticipate that we are all on the same page, trying to make our patients better. In my heart, altruistically, I feel that we are trying to help people. I believe that a lot of treatments have merit, and some of these are treatments that I don't entirely understand, but if they are modalities that have positive effects upon people, then I'm not going to criticize them just because I don't understand them. In allopathic medicine, however, we tend to not be open to other treatment modalities. If a treatment doesn't fit our guidelines of thought, we criticize it and five or ten years down the road, we suddenly learn that it has merit. This sort of thing happened with snake oil. People today call remedies that don't work "snake oil," but most people don't know that real snake oil happens to have the highest concentration of omega-3 fatty acids of any substance! So snake oil really was a valid treatment; it lowered inflammation, because of its high EPA/DHA content. Lyme disease is a challenging condition to treat and we are too premature in our understanding of treatment options to arbitrarily dismiss other approaches just because they are unfamiliar to us.

Healing Is All About Reducing the Body's Total Stress Load

Finally, and as mentioned in the Functional Medicine Matrix section, I believe that healing is all about reducing the body's total stress load. All that we (the practitioner and patient) are really doing when we treat infections is leveling out the playing field so that the body can, at some point, take over in the healing process. No one will ever convince me that we have a pharmaceutical drug that is more powerful than anything that we have in our own bodies. So we have to optimize our team, so to speak, and in order to do that, we have to reduce our bug counts. If you talk to any Lyme-literate physician, they will tell you that once you have chronic Lyme disease, it never goes away. You've got it for life. But I prefer to reframe the situation and prognosis and encourage my patients to say, "Okay, I have this disease. That means I can't trash my body. I will use herbs, vitamins, supplements and other therapies to support and maintain a strong immune system. And doing these things can, collectively, provide me with a greater and longer quality of life than if I had never had Lyme in the first place". Lyme disease can be the catalyst for teaching us to honor our body's natural blueprint for health by showing us how to reduce its overall stress load.

Last words

The most successful practitioners maintain an open mind and eye, and listen to their patients, whose experience holds the keys to health. The most successful patients fully participate in their care, while supporting their natural, integrative capacity for health, which in turn increases their chances for healing.

How to Contact Peter J. Muran, M.D., M.B.A.

Longevity Healthcare
1405 Garden Street
San Luis Obispo, CA 93401
Telephone: (805) 548-0987
Toll Free: (888) 315-4777
E-mail: info@longevityhealthcare.com

Chapter References

[1] *Joseph J Burrascano. Diagnostic Hints and Treatment Guidelines for Lyme and other Tick-Borne Illnesses ILADS.org, Updated September, 2005.*

[2] *Institute of Functional Medicine. Applying Functional Medicine in Clinical Practice, Course Syllabus March 2005. Web site: www.functionalmedicine.org*

[3] *Jones, D. (editor). Textbook of Functional Medicine. Gig Harbor, Wash: Institute of Functional Medicine; 2005.*

[4] *Ester Sternberg. The Balance Within: The Science Connecting Health and Emotions. (W.H. Freeman :NY) 2000.*

[5] *Candace Pert. Molecules of Emotion. (Simon &Schuster, NY) 1997.*

[6] *H. Mielants et al., Reflections on the link between intestinal permeability and inflammatory joint disease. J. Rheumatology 1990;8:523-524.*

[7] *RS Pinals. Arthritis associated with gluten-sensitive enteropathy. J Rheumatology 1986;13:201-204.*

[8] *F Velluzzi, A Caradonna, and MF Boy, et al. Prevalence of Celiac Disease in Patients with Thyroid Autoimmunity. Am J Gastroenterol. 1998;93(6):976-979.*

[9] *Jeffery Bland Seminars: 2000 Syllabus (Chapter 3)*

[10] *ILADS verses IDSA treatment profile.*
http://www.ilads.org/guidelines.html

[11] *Paul Cheney, Balancing the Th1/Th2 immune system.*
http://www.anapsid.org/cnd/diagnosis/cheneyis.html

[12] *Richie Shoemaker. Mold Warriors (Gateway Press, Baltimore, MD) 2007.*

•CHAPTER 10•

Nicola McFadzean, N.D.
SAN DIEGO, CA

Biography

Dr. Nicola McFadzean is the founder and owner of *RestorMedicine* in San Diego, CA. Originally trained as a nutritionist and traditional naturopath in her native country of Australia, she later went on to receive her Doctorate of Naturopathic Medicine at Bastyr University in Seattle, WA. Dr. McFadzean is a Lyme-literate naturopathic doctor who combines conventional and integrative medical approaches to treat tick-borne illnesses. Dr. McFadzean is a member of the International Lyme and Associated Diseases Association (ILADS) and has completed the ILADS training program under the mentorship of Dr. Steven Harris. She is also affiliated with Dr. Yang's Family Care in Santee, CA.

Treatment Approach

My treatment approach is multi-faceted, broad-based and holistic, which comes naturally to me because of my training as a naturopath. Hence, I believe that treating Lyme disease with antibiotics alone is insufficient for obtaining a cure. Practitioners must address their patients' healing on multiple levels, taking into account issues such as immune and hormone dysfunction, environmental toxicity, and other problems. As well, they must address any psycho-emotional factors that are contributing to their patients' illnesses, because the Lyme "bugs" mess with neurotransmitters and bioche-mistry, which in turn can cause depression and complicate healing.

Treatments for Lyme and Co-Infections

Borrelia/Candida

Through my experience in treating Lyme disease, I have learned that it's sometimes beneficial to first address any Candida problems that patients might have, before doing any other type of treatment. First, because this almost always helps to ameliorate their symp-toms, and secondly, because it prevents them from having problems with yeast further along in the healing journey.

Also, this approach allows me to get started on treating them while we are waiting for their other lab test results to come back. So when I get new patients who are reporting brain fog and other Candida-like symptoms such as gas and bloating, I will start them on an immune support product such as transfer factor, along with Diflu-can, Nystatin or an herbal antifungal.

I tend to keep patients on a higher dose of Diflucan for only the first two to three weeks of treatment, and then lower their dose once I start treating their other infections. I have found that two to three weeks of Diflucan doesn't usually get rid of their yeast problems entirely, but after a few weeks, I can usually reduce the dose. So I might prescribe them 100-200 mg twice a day for a week, then reduce that to 50-100 mg twice a day, and by the time they start antibiotics for other infections, they might be taking just 50 mg per day. For others, I might recommend a pulsed regimen of Diflucan, 100 mg per day, to take on weekends only.

If I suspect that my patients' yeast is primarily in their gastrointes-tinal tract and if they aren't presenting with systemic symptoms, then I will prescribe them probiotics, along with a gentler medication like Nystatin or a natural remedy such as grapefruit seed extract. I find Nystatin to be a safe and reliable agent for treating intestinal yeast.

Once my patients are on a Candida protocol, I will then start treating them for the cyst form of Borrelia. I generally start by prescribing tinidazole, which I prefer over Flagyl (metronidazole) because patients tolerate it better. Flagyl is hard on the digestive system. I recommend Flagyl only when tinidazole is cost-prohibitive for patients, because the latter isn't always covered by insurance. Grapefruit seed extract and Alinia (nitazoxanide) can also be used to treat cyst forms. If I treat my patients with intracellular drugs first (which attack active forms of Borrelia), then we run the risk of the cysts constantly rising up and replacing them like a new army of soldiers. By treating cysts at the same time as active forms, we minimize the creation of new "baby" Lyme disease spirochetes, and that's important.

If my patients have both Babesia and Borrelia infections, and their medications are covered by insurance, after starting them on a cyst-busting drug, I may add Zithromax (azithromycin) to their protocol, with the idea of adding Mepron (atovaquone) a few weeks later. If my patients don't have Babesia, I may instead prescribe doxycycline, Biaxin (clarithromycin) or Omnicef (cefdinir) for Borrelia. There are many different antibiotics that can be used for Lyme and Lyme-related infections, and my decision regarding which ones to use is usually based upon the combination of co-infections that patients present and the combinations of medications that work well for all of these infections. Doxycycline and rifampin work well together for the treatment of Lyme and Bartonella, for instance, while Zithromax and Mepron are frequently used for Babesia. Other medications that I use less frequently include amoxicillin and Alinia (nitazoxanide).

If my patients don't test positive for Babesia but I am yet suspicious that the infection is present and causing them symptoms, then I may start them on 500 mg per day of artemisinin, an herbal extract that is effective against Babesia. If they experience either improvement, or a worsening of their symptoms (as a result of a Jarisch-Herxheimer or "Herx" reaction) after their treatment, then they may still be infected with Babesia despite their negative lab test results.

Also, I try to start them on only one new medication per week, so for instance, I might send them away with a prescription for tinidazole, Zithromax and artemisinin, while instructing them to start just one of these at a time, in a specific order. I space out the timing of new medications so that if patients have a negative reaction to a medication, then they will know right away which one it is. I also do this so that they won't "Herx" too much. That said, some people don't "Herx" until three or four days after taking a medication, which means that their Herxheimer reactions may not yet be well cleared after a week. If this happens, then I wait until they are over the worst of their Herxheimer, before starting them on a new medication.

I am a little less aggressive about prescribing antibiotics than some Lyme doctors, perhaps due to my naturopathic background, and fears about the negative long-term effects that multiple antibiotics can have upon the body. I know that some doctors prescribe four or five medications for Borrelia alone, before they even address co-infections. I believe that using natural agents and herbal antimicrobials in combination with the antibiotics allows me to achieve a similar efficacy with fewer medications. The tolerability of medications, side effects, costs and benefits must all be weighed when formulating an effective, yet balanced protocol.

I also don't actually prescribe IV antibiotics, as this is outside my scope of treatment as a naturopathic doctor; however, I am affiliated with an M.D. who can prescribe intravenous therapy for patients that need it. I tend to recommend IV's for patients who have long-standing infections and/or very severe symptoms, especially neurological symptoms, and for those who have not responded well to oral medications.

Babesia

I tend to use artemisinin as a starting point for treating Babesia. It's a good "stepping stone" to other treatments, and for people who don't have insurance, is much more affordable than the Babesia medications. Mepron (atovaquone), one of the primary Babesia medications, costs over $1000 per month, and Malarone (atovaquone plus proguanil) isn't much cheaper. In contrast, artemisinin costs less than $50 for a three-month supply. Also, I am comfortable integrating artemisinin into a protocol with other medications, and am less concerned about it causing liver toxicity, as Babesia medications often do. Furthermore, when patients start with artemisinin, they tend to have less of a Herxheimer reaction than with Mepron, and by taking artemisinin first, their parasitic load is reduced somewhat so that when they do start on Mepron, their Herxheimer reactions aren't as strong.

Unfortunately, Mepron, while a useful medication for Babesia, doesn't always get the infection out of the brain. For this reason, I sometimes transition my patients to Lariam (mefloquine), which gets into the brain better. It's a very strong medication though, so I never start out with it and instead wait until my patients stabilize on Mepron or Malarone for a couple of months before transitioning them to this medication; otherwise, their "brain Herxes" may be too severe.

Still, a lot of people do well taking a combination of Mepron, Zithromax and artemisinin for the treatment of Babesia. Like all Lyme protocols, it doesn't help everyone, but it's probably the best combination of medications that I have come across for treating this infection.

Bartonella

I use some of the same medications for Bartonella that I do for Borrelia, such as doxycycline, along with Levaquin (levofloxacin) or rifampin, with good success; however, there is some speculation within the Lyme-literate medical community that there are strains of Bartonella that become more virulent when exposed to doxycycline. So if my patients get worse taking doxycycline and this feeling worse goes beyond what would be expected from a Herxheimer reaction, it might be that they are infected with one of these strains of Bartonella. If I suspect this to be the case, then I re-think the medications that I give them.

Also, I typically try rifampin before Levaquin, because there is a potential for tendon damage with Levaquin. I have had some patients experience tendon pain with Levaquin, although thankfully no ruptures or permanent damage, and that is a statistic that I would like to maintain! In any case, these two medications are among the most specific for Bartonella.

Mycoplasma

Lab testing for Mycoplasma is problematic, since standard labs such as Quest and LabCorp only test for Mycoplasma pneumoniae and not some of the other strains, such as M. fermentans and M. hominis. Several private labs offer more comprehensive testing, however. Doxycycline and rifampin are among the medications used to treat Mycoplasma, but I also have success with natural agents such as colloidal silver.

Ehrlichia

Only about 20% of my patients test positive for Ehrlichia. Often, the infection will get eliminated when I treat patients with the same antibiotics that I use for Borrelia, such as doxycycline, rifampin or Levaquin.

Opportunistic Viruses

I test my patients for viruses such as EBV (Epstein-Barr virus), HSV 1&2 (Herpes simplex viruses 1&2), HHV-6 (Human Herpes virus), as well as CMV (Cytomegalovirus). While I think that these viruses put one more stress on the immune system, I haven't had a lot of success treating my patients with anti-viral medications. Personally, I'm wary of Valcyte. I think it's a more effective remedy for HHV-6, but it's definitely toxic to the liver. Valtrex is helpful to a subset of patients and is somewhat less toxic than Valcyte.

My patients have responded well when I treat them with an herb called larrea tridentata, in a product called LarreaPlus by Biogenesis. It's especially beneficial for treating Herpes viruses, and is preventative for those who get outbreaks of HSV-1 and/or HSV-2. I think that this herb is at least as effective as Valtrex, but is less toxic to the body, and is also anti-inflammatory. LarreaPlus also contains bee propolis, Melissa officinalis, olive leaf, L-lysine, zinc and Vitamin C.

One of my challenges when treating opportunistic viruses is discerning whether my patients' IgG antibodies on lab test results reflect the presence of a chronic viral infection or simply a past exposure to a virus. It's hard to discern how much of a role chronic viral load plays in their symptomatology. My experience has been that many with Lyme are co-infected with viruses but anti-viral treatment does not significantly alter their symptoms.

Herbal Protocol for the Treatment of Lyme Disease

I have formulated an herbal blend remedy called Dr. Nicola's Lyme Formula. This product contains samento, teasel, smilax (sarsaparilla), guaiacum (an anti-spirochetal herb used in Europe but which is not very well known in the United States), and astragalus (which is used to boost the immune system).

When I started using this formula on my patients, I found that they often had severe Herxheimer reactions at the beginning of their treatment. So I now start off by giving some of them a teasel tincture instead, which I have found to be effective, but gentler on the body than the combination product. I have also isolated the smilax from my formula to give to them separately. Smilax is somewhat like a neurological cleanser, and helps them to deal with the neurotoxin aspect of Lyme. So for my patients who have strong neurological symptoms, I recommend that they start off by taking smilax and teasel, and then work up to the more potent herbal formulas.

I also use Transfer Factor Multi-Immune from Researched Nutritionals as part of my protocol, which is an excellent formula. I may start my patients on this product, then add teasel root tincture to their regimen. I will usually do this prior to administering antibiotics, and depending upon the patient. So the first few weeks of a typical Lyme disease protocol might involve patients taking Diflucan and/or Nystatin, along with smilax and transfer factor the first week, adding teasel to the protocol the second week, and then adding samento or guaiacum, or my herbal Lyme formula the third week. At week four, patients start antibiotics while continuing to take the other supplements, because I believe that combining herbs with antibiotics is much more effective than just doing antibiotics alone.

Also, it's important to note that while antibiotics kill bugs, they also weaken the body. They aren't selective about what they kill; they will knock out bad stuff, but also the good, because they don't discriminate against microorganisms. Herbs work synergistically with antibiotics by making them more effective, but they also protect the body, by providing support to the liver, other organs and tissues. Antibiotics take a greater toll on the body if people don't take supportive herbs, nutrients and probiotics.

Supporting the Immune System

To support the immune system, I recommend transfer factor, beta glucan, astragalus and colostrum, as well as intravenous vitamin cocktails. I'm a fan of Myer's cocktails, which are intravenous cocktails containing calcium, B-12 and other B vitamins, Vitamin C, magnesium, and trace minerals. When my patients do these once per week, it helps to alleviate their symptoms, because they receive the vitamins and minerals that they need in higher concentrations than if they were to take them orally. Also, the nutrients get pushed into their cells more easily with an IV. For example, people with

Lyme have magnesium deficiencies, and I suspect that many take this mineral orally but that much of it doesn't get into their cells. Unfortunately, intravenous cocktails can be costly and hard for patients to access, especially if they live in more remote areas.

Treating Hormonal Dysfunction

I advocate a lot of adrenal and thyroid support for my patients. To help determine what their hormonal needs are, I run a saliva cortisol test, which measures adrenal function. Along with that, I run blood tests for the thyroid. I find that many of my patients have thyroid hormone test results that fall within the "low-normal" range, which actually means that they have sub-clinical thyroid hormone deficiencies. To make up for such deficiencies, people often think that they must supplement their thyroid with either synthetic thyroid hormone or Armour (which is sourced from pigs), but they can also take bioidentical thyroid hormone, which mimics human thyroid hormone exactly and is my preferred method of supplementation. Adding iodine, zinc and selenium to the diet—nutrients needed by the thyroid gland to produce thyroid hormone—is sufficient for giving some patients the boost that they need.

I also believe that if I give my patients supplements for their thyroid without supporting their adrenals, it's akin to putting one foot on the gas pedal of a car while the hand brake is still on. This is because thyroid supplementation speeds up the body's metabolism but when the adrenal glands are weak, the body doesn't have the constitutional strength to support this accelerated metabolism. So treating the thyroid alone can wear the adrenals out even more.

For that reason, and because most of my patients suffer from adrenal depletion, I also give them a lot of nutrition and natural support for their adrenals, such as the herbs ashwagandha, rhodiola and Cordyceps, and nutrients such as vitamins B-5 and B-6. I also recommend licorice if their cortisol levels are low and their adrenal glands need re-building, and as long as they are not hypertensive or estrogen dominant, as licorice use is contraindicated in these conditions. I don't recommend a lot of glandular formulas because I don't believe that they are all that natural for the body, but that is just my preference. If my patients have really low cortisol, I may prescribe them hydrocortisone for a short period, but I avoid doing this whenever possible.

In addition, I recommend DHEA and pregnenolone supplementation to support the adrenals, both of which can be quite effective. It's important to ensure that the body's ratios of cortisol to DHEA are balanced, because DHEA protects against some of the catabolic effects of cortisol. Cortisol is, in a broad sense, a catabolic hormone, so when patients are deficient in DHEA, their cortisol levels can get out of control. But cortisol is a very important hormone that regulates blood sugar, metabolism, immune function and detoxification, as well as other functions, and when the body's levels of this hormone are out of whack, then the reproductive and other hormones are generally out of whack, too. Pregnenolone is the "grandmother" hormone that the adrenals use to make other hormones, so if the body has a high demand for cortisol due to a chronic stress response, then it needs more pregnenolone to supply that cortisol. This then leaves less pregnenolone for the production of other hormones such as estrogen, progesterone and testosterone. For this reason, I sometimes prescribe bioidentical hormones to my patients to make up for any hormonal deficiencies. When women take bioidentical progesterone during the second half of their menstrual cycle, it can counter a lot of their PMS symptoms and even reduce the flares that they get around this time of the month. Testosterone gel can help both men and women to maintain strength, lean muscle mass, energy and libido.

Healing the Gut

I try to get my patients to eat foods that support their guts, such as kefir, kombucha tea, and aloe vera juice. It's also important that they take a lot of probiotics, anywhere from 50-100 billion microorganisms per day. Researched Nutritionals has a great formula called Prescript-Assist which is a soil-based organism product that I really like because the types of organisms in it are resistant to stomach acid, and it does not require refrigeration. In general, I recommend a combination of three types of probiotics: soil-based, an acidophilus-bifidus blend and saccharomyces boulardii.

Treatments for Symptomatic Relief

Insomnia

Insomnia is a major problem for people with Lyme. I don't prescribe sleep medications in my practice and instead recommend a lot of natural remedies to help my patients sleep. 200 mg of 5-HTP often works well, as does 5-10 mg of melatonin (the sustained release kind is good for those who can't stay asleep). Hot baths before bed can also be beneficial. 100 mg of oral progesterone before bedtime helps women to sleep, especially if they are peri-menopausal. Also, I have some pre-menopausal patients whose insomnia gets worse during the second half of their menstrual cycle because their progesterone levels are low, so supplementing with progesterone during this time can be beneficial for them. Fixing thyroid problems can also resolve insomnia. Finally, Eschscholzia californica (California poppy) is an herb that helps with pain and is also a good sedative at night.

Pain

Treating nerve pain is difficult. As mentioned previously, California poppy can help to relieve pain, as can Vitamin B-12. The supplement that I recommend most for pain is called Soothe and Relaxx, from Researched Nutritionals, which is a company that makes useful formulas for conditions found in chronic illnesses such as Lyme. This product contains glucosamine, MSM, chondroitin, and hyaluronic acid—all of which protect the connective tissue and joints—along with magnesium and malic acid, which are good for the muscles. In addition, it contains 5-HTP, lemon balm, valerian root, and passionflower, all of which sedate the nervous system. Finally, it has holy basil, curcumin and other anti-inflammatory substances. I find that it helps nine out of ten of my patients who have pain, muscle spasms, anxiety and insomnia.

The herb smilax can also alleviate pain since it cleanses neurotoxins from the body. I use this herb extensively in my patients who have neurological symptoms. Also, magnesium, when applied topically as a cream, is a great muscle relaxant and can improve sleep; when combined with GABA, it aids in lowering anxiety.

Anxiety and Depression

As other symptoms, I treat my patients' anxiety and depression with natural remedies. I understand that some patients have good results with anti-depressants, and I think that it's okay for them to take these at the beginning of their treatment regimen, to manage symptoms while we are getting their Lyme protocol rolling, but they are not beneficial long-term.

I sometimes recommend L-tyrosine to my patients for the treatment of depression, since this amino acid supports the production of epinephrine and norepinephrine. Some people get adverse affects from L-tyrosine, though; for example, they might feel wired, as if they have had too much coffee, but others have good results with it and it helps them to overcome depression as well as problems with focus, concentration and low energy. Conversely, 5-HTP, L-tryptophan, GABA, L-theanine, and amino acids of the like support the production of soothing, inhibitory neurotransmitters, so these are good for those who suffer from anxiety. If my patients end up needing anti-depressant medications, then I will refer them to their primary physician or psychiatrist for a prescription.

Headaches

The herb smilax glabrae (Chinese sarsaparilla) can be beneficial for relieving headaches and migraines (since it is a neurotoxin cleanser), as can B-12 and folic acid. Also, avoiding foods that cause inflammation can reduce neurological symptoms and headaches, because a lot of symptoms (in general) are caused by inflammation. In addition, I recommend any of the anti-inflammatory herbs that I mentioned in earlier sections, along with a lot of proteolytic enzymes. All of these things can calm the nervous system and reduce headaches.

Detoxification

I don't have a set detoxification protocol for my patients. There are so many different types of detoxification regimens to address different toxic assaults on the body, but if I had to recommend one substance alone for detoxifying the body, it would be glutathione, especially IV glutathione, which has amazing benefits. It increases energy, lowers pain levels, improves neurological function and decreases the frequency with which people get headaches and migraines. Also, the results are quite immediate and dramatic and can last several days. I have seen patients who have had great pain and debility walk out of my office much more comfortably after a glutathione IV. So I like to use glutathione as my starting point for detoxification; for its symptomatic benefits, because it's a key anti-oxidant and helps to support the healing process.

If they can't do IV glutathione, then I recommend that they use a transdermal form of this substance, or lipoceutical glutathione, which is a liquid that is formulated so that it can be absorbed through the mucous membranes of the mouth. Some practitioners recommend taking NAC (N-acetyl-cysteine) to increase glutathione in the body. NAC is a precursor to glutathione, but I am concerned that it can flare up intestinal yeast, so I am careful about recommending it to my patients.

The other supplement that I recommend as a starting point for detoxification is methylcobalamin (methyl-B12 or MB-12). The "methyl" part of the methyl-B12 supports the body's detoxification pathways. The B-12 supports the immune system and is also energizing.

For detoxifying heavy metals, lately, I have been giving EDTA and glutathione suppositories to my patients. When these two supposi-tories are used together, it has been demonstrated that the body dumps triple the amount of metals than if the EDTA had been used alone, so it's a nice combination. Some people don't like the idea of suppositories however, and instead prefer oral chelators.

I used to prescribe oral DMSA on a rotating schedule of three days on, eleven days off, but some people with Lyme don't cope well with this chelator because it causes too much of a detoxification reaction and the dosing schedule is too difficult for them to maintain. Lately, one Lyme-literate doctor has been advocating 100 mg of DMSA every three days, along with NAC and alpha lipoic acid, which may be a more manageable and gradual heavy metal chelation program. I have been using this protocol also, but so far, it's too early for me to know whether I can report the same success as this doctor. In general, EDTA is known to be a better lead chelator, while DMSA and DMPS are more specific for mercury.

Finally, I tend to treat the body for infections before heavy metals. Once patients are either stable and doing well on their anti-microbial treatments, or if they reach a plateau in their progress and I suspect that heavy metals might be getting in the way of further progress, then I will start them on a heavy metal detoxification protocol. Other doctors believe that it's important to clear the body of heavy metals before attempting treatment for infections. In the end, these decisions are made on a case-by-case basis. It is often difficult to prioritize patients' health issues and know which ones to treat first!

Treating Detoxification Problems

Taking amino acids and trace minerals can help those with compromised detoxification mechanisms, but some patients are so chemically sensitive that I can't even give them supplements, so I might start by recommending that they take a homeopathic detoxification formula, in order to open up their detoxification pathways. I will also sometimes recommend products like Cell Food to feed extra oxygen into their system, or lipoceutical glutathione, to help their bodies to get rid of toxins. Unfortunately, some people have impaired sulfur metabolism and glutathione and methyl B-12 can actually make them worse. Such people don't do well on a lot of remedies, so they are a challenging population to treat.

Sometimes, detoxification problems can be corrected by simply opening up the body's phase one and phase two liver enzyme pathways. I recommend medical foods like Ultra Clear by Metagenics to help open up the phase two pathways. Most of the time, people have more trouble with phase two than phase one pathways. I also use artichoke and dandelion root (which I import from Australia) for improving phase two pathways. Dandelion root can be made into a coffee-like beverage. I can't find anything in the United States that compares to it, so I bring it home by the jarful whenever I go to Australia. It's great because it looks like coffee, is made in a French press like coffee, and tastes fantastic. It's a wonderful way for patients to have a coffee-like ritual without the caffeine, and it's good for their livers.

Diet

People with Lyme disease should not consume gluten. This is vital for healing. I know that it's not easy, especially because, to be truly gluten-free, people must be well educated on the issue of which foods contain gluten. Yet it's important, because those who eat a lot of products containing dairy, sugar and gluten are the ones who seem to fare the worst with their treatments, most likely because these are pro-inflammatory substances. I don't mind my patients eating brown rice and potatoes, but if yeast is a problem for them, then any carbohydrate can make this problem worse. If they don't have too many problems with yeast, then they might be able to eat some grains.

In addition to not consuming gluten, people with Lyme should avoid refined sugar. One study has demonstrated that one teaspoon of refined sugar suppresses the immune system for sixteen hours. Knowing this might help people to stop and think, "Gosh, maybe I shouldn't have that dessert!" Dairy products are likewise inflammatory.

I emphasize fruits and vegetables for my patients, as well as healthy fats, such as flax oil. I have a breakfast smoothie recipe that I recommend, which contains almond milk as a base. It also has protein powder for the adrenals and to balance blood sugar; ground flax seed for the bowels, a tablespoon of flax oil to provide essential fatty acids, and a bit of fresh fruit can be added if yeast is not a problem for patients. Some of my patients also like to add a healthy "green" powder to the mix, such as NanoGreens.

It's also important for people with Lyme to get their bodies into an alkaline state as much as possible, especially when they are Herx-ing. Drinking lemon juice in water helps to accomplish this, as does adding a product like NanoGreens to beverages, since it contains concentrated fruits, vegetables and other alkalinizing nutrients.

In addition to fruits, veggies and healthy fats, I recommend that my patients eat a lot of lean proteins, such as organic chicken, turkey and wild-caught fish.

Also, instead of telling them what they can't eat, I try to focus on what they can, and make food recommendations to help them with this, such as the smoothie recipe mentioned above. As another example, I might recommend cashew butter, raw nuts, hummus or corn chips for a snack.

Finally, I encourage my patients to eat small, frequent meals throughout the day, instead of infrequent, larger ones, because the former regimen is much easier on the adrenals and the body's blood sugar regulatory systems.

Addressing Food Allergies

I recommend doing IgG allergy tests for foods, because I find that a lot of my patients have sensitivities to foods that they wouldn't ordinarily imagine to be a problem (such as blueberries, bananas and garlic). The food sensitivity test involves a finger prick test, which I do in my office. The blood from the finger prick test is then sent to a lab, where it is analyzed for sensitivities to more than ninety-six different foods.

I find that eggs often come up as a sensitivity for my patients, but not everyone is the same. I also find that a lot of them don't do well consuming cow dairy but can tolerate goat dairy, so this leaves the option of goat milk, cheese and yogurt open to them. In general, I try to discourage the consumption of dairy products, but goat dairy is the lesser of the evils. Kefir is the exception to the rule, because, while it's a fermented milk product, it contains active cultures and beneficial enzymes, is much easier to digest than yogurt, and can help to maintain healthy gut flora.

Exercise

The amount of exercise that people with Lyme should do depends upon the severity of their illness. In general, I don't push my patients to do too much physical exercise, especially if they are really tired and sick, or their adrenals are depleted, but I try to encourage them to go outside, get some sunshine and take walks. I especially don't push them to do aerobic exercise. Gentle stretches are better, or, if they are stronger, they can do yoga and Pilates. I believe that it's important, even for bed-bound patients, to incorporate some movement into their daily routine—even if it just means doing a few gentle stretches to enhance circulation, move the lymphatic fluid and maintain movement in the muscles.

It's easy for those with Lyme to "cross the line" when it comes to exercise. When they start getting better, they try to do all of the things that they missed out on when they were ill, and before you know it, they have pushed themselves too far and are flat on their backs or in pain again.

Patient and Practitioner Challenges in Treating Lyme Disease

As a practitioner, one of my biggest challenges of treating Lyme disease is that I can't put my patients on every single supplement or therapy that they need. Financially, logistically, and because of what their bodies can handle, it's impossible for them to do or take everything!

Therefore, I try to put together their protocol in a manner that's beneficial but manageable for them. I'm not a big believer in sending people home with dozens of bottles of vitamins. I don't feel that this is realistic, so I'm always trying to streamline and pick the most relevant remedies for each patient, which is also a challenge. The remedies that I tend to recommend the most (besides antibiotics) are Soothe and Relaxx (Researched Nutritionals), transfer factor, teasel, smilax and my herbal Lyme formula. Those are my five favorites. Also, I always recommend probiotics.

Another challenge for patients and practitioners is that unless a protocol is all mapped out for the patients, "Lyme brain" makes it easy for them to lose track of which therapies they need to do, and which remedies they need to take. Often, patients will start out "gung ho" with their treatments, but if they are not significantly better after a month, then they get discouraged and quit. I try to prepare them for the fact that treating Lyme can be a long, slow road—a marathon and not a sprint, and that they may get worse before they get better.

Herxing is a challenge for patients, but it helps, I think, when they are educated to recognize and understand the process. Also, there are definitely people who take greater responsibility for their healing and treatment course and who educate themselves on their options and what to expect during treatment. I believe that these people tend to fare the best in their healing journeys.

Limited financial resources can also be an obstacle to healing. Lyme disease is a very expensive illness, and many people are not able to work, which makes the financial burden even harder to bear. I have seen many of my patients deplete their savings, sell their houses, borrow money and live in the most frugal ways just to maintain their treatment regimens.

How Long Does It Take To Heal from Lyme Disease?

The time frame for healing from Lyme disease depends upon the person. I have patients that I have worked with for a year or two or more who are making progress but who are not "out of the woods" yet. Then I have patients who are faster responders who heal in six to twelve months. In general, I notice that men tend to respond faster to treatments than women. It may be that women's hormonal imbalances create an obstacle to healing, as may their Vitamin D deficiencies, because Vitamin D is important for proper immune function, and such deficiencies are more common in women.

EFT (Emotional Freedom Technique) for Healing Emotional Trauma

To address the emotional component of healing, I recommend EFT, Emotional Freedom Technique. I find this to be a very powerful strategy for clearing blocks to healing.

Counseling, while it can be beneficial in many situations, does not as effectively access the subconscious mind. For that reason, I find EFT to be effective for breaking through into those deeper places. Also, a lot of patients don't have the money and energy to go to counseling appointments every week, and one of the great things about EFT is that it is inexpensive and people can do it at home, once they learn the techniques. So initially, I might refer my patients to a well-trained energy psychologist, who can teach them the EFT techniques, and after that, they can do these on their own. I find this strategy to be particularly helpful for those who have anxiety.

The Role of Spirituality in Healing

I think people who have strong spiritual beliefs have an easier time in the healing journey, because spirituality provides an outlet outside of themselves upon which they can cast their worries and through which they can draw hope. I find that more and more, I am talking to my patients about their spiritual beliefs and practices, and I integrate prayer into some of their visits.

While I am certainly respectful of others' spiritual beliefs, if my patients have not integrated some type of spiritual practice into their healing regimen, I might at least introduce them to the concept of meditation or teach them deep breathing techniques. Spiritual practices may not involve God for some people; they might involve relaxation techniques or a daily routine that enables them to tune into the universe or their own inner healing capacity. I think that people who have faith have a more positive attitude and more gratitude in their daily lives. They don't tend to fall into a negative mentality as easily. Don't get me wrong—people with Lyme have a hard time and recognition of that is necessary, but those who are spiritually grounded tend to have more acceptance of their situation, which is beneficial for healing.

Is Lyme Disease Always Primary in Patients' Overall Symptom Picture?

In my practice, I see a couple of different scenarios. I have patients that seemed to be doing fine before they had Lyme disease. They were healthy and active, and then everything went haywire! They may or may not be able to track the date of their tick bite, but in any case, it was an "all of a sudden" type of thing. The Lyme infection(s) are probably primary in these patients' overall symptom picture. Then there are other patients who have never felt well throughout their entire lives. They were ill as kids; they had asthma, eczema, or frequent colds, and they may now have immune weakness due to a genetic predisposition, or because they just have so many toxins and infections that got piled up along the way. I believe that for these types of people, Lyme may have been "the straw that broke the camel's back." Also, some may have a methylation defect that doesn't allow them to detoxify and which has contributed to the impact that Lyme has had on their bodies. I think that there must be a plethora of other people out there who have been exposed to Borrelia, but whose immune systems have effectively dealt with the infection, and so they therefore aren't manifesting symptoms.

Hyperbaric Oxygen Treatments (HBOT) as an Adjunct to Healing

HBOT can be hugely beneficial for those with Lyme. If my patients do this therapy, I try to simultaneously support their detoxification pathways, mitochondrial function and cellular energy production so that they receive maximum benefit from the therapy. At the same time, I try to ensure that their nutritional status supports anti-inflammatory pathways. HBOT accelerates cellular healing and creates an environment that is unfavorable to microorganisms, due to the high concentration of oxygen that it creates within the cells. If my patients have Babesia, then I treat them for this infection prior to having them start the hyperbaric therapy. It is believed by some that HBOT can make patients worse if they have untreated Babesiosis infections. In general, I support HBOT, because while it is definitely a commitment of money and time, the rewards from its use are often great.

Beneficial Lifestyle Habits

I think that connection with other people is really important, and those with Lyme disease can benefit from spending time with others who have Lyme. Lyme disease support groups can be beneficial, as long as they don't serve as forums for negative thinking and are instead used to share hope and information. Lyme sufferers must surround themselves with as much positivity as possible.

I also encourage my patients to journal, and if they spend a lot of time in bed or are not very active, I encourage them to read positive books that are food for the brain and spirit, so that they are using their time productively. Again, prayer and meditation can be really beneficial, as can trying to maintain a balance in their life's activities, so that they don't feel completely deprived and disconnected from life. That may mean inviting friends over and having them bring take-out food to the house. Disconnection from others can be an obstacle to healing.

Getting outside of oneself can also be important for healing. Serving others, for example, is a good way to do this. Sometimes, I encourage my patients to provide an ear to others who are discouraged, even though they may not think that they have anything to offer, because just being there for others who are suffering can be helpful.

How Family and Friends Can Help the Sick

There is a lack of understanding about Lyme disease in general, and I think that while friends and family may try their best to understand their loved ones with Lyme, it can be challenging to know what to do for them.

Helping the chronically ill to stay hopeful is important. Family and friends shouldn't take pity on their loved ones, but instead encourage them. Doing little favors for them makes all the difference in the world. When they aren't feeling well, making a bowl of chicken soup or rubbing their feet can be wonderful. Gift certificates for massage, pet sitting or errand services are welcomed by most!

I have a patient whose wife accompanies him to all of his appointments. He has Lyme disease, so she brings along trivia cards and crossword puzzles to keep his brain alert and to keep him busy in the waiting room. It's so great to always see her there, supporting him. I like to see partners getting involved in their loved ones' recovery, and doing things such as accompanying them to their doctors' appointments, so that they can, for example, help them to recall what was discussed during those appointments, and provide moral support to them.

I had another patient who was sick due to chronic mold exposure. She and her husband had moved into a new house that had a lawsuit against its builders, and she got sick as soon as they moved in there. Her husband, however, didn't believe that she was that ill. I thought, *The poor lady will have a hard time getting well, because not only does she feel like death warmed over, her husband doesn't even believe that she is ill!*

But then you have the others; the husband who is there with his wife during her doctors' appointments, taking notes, and telling her, "We will find a way to pay for treatments. We'll get you better, don't worry." I think that those people are the ones who have an easier time healing. The role of emotional support in healing is tremendous.

Last Words

Lyme disease can have devastating effects upon a person's life, and the road to recovery can be long and strenuous. However, recovery is possible and those with Lyme should never give up hope for a full recovery. I strongly believe that antibiotic therapy by itself is insufficient for obtaining a cure—instead, a holistic program incorporating nutrition, immune support, detoxification protocol, strategies for digestive health, herbal antimicrobials and lifestyle modification puts people in the best position for healing.

How to Contact Nicola McFadzean, N.D.

RestorMedicine
1111 Fort Stockton Drive, Suite H
San Diego CA 92103
Telephone: (619) 546 4065
Fax: (619) 270 2582
E-mail: info@drnicola.com

•CHAPTER 11•

Marlene Kunold, "Heilpraktiker"
(Health Care Practitioner)
HAMBURG, GERMANY

Biography

Marlene works in Hamburg, Germany as a "heilpraktiker," which, in English, might be translated as "healing practitioner," but in Germany, this title encompasses a broad range of training programs and qualifications. Some practitioners with this title are only qualified to do reflexology massage, for example, while others do the kind of work that Marlene does, which is similar to that of a naturopathic doctor. To obtain her certification as a heilpraktiker, Marlene had to undergo medical training and take a written and oral exam, the latter of which involved standing in front of doctors who asked her difficult questions in an attempt to make her fail the exam! This practice of asking difficult questions, however, is quite common, and is done in order to separate the "good from the bad".

The education and training of a heilpraktiker is shorter than that of a physician's, but is more holistic, although the time that it takes to finish a particular program depends somewhat upon the student's initiative and how much he or she wants to learn. Marlene has also completed a lot of seminars, studying and teaching on her own, in addition to what she learned through this program. That she is able to work as a holistic heilpraktiker is no small feat, since 90-95% of those who wish to obtain this title don't pass the certification exam, because it's so difficult. Those that do, however, can then choose the areas of medicine that they want to specialize and work in. It's also up to the individual heilpraktiker to decide how deep he or she wants to get into the healing arts.

Today, Marlene maintains a practice in Hamburg. About 40% of her cases involve patients with Lyme disease.

How I Became Involved in Treating Lyme Disease

I had Lyme disease myself for twelve years. At the time that I caught it, knowledge about the disease was scarce, and I didn't have the typical signs and symptoms. I caught it in 1995, while at an open-air event. I was lying around in the grass and two or three days later, discovered an eczema rash on my belly. I didn't remember getting bit by a tick, but it was not known at that time that eczema could be a sign of Lyme disease. I also had a slight fever, sore lymph nodes, and thought that perhaps these symptoms were due to an allergic reaction from a bee.

In the following years, I developed persistent bronchitis, as well as frequent sinus problems. I went to a friend who was a doctor, and he gave me antibiotics (doxycycline), which, overall, made me feel worse! Years later, I became so sick that I couldn't continue my work. I had a successful PR office at that time, and was a music journalist. I even had my own TV show (the videos of which I keep stored away, because I think the show was quite bad!).

I started detoxifying my body and doing other things to improve my health, and meanwhile, moved to Hamburg from Berlin. Shortly thereafter, I became pregnant, and after I had my baby, I started getting muscle weakness in my body. Every time that I would kneel down to pick up my baby, I couldn't get back up again. Climbing stairs became almost impossible. Whenever I tried to carry something, it just slipped out of my hands. My joints ached and my mental state was quite miserable.

I went to see a few different doctors, and I told them to test me for Lyme, and they did the usual antibody blood tests, which always came out negative, so they not only refused to give me antibiotics, but also believed, I think, that I was weird! They said that the symptoms were "all in my head", and that I was under too much stress.

Yet suspicious that I had Lyme, I began investigating alternative ways of testing and detecting what was wrong with me, and I was eventually able to confirm my Lyme disease diagnosis through these tests. At that time, however, there was still no such thing as a lymphocyte transformation test (which is an important test that is currently used in Germany to test for Borrelia).

I tried different healing remedies, including Rife machines, Clark frequency zappers and colloidal silver, but nothing really worked. Then I used ozonides, which are very powerful remedies that also turned out to be beneficial for treating intracellular microbes, and as a result, my symptoms began to disappear. I also started working with a device called the QXCI, which is precursor to the electro-physiological biofeedback SCIO system that is more commonly used today. This device, along with the ozonides, enabled me to become symptom-free.

For awhile, I was optimistic that my Lyme disease was gone, but two or three years after these treatments, I was invited to see a Philippine healer and attend a "clearing" session. Curious, I went to see the healer, who performed a treatment on me that compromised my breathing and caused my head to become plugged within minutes following the treatment. I then developed a heavy fever that stayed with me for months. It eventually dropped to a lower level, but its presence continued for years.

At some point, I went to see another colleague and he diagnosed me with liver cancer! I was quite shocked to receive this diagnosis, and I started doing every single therapy that I had learned about up until then for treating cancer because I wanted to live. Around the same time, I came across more current information on Lyme disease, which described how cancers of different organs some-times result from Lyme disease. So I learned how to give myself shots and intravenous infusions, and did literally every therapy that I knew of in natural medicine for treating cancer. Such therapies included Cell Symbiosis (Dr. Heinrich Kremer), and taking protein-omega 3 oil (Dr. Budwig). My son was six or seven years old at the time and I was really struggling. To this day, I don't know how far the cancer had developed because I never wanted to see the tumor that the doctor had found on my liver.

Some time after that, a colleague convinced me to do a lymphocyte transformation test, so that I could determine once and for all whether I had still Lyme disease. I agreed, and after more than ten years of negative lab test results, this one finally came out positive. As I held the results in my hands, I said, "Yep! It's Lyme disease." That got me investigating again other therapies that would get rid of Lyme disease. Finding a real solution, however, took awhile.

At some point, I discovered Dr. Woitzel's biophoton therapy for Lyme disease. I combined this with a protocol that I had developed, and it ended up being the perfect treatment solution for me. Fol-lowing treatment, my LTT test came up negative, and has remained so, up to this day.

While living in Hamburg (and still having Lyme) I opened a well-ness center and shop called Catch a Dream, where I sold a variety of herbal and other remedies, as well as nutritional supports from all over the world. At the time, I was the only one in Germany who owned a shop of this kind. I had a lot of clients with Lyme, allergies, drug addictions and other health problems who would visit the wellness center. Also, I still hadn't received my certification as a heilpraktiker, so I couldn't treat them, but they could consult me and I could give them advice, based on my own experiences with different treatments. This was in some ways beneficial, because whenever I discovered a remedy that worked for me, I would share it with those who came into my shop.

Subsequently, at the beginning of the millennium, I received my certification as a heilpraktiker, and was then able to open a practice and start treating Lyme patients as well as others that were suffering from unexplainable illnesses. By that time, I had also gone through a lot of extra training in immunology, endocrinology, neurology, and other disciplines, which helped to improve and expand my work as a heilpraktiker.

Initially, I treated my patients' Lyme disease (Borreliosis) using stabilized oxygen and glutathione. This helped to reduce their symptoms, but it didn't eliminate all of the borrelia from within their cells nor did it heal them 100%. Subsequently, I began to use biophoton therapy in my practice. I administered treatments to my patients using a device called the Bionic 880, which proved to be very effective for eradicating borrelia. In fact, ever since I have used the Bionic 880 in conjunction with my own specific healing protocol (which I have worked out over the years), I have been able to claim that I have found a successful treatment for Lyme disease (Borreliosis).

Healing is about more than just simply getting rid of Borrelia, however, because most patients are also confronted with all kinds of co-morbidities, opportunistic infections and immune system challenges such as systemic inflammation, which must also be dealt with if they are to completely heal.

I am currently in the process of writing a book in German about how chronic, multi-system and autoimmune diseases come about. In this book, I discuss the factors that play a role in the development of disease, including chronic infections. I have found that certain chronic infections have been underestimated or forgotten by the scientific community, even by people whose work I respect a lot, and I think that this is a problem. For example, many healthcare practitioners will say that Chlamydia doesn't play a role in chronic illness, and that antibodies that patients present to this infection are really indicative of old infection. I think, however, that such antibodies may reflect the presence of an active, chronic infection, which can play just as much of a role in the development of symptoms and chronic illness as Borrelia. This is one of the ideas that I emphasize in my book, among others. On the other hand, antibody testing doesn't necessarily provide all of the answers. Patients can test negative on antibody tests, even if they have an active infection, and they can also test positive on antibody tests when their infections aren't active anymore. Therefore, it can be difficult to discern the status of their infections. For that reason, only the LTT (lymphocyte transformation test) can actually determine whether an infection is active and if the treatments used for that particular infection are successful. This is, unfortunately, the only accurate blood test for many types of infections, especially intracellular infections. Also, it is far more expensive than antibody tests and offered only in a handful of practices.

Healing Philosophy/Treatment Approach

Whenever I suspect that my patients have Lyme disease (or Borreliosis, as it is called here in Germany), the first thing that I do is send them out for a LTT, or lymphocyte transformation test (as mentioned previously). This test looks for a specific cellular immunological reaction to Borrelia, and is about 90% accurate for detecting active infection.

I then have them do other blood tests so that I can determine the state of their immune system as well as what is happening in their cells. Such tests include:

- Homocysteine (to determine how well cell symbiosis is taking place)

- Zinc and selenium (to determine the body's toxic load, as well as how strong and adequate immune responses are)

- Vitamin D (the levels of which are almost always low in those with chronic disease. This vitamin is essential for combating infection and inflammation, as well as for building hormones)

- Inflammatory cytokines (TNF alpha, IL-10, IL-1ß, Interferon gamma)

- Natural killer cell function

- Cortisol circadian rhythms. (This is actually done using a saliva test. If patients' cortisol levels are low, then these must be corrected before they can begin treatments for Borrelia, as the treatments will be unsuccessful otherwise.)

- Nitric oxide stress (to determine mitochondrial stress)

- Intracellular glutathione

I then use the results of these tests to help me to formulate a treatment protocol for my patients.

My main treatment for Borrelia is biophoton therapy using the Bionic 880 device. This therapy involves placing homeopathic nosodes on the patient's solar plexus while administering biophotonic light to different points on his or her body. The homeopathic nosodes contain the energetic imprint of the borrelia organism or whatever infection I happen to be treating, and give the body the information about what it must do, which is, in the case of borrelia, to expel the organism from the cells.

I accompany these treatments with intravenous infusions of stabilized oxygen, which are given in a saline solution. The stabilized oxygen helps to oxidize floating microbes in the blood, and is a helpful adjunct to the photon therapy. It eliminates borrelia or whatever other oxygen-sensitive microbes are floating around in the blood, and acts as a blood cleanser of sorts.

My patients usually require eight biophoton treatments in order for their Borrelia infections to be put into remission. From their second or third treatment on, I also give them homeopathic Borrelia no-sodes to take orally, which are of the same type that I place on their solar plexus for use in conjunction with the biophotons.

Most of the time, I also give them intramuscular B-12 shots after the therapy, because it gives them a little more neurological stability, and helps their bodies to heal on many levels.

It is important to note here that biophoton therapy does not kill the borrelia organism. It supports the immune system, so that the immune system can accomplish this itself via increased natural killer cell activity, which happens as a result of more efficient ATP production.

A scientific explanation is appropriate here. The human body has a highly sensitive, yet extremely effective way of producing energy by using oxygen. This energy—ATP—is so important for the body, that it produces around seventy kilograms, or approximately 145 pounds of it per day. If this energy were not present, then the body would die within seconds. At least a thousand mitochondria are present in every cell, and these mitochondria carry out the work of energy production. The process of ATP formation is a cycle, which is carried out in five steps, or five complexes, in which electrons are transported from one complex to the next. Complex IV (or the fourth step) in this chain absorbs about 90% of the body's inhaled oxygen. This absorption occurs within a wavelength range of 600 to 900 nanometers. Chronic illness is accompanied by a dysfunction in complex IV. The implication of this is that the electron transport process gets "stuck", which then creates dysfunctional mitochondria that are unable to adequately produce ATP. The Bionic 880 happens to emit photons at a wavelength of 880 nm, which falls within the body's range of complex IV-absorbing photons. The body can therefore use the photons from the Bionic 880 to eliminate the blockages in its electron transport system. In turn, the natural killer cells benefit from the increased ATP that is produced as a result, and become more effective to the body in its fight against borrelia. Curcumin may also assist with this process. So with the help of the Bionic and a little curcumin, the body is enabled to eliminate intracellular microbes by means of its own resources.

That said, if photon therapy is undertaken without supporting other systems in the body that may be "out of tune", then it may trigger a systemic inflammatory response. If this happens, patients will feel very bad after treatments. Their body's inflammatory response, nitric stress levels, and even allergic or aberrant neurotransmitter reactions can all be triggered.

After administering stabilized oxygen to my patients following their biophoton treatment, I then give them a glutathione fast push, in order to support their body's cellular antioxidant system, which is "run" by glutathione. After the body starts to kill cells that are contaminated by borrelia, it needs an anti-oxidative support to detoxify the debris from these cells as well as from the borrelia neurotoxins, and this can be partially accomplished with gluta-thione. So glutathione acts as a kind of support for the cellular system.

Finally, it's vital to support the body in other ways during photon treatment. I advise my patients to maintain a low-carbohydrate diet that is high in protein and omega-3 fatty acids. Taking high doses of coenzyme Q-10, magnesium, B-vitamins, Vitamins D and C (which are anti-inflammatory), probiotics and certain amino acids that are precursors to neurotransmitters are also a must during treatment. I recommend that practitioners test their patients for deficiencies of these before supplementing with any of the above, however.

Author's note: For more information on how the Bionic 880 works, see the chapter on Dr. Woitzel, who also uses biophotons for the treatment of Lyme disease

Diagnostic Procedure

When new patients come into my office, I first ask them to fill out a long questionnaire. We then have a conversation to discuss their responses, as well as any other personal information. I use this information, as well as their lab test results, to establish their treatment regimen. Then I use energetic testing devices such as the biotensor to confirm the treatments that are the most appropriate for them.

So I not only treat my patients for borrelia, but for other problems that they may have, as well. It's important that I test the function of the entire body. If I don't, then I make mistakes in patients' treatment.

The elimination of borrelia should be at the forefront of any treatment protocol for Lyme, however. If the body doesn't get rid of borrelia, then any other treatment is more or less useless.

It's also important for me to determine my patients' adrenal gland function, because the success of any treatment regimen depends upon the adrenal glands working properly. If adrenal function is low, and cortisol levels are low, then as a practitioner, I will not succeed in anything that I do for my patients until I can improve the functioning of their adrenals.

Symptoms of adrenal fatigue include extreme fatigue, depression, insomnia or oversleeping; for example, having to sleep for twelve or fifteen hours, or not being able to sleep soundly at all. Also, those with adrenal fatigue tend to catch every infection around, are often underweight and lack muscle strength. They may also have a pale complexion. The exhaustion in those with adrenal fatigue can be so profound that they get what is called "burnout syndrome", which means that they lose complete interest in their social obligations and in life. Having to call people or get things done by a certain time becomes overwhelming for them. They are basically able to sit or lie around, and are not able to do much else. Their tolerance to stress, noise or fragrances is also low.

318

So therapy for Borrelia and other conditions may not be effective unless the adrenals are adequately supported, because when the adrenals are weak, the body simply won't respond to treatments. This I learned after treating many patients, because there were some for whom the LTT test would not turn negative, even after they had received multiple photon treatments for Borrelia, and I would ask myself, *What's stopping us here?* After doing a few tests, I learned that poor adrenal function was what was hindering these people's healing, and I've seen this scenario happen quite a few times ever since.

In addition to the adrenals, thyroid function must also be carefully tested and treated, when necessary. Triiodothyronine, T-3, as well as TSH, are among the tests that I do to determine patients' thyroid function. If I suspect that they have autoimmune disease, as well as high levels of nitric stress (nitric oxide and peroxynitrite) in their urine, then it may also be necessary to test them for thyroid antibodies.

In summary, when the adrenal and thyroid glands aren't functioning properly, it's very difficult for patients to heal, and I often see low thyroid and adrenal function in those with Lyme disease.

In general, it's good for practitioners to look at the function of all of their patients' hormones when treating them, because the hormonal system functions by a reverse feedback system. The implication of this is that if practitioners "push" one gland without addressing the others, then they may seriously disturb homeostasis in their patients' bodies.

Hormone, Neurotransmitter and Other Types of Testing

I do saliva and urine tests on my patients to check the functioning of certain hormones, such as the catecholamines, which are the "fight-or-flight" hormones. These include epinephrine, norepinephrine and dopamine, which are released by the adrenal glands in response to stress.

319

The Neuroendocrinological Stress profile is another test that I often have my patients do. There is a lab in Munich (Lab4More), as well as one in Augsburg (Biolabs) that does this. These labs specialize in the testing of neuropeptides, neurohormones, catecholamines and other hormones, as well as neurotransmitters like GABA, glutamate, serotonin and dopamine. Through such tests, I am able to formulate a treatment protocol to correct my patients' hormonal and neurotransmitter imbalances.

For instance, yesterday there was a young woman that I needed to do the Stress profile on. This woman is thirty-one years old and hasn't had her period for six years. She has anger problems, as well as a tendency to hurt herself physically in order to feel better emotionally. In addition, she has neuroborreliosis. This type of patient requires a complete panel of tests to determine what hormonal and neurological imbalances are playing a role in her illness. I can then correct these, for instance, with the use of amino acids and other neurotransmitter precursors, or homeopathic remedies that support the functioning of her whole body.

Also, here in Germany, practitioners have the opportunity to use injections containing real organ extracts to balance their patients' hormones. By law, such extracts must be prepared by practitioners and can be used only in their practices. These extracts are of extremely high quality and safety, however, and are effective because they stimulate millions of potent, multi-purpose stem cells in the body. (See below for more information on their use in correcting adrenal dysfunction).

My patients' treatment is always very individualized, though, because they don't come to me with "just" Lyme disease. They have a wide variety of problems, and everyone with Borreliosis has a different set of symptoms. Getting rid of Borrelia first is important, but balancing everything else in the body is, too. If we (the patient and I) miss out on an important issue, we might not reach our goal of health.

Another test that I do involves measuring my patients' homocyste-ine levels. If these levels are too high, then I know that they have a problem with ATP production. They might have, for instance, a problem with methylation, which is involved in ATP synthesis. I must discover the cause of their high homocysteine levels and regulate its production so that their cellular metabolism functions properly.

I also check Vitamin D levels, because this nutrient protects the body against infections; it is both anti-inflammatory and anti-microbial. Just about everyone who is chronically ill has a Vitamin D deficiency. Also, Vitamin D isn't really a vitamin, it's a hormone that helps to keep the other hormones in balance. For these rea-sons, its role in the body is vital for maintaining health.

It's interesting that nowadays, there are about twenty percent less photons from sunlight that reach the earth than from years past (the sun emits photons, just as the human body). This was meas-ured and investigated in a research project on global warming, but since photons are light, I think it's more accurate to call this phe-nomenon of reduced photon activity global *darkening*, instead of global *warming*! This may be one reason why so many people these days are lacking in Vitamin D, especially in northern Europe, where people tend to stay inside the house during winter when there is less sunlight, anyway.

Treating Hormonal Dysfunction

I support my patients' adrenals with a glandular formula that also contains licorice, Siberian and Korean ginseng, Vitamin B-5 and other micro-nutrients. Also, I have recently produced an adrenal extract that is made from the adrenal glands of organically-raised animals. Preliminary results from using this extract have been promising, but so far I have only had a few experiences with it. It seems that caution must be exercised when using it on those who are extremely fatigued and cortisol-deprived. The extract regene-rates the adrenals at the same time that it supplies cortisol to the body. It is quite difficult to produce, and in Germany, health care practitioners and medical doctors must make it themselves for use only in their patients. The organ extracts are administered via injection twice a week, and it's important to combine the injections with thymus extract, because the immune system needs to be supported at the same time. If the adrenal organ extract is administered alone, then the adrenals might overreact to it. An overstimulation of the adrenals can lead to peaks in adrenaline, accelerated heartbeat and circulation problems. The thymus extract helps to prevent this reaction.

Another supplement that I recommend which is beneficial for helping the adrenal glands to recover is omega-3 fatty acids. People with Lyme should consume—or rather, drown their bodies in this stuff! Omega-3 fatty acids are also important for recovery of the neurological system, and especially the myelin sheath that covers the nerves, as well as for the body's cell walls. Also, omega-3 fatty acids help the body to get rid of borrelia neurotoxins. For this reason, I recommend high dose omega-3 fatty acids to my patients, as part of the baseline of their therapy. And when I say "high dose" that might mean 3-5 tablespoons of linseed oil, along with two 3,000 mg doses of omega-3 fish oil per day.

For treatment of the thyroid, I might give my patients selenium, if their test results show that they are deficient in this mineral. Because zinc supports the basic building blocks of thyroid hormone, I might also recommend zinc supplementation. If the thyroid requires more support than this, then I might ask a medical doctor for further advice and support, which may include a prescription for thyroid medication that contains active T3 and T4 hormones. (In Germany, health care practitioners that are not medical doctors cannot prescribe thyroid hormone, nor are they allowed to prescribe any other kind of hormonal treatment).

Another hormone that I test and treat in my patients is DHEA. When I look at their DHEA and cortisol lab test results, then I can determine to what degree they are stressed or exhausted. It sometimes happens that before patients' cortisol levels drop (as a result of stress), their DHEA levels go up. This scenario occurs when the body is under constant stress, whether that stress comes from one's job, disease or environment. If this stress continues, however, then at some point, the body's DHEA levels will also eventually drop, so that both cortisol and DHEA levels become low. Whenever I see this scenario in my patients, I recommend that they request a DHEA prescription from their primary care physician, since in Germany, only physicians are able to prescribe this hormone. Fortunately, I work with some well-respected and excellent doctors, who collaborate with me on this issue.

Supplementing with bioidentical transdermal progesterone and/or estrogen may be a good idea for women, if they are deficient in these hormones. I never, ever, advise them to take synthetic hormones, only natural ones that balance the endocrine system. Once their hormones are balanced, I may recommend that they switch from bioidentical to phytohormones, or plant hormones, which contain some of the same hormone-balancing properties as the bioidentical hormones, but which also supply holistic plant information to the body. Plants contain multiple constituents that function synergistically to benefit the body, whereas synthetic medications, which are made from plant extracts, isolate only one or two of these constituents so that the body doesn't have the full benefit of all of them working together. Soybean, red clover, Dong quai, and black cohosh are examples of plants that are beneficial to the female endocrine system.

Treating Inflammation

People with Lyme disease have systemic, chronic, silent inflammation in their bodies. Pain is one indication of inflammation, and when I see patients who are in a lot of pain, then I know that they have a lot of systemic inflammation that I need to treat. If I don't, then their recovery will be more complicated and strenuous.

To determine the degree of inflammation, I test their cytokines, such as TNF alpha, interleukin 10 and 6, interferon gamma, and, if necessary, interleukin 1-beta. The results of these tests also help me to determine other things, such as, for instance, whether their bodies are having an allergic reaction to something.

There are four or five good remedies which are known to lower TNF alpha and inflammation. The lab that I work with in Berlin determines which of these is best for my patients, through use of a specific test that analyzes how their TNF alpha reacts to certain agents such as boswellia, curcumin, artemisinin or a remedy called TNF Direct.

My wonderful friend and colleague Thorsten Hollmann, who is based in Wuppertal, Germany, established this test. He always comes up with interesting new ways of discovering which remedies and lab tests work and which ones don't. He is also an expert in diagnosing and treating CFS (chronic fatigue syndrome). CFS, by the way, is often a manifestation of chronic Lyme disease, which is often accompanied by other problems such as Epstein-Barr and Herpes' viruses, Candida and heavy metals. A tremendous range of scientific material on this, and many other interesting subjects can be found on T. C. Hollmann's website at: www.cfs-center.de.

Thanks to Thorsten Hollmann and his scientific approach to holistic medicine, I have had to advance my knowledge in certain areas of medicine at the speed of light in order to keep up with his expert knowledge on chronic illness. Four eyes see more than two, as we say in German! And when we health care practitioners throw our findings together, the outcome can be quite enlightening at times.

Hence, the TNF inhibiting test can help practitioners to discern the most appropriate anti-inflammatory remedies for their patients, based on individual test results. Also, and in general, it is wiser to use the micronized form of these agents, because a lot less is needed (than the other forms) to achieve the same results.

When my patients' joint and pain symptoms get worse following photon treatment, then this indicates to me that their body's inflammatory response hasn't been adequately addressed. When practitioners work "anti-infection," then they are also working "pro inflammatory", because inflammation is the normal physiological response of the immune system when eliminating infection. Whenever there is systemic inflammation, however, it's important to be mindful of immune system overreaction, but there is a fine line between balancing optimal immune response and adequate treatment of microbes. That's why, when practitioners are dealing with both inflammation and infection in their patients, which is usually the case, they need to balance their patients' anti-infection treatment with some type of anti-inflammatory treatment. If they neglect either one of these, then their patients will get worse.

Treating Other Infections

I treat my patients' other infections after Borrelia using photon therapy, but I also support getting rid of microbes with herbal remedies.

Examples of anti-microbial herbs that I use in my practice include Kardenwurzel, which is a type of thistle, as well as olive leaf, cat's claw and artemisia (the latter I use for intracellular microbes). But the most promising remedies for eliminating unwanted microbes are ozonides, because they oxygenate the body while killing bugs. These are made in a base of ozonated castor oil, using the essential oils of potent plants. They are water and fat soluble, which means that they can go everywhere in the body. They are a potent treatment to use along with biophotons.

One of the reasons that I use herbal remedies in conjunction with biophotons is because patients may have infections that I haven't been able to detect and if I use only the nosodes and photons to treat these, then I might miss one of them. Using the blood as a homeopathic nosode, however, will usually mop up any undetected infections, but this should be applied only after the body has had the chance to build up its capacity to recover. Otherwise, patients' Herxheimer reactions may be quite strong.

In any case, I think that we sometimes have to come at the infections from different angles in order to get rid of them all. For this reason, I may recommend that my patients take herbs at the same time that they do photon treatments.

Some of my patients are sensitive to strong remedies, so once I have "worked off" some of their more important infections, like Borrelia, Chlamydia, or Candida, I may then treat them for other undefined infections or stressors, using a drop of their blood as a homeopathic nosode. The blood nosode functions as a kind of natural vaccination when used along with the biophotons, and treatment with both usually takes care of any remaining infections in the body. This is because every human cell (including those in the blood) contains all of the body's information, so even though a particular pathogen may not be present in the blood, the blood yet contains information about that pathogen's presence, whether the actual pathogen is in the tissues or elsewhere.

I must warn people against believing that photons and nosodes are the solution for everything, however. The photon therapy only donates photons to the body, to assist the body in what it needs to do. This is physics, but there is a biochemical side to the body, too, which requires its own support. If patients don't get this support, then one system in the body may be activated, while another is neglected, which means that patients can get worse, instead of better, as a result of photon therapy. This does happen, so I caution readers to not underestimate the power of this therapy.

Photons, however, are extremely effective for getting rid of infections. Some patients that I have treated only with nosodes, detoxification and anti-inflammatory agents, as well as TH1 and T2 balancing agents, have improved significantly through these things alone, but others need more support.

Detoxification

It's crucial to support the body in its detoxification processes, and to do this in conjunction with Borrelia treatments, because once the body is activated by photons, then the cells start spitting out toxins by themselves, and the body must be able to deal with these toxins. Also, immune cells lead diseased cells to apoptosis, which is programmed cell death, and cells with Borrelia inside are marked for this type of destruction. So this waste needs to be processed and leave the body, too, or else it will harm the body, which is why it's good to have a detoxification program in place to deal with all these neurotoxins.

My detoxification protocol involves using substances such as glutathione, selenium, cysteine, zeolites, alpha lipoic acid, omega-3 fatty acids and sulfur-containing agents to chelate, bind and dispose of the toxins generated by biophoton and other treatments. All of these detoxification substances need to be tested on each patient though, because not everyone can use the same ones. The choice of toxin binder or detoxification agent also depends somewhat upon the types of toxins that patients have collected in their bodies. For example, I must determine whether solvents, chemicals, heavy metals, or medications are significant problems, and to what degree they influence my patients' physiology. It may also be important to check patients' genes to determine what their detoxification capabilities are.

Another substance that I find to be beneficial for detoxification is broccoli extract. A chemical in this extract supports phase two detoxification in the liver, which often doesn't function properly in the chronically ill, especially in those with glutathione or SOD enzyme deficiencies. So broccoli extract makes it much easier for the liver to get rid of toxins.

Zeolite is beneficial for binding toxins but it doesn't touch neurotoxins or stored toxins. Lecithin and omega-3 fatty acids are better for detoxifying fat-soluble toxins and those that are in the brain. They also protect the lipid part of cell walls.

For the detoxification of heavy metals, I use a remedy called Biolo-go Detox. This product contains micronized chlorella, coriander and healing mushrooms. It's quite powerful, and I use it often in my patients. Another remedy that I use is Sporopollein, which is also a chlorella algae extract. It's very strong and can remove large toxic burdens from the body. For severe cases of heavy metal toxicity, intravenous chelation with EDTA might be the best type of therapy, but it's powerful, and most of the time, I prefer to walk a softer path with my patients. If they respond well to this therapy, however, then the greatest benefits occur when the therapist is able to administer ten one and a half -hour sessions. Chelation therapy is also quite expensive.

Finally, I don't advise patients or practitioners to detoxify heavy metals using nosodes and photon therapy! This is dangerous and harmful, because while the photons mobilize metals, they cannot bind them, and will instead invite them into the nervous system, which is dangerous. Whenever I speak to doctors and therapists, I emphasize that the detoxification of metals with homeopathic and energetic strategies is not a good idea, because such strategies mobilize metals but don't carry them out of the body. It's important to use a substance that also binds with the toxins and which can assist the body with their excretion, otherwise they will circulate in the bloodstream and eventually settle down again someplace else in the body.

Patient and Practitioner Challenges to Healing

Adrenal problems are my patients' greatest obstacle to healing, and problems with other hormones or glands are the next greatest. Those with compromised detoxification also have trouble healing, as do those with certain emotional problems.

It's sometimes important for patients to ask themselves questions like: "Do I want to heal? Am I able to work for my healing? Do I believe in my healing? Am I a positive person?" And if the answer to any of these questions is No, then they must work to change those answers. Lyme disease can completely change a personality, and make people miserable, aggressive, childish and hurtful, as well as many other things, and it takes discipline to change one's thinking patterns or ways of being.

I assist my patients with this aspect of healing by trying to discern what their emotional issues are and then giving them exercises, affirmations and other suggestions for dealing with those. I might, for example, give them homework that involves standing in front of the mirror every day and saying things like, "I am the boss in my body. I am the boss of my life. Problems must take a backseat for now!"

Sometimes, I will also teach them strategies for dealing with any leftover childhood trauma, but I usually prefer to start by doing a therapy called Life System with them. This therapy utilizes biofeedback to provide me with a deep look at the bottom of the soul, along with different strategies that are helpful for discovering the root causes of their problems. Using biofeedback strategies involving sound, light and energetic frequencies, I can then balance their fear, or whatever negative emotional or thinking patterns that may have built up inside of them which are keeping them from wellness.

Other people need to forgive in order to heal, but before they can do that, they need to know what this means. To me, forgiveness involves a belief that our souls have contracts with other souls and that we are here to fulfill those contracts. Let's say, for instance, that a lady's husband makes her learn some very painful lesson. When looked at from a universal angle, it may be that both she and her husband agreed to the situation that led to the painful lesson, and that such a situation was necessary in order for her to take the next step in her journey of personal growth.

When looked at in this context, it becomes much easier for people to forgive, because then they can say, for instance, "He and I both needed this situation in order to learn a certain life lesson." We can then be grateful that a dear person was willing to "play mean," just so that our stubborn heads could learn this lesson. Consequently, saying "Thank you" to the person that hurt us, instead of whining, "You are so mean, and you are the reason why I feel bad!" can be beneficial, because we have learned something as a result of the experience, and perhaps the other person did, too. We were divine tools for the growth of one another.

Lifestyle and Dietary Recommendations for Healing

Sleep Hygiene

If I suspect that my patients have weak adrenal glands or immune problems, then I advise them to go to bed early, before 10 P.M. I may also recommend that they take melatonin before bedtime. Only when they get very sound sleep is it possible for their immune systems to regenerate.

Dietary Recommendations

People with Lyme disease should maintain a diet that is rich in EFA's (essential fatty acids), as well as protein. Carbohydrates should be kept to a minimum, because they can feel "heavy" for those who are very ill, and can exacerbate inflammation. Apart from these guidelines, people with Lyme should eat things that they know they can tolerate, because some have food intolerances and immune reactions to certain foods. Most of the intoxicated and chronically ill can't tolerate dairy or wheat, for example, and I will sometimes recommend that my patients go a week without consuming any dairy products, to see how they feel. If they don't notice any difference in their symptoms, then it may be okay for them to continue consuming a particular dairy product. In any case, milk should not be part of anyone's diet, since we are humans and not baby cows!

If patients feel worse after consuming certain foods, then they should stop eating those foods. If their adrenals aren't functioning well and their cortisol levels are low, then you can bet that they have food intolerances and allergies. Also, it's much easier for their immune systems to recover when they avoid the foods that they react negatively to, as well as those foods that don't match their blood type. In general, avoiding milk and dairy products, wheat and refined carbohydrates, and especially white sugar or flour, is most important. The worst possible diet for Lyme sufferers would include white flour, white sugar, heated fat and animal protein. So burgers should be a thing of the past!

Exercise

I recommend that my patients do mild aerobic exercise, and certain sports, as long as these activities don't leave them exhausted. They should avoid any type of "heavy" movements. Weight training or exercise that increases the pulse beyond 125 beats per minute isn't beneficial, because it puts the body into a catabolic state. Lyme sufferers should not get into a catabolic state because this causes pain in their bodies the day after they exercise and hence more oxidative stress, which is not beneficial for healing. Exercises such as walking and cycling are better.

The Role of Nitric Oxide in Disease

Nitric oxide and peroxynitrite are two chemicals that those with Lyme disease often have in abundance in their bodies. Quite simply, whenever the body is bombarded with intracellular microbes, it fights against them by producing nitric oxide within the cell. Chronic intracellular infection raises nitric oxide levels for a rather lengthy period of time when compared to other causes of excessive nitric oxide output. Therefore, I believe that intracellular infections have a lot to do with elevated nitric oxide levels in the body. Elevated nitric oxide levels can then cause peroxynitrite to be produced, which is a substance that is very toxic to mitochondria. When people with Lyme have elevated inflammatory levels, then this causes nitric oxide to upregulate (hence also creating more peroxynitrite) which in turn increases their inflammatory levels, and it becomes a vicious cycle. So if patients have nitric stress in their bodies, which can be ascertained through a urine test, then their practitioners must help them to interrupt this cycle, as well.

Interrupting the cycle can be done in a few ways. I give my patients high doses of Co-Q10. Co-Q10 plays an important role in interrupting nitric acid production, as do hydroxycobalamin (Vitamin B-12) injections, alpha lipoic acid, magnesium, L-carnitine, Vitamin D, and intravenous Vitamin C in high doses. Checking and balancing any other nutritional deficiencies can be helpful, as well.

Scientist Martin Pall wrote an excellent book called *Explaining Unexplained Illnesses*. His discoveries and findings on nitric stress have been amazing. And over the last year, even more information has come out on the subject. Such findings are important, because nitric stress is one key factor in the development of autoimmune and multi-system illnesses such as PTSD, CFS and MCS, as well as in neurological illnesses such as MS and Parkinson's.

I am convinced that intracellular microbes play a role in the development of autoimmune disease. They may switch on the nitric stress cycle in people who have been suffering from long-term inflammation, and there's no way that the body can shut this cycle off unless we help it to do so. This is another reason why I believe that it's dangerous to claim or even hope (as some do), that one machine (the Bionic 880, for example) can heal everything. The Bionic can light up the body where it's dark; it can support the body, but it's not a machine that can heal everything. There are so many reasons why chronic illness happens, and practitioners must determine which areas of their patients' bodies need to be upregulated as well as which ones need to be downregulated, and choose the most appropriate methods for re-achieving balance. People tend to want to have just one tool that they can build a house with but that is a dream; it can't happen. Human beings are more subtle and complicated than that. If patients have a dramatic vitamin B-12 deficiency, for instance, then how in the world do they expect to balance that with biophoton therapy? It just doesn't work. They must instead give the body supplemental Vitamin B-12.

Last Words

As a practitioner, if you have ever had to battle illness, then you have a different kind of compassion when you work with patients who are going through similar experiences, because you have felt what they are going through and can empathize with them. I am one of these people. My Lyme patients don't need to explain to me how they are feeling, because I have experienced many of their symptoms myself.

Many people with Lyme have been given the impression by previous health care providers that their illnesses are "all in their head," yet deep down inside they know that this isn't true. They suffer from severe immunological disease. And I feel blessed that I can assist such people in realizing what is actually wrong with them, and support them in getting well again.

How to Contact Marlene Kunold, "Heilpraktiker"

Naturheilpraxis Marlene E. Kunold
Torstr. 40
D-22525 Hamburg-Germany
E-mail: hp-mek@gmx.de

•CHAPTER 12•

Elizabeth Hesse-Sheehan, DC, CCN
KIRKLAND, WA

Biography

Dr. Hesse-Sheehan is a Holistic Chiropractor, Quantum Neurologist and Certified Clinical Nutritionist. She has the exceptional ability to learn about and integrate the newest, cutting-edge healing techniques into her classic holistic healing background. Her scientific approach and intuitive heart have allowed her to be an innovator in various fields of kinesiology, as well as in chiropractic and light therapy. She is extensively trained in a variety of healing modalities including multiple chiropractic techniques, Autonomic Response Testing and Quantum Neurology. She utilizes the teachings of Drs. Dietrich Klinghardt, M.D., Ph.D., John Brimhall, D.C., Dominique Richard, M.D., W. Lee Cowden, M.D., George Gonzalez, D.C., Q.N., and Louisa Williams, D.C. She has been in practice since 2000, and specializes in the care of complex disorders including chronic immune dysfunction syndromes, Lyme disease and autism. She has offices in Kirkland and Spokane, Washington.

Healing Philosophy

I try to discover and remove the obstacles that hinder the body's innate capacity to heal and overcome disease. It's important to find these obstacles since they are what prevent Lyme disease patients from overcoming their health problems. This means finding and putting together as many pieces of their healing puzzle as possible, so that they are able to heal from within.

I perform Applied Kinesiology or ART (Autonomic Response Testing) and laboratory tests (including orthopedic and neurological tests), along with a physical examination, to discern the imbalances that are present in my patients' bodies.

After working with the chronically ill for several years, I have come to the conclusion that where many doctors may be missing the boat is in their lack of immune system testing. They seem to concentrate on treating infections, and while it's important to treat or manage patients' infections, it's also important to address their immune dysfunction. Yet, I don't observe many doctors (at least in my geographical area) running immune system tests, such as lymphocyte subset tests and immunoglobulin panels to determine the state of their patients' immune systems. Neither do I observe them asking questions such as, "Is the immune system suppressed, and if so, how much? Is the patient having autoimmune, or hyper-immune responses?" Consequently, I don't see practitioners doing targeted therapies to effect and re-modulate the immune system, and I believe that this should be an important part of any treatment protocol.

Also, some practitioners fall into the trap of thinking that if they just kill the bugs, then their patients' immune systems will kick back in on their own, but I don't think that this happens in all cases. It's important to eradicate infections, but practitioners must strengthen their patients' immune systems, as well. Or sometimes practitioners think, *Let's throw some mushrooms or colostrum at the patient!* These substances might be problematic for people who are having hyper-immune or autoimmune responses, because they can stimulate the wrong part of the immune system. So it's important for practitioners to run immune system tests on their patients. Also, while performing ART testing can tell practitioners a lot of things about their patients, it doesn't reveal everything, such as, for example, what their lymphocyte sub-populations are or what their ratios of NK killer cells to CD3, CD4 or CD8 cells are.

That said, Applied Kinesiology or ART should be used to test for infections, organ stresses, and toxins in the body, since lab testing is notorious for not being able to discern such problems. After all, we get so many false negatives on Lyme and co-infection tests.

Hence, I combine ART and Applied Kinesiology techniques with lab testing in order to achieve the best possible testing outcomes with my patients.

Plant Stem Cell Extracts for the Management of Lyme and Immune System Dysfunction

My current biochemical remedies of choice for addressing infections, biofilms, and immune system dysfunction in those with Lyme disease are several types of herbal remedies, including embryonic herbal extracts, or plant stem cell extracts. While this type of therapy is new to the United States, plant stem cells have been used extensively in Europe over the past thirty years, and I believe they are a powerful healing modality, with much potential and promise for healing people of Lyme disease. The two main companies that distribute stem cell products in the United States are Herbal Gem (from Belgium) and PSC Plant Stem Cells (from Italy).

Plant stem cells are herbal medicines that are made by harvesting plants when they are in their embryonic form and creating extracts from their shoots, buds, rootlets and seeds. Extracts made from embryonic plants have a dramatically different biochemical composition than extracts made from adult plants. The embryonic herbal extracts contain actual plant stem cells (which serve to detoxify, rejuvenate and regenerate human tissue), and hormones (which modulate the immune system) and are much higher in phytochemicals than the adult plants. Adult plants are touted for having high levels of phytonutrients, but I've observed that often, they don't seem to benefit my patients much. Take ginkgo and bilberry, for instance. I have witnessed many people take these herbs and derive no real beneficial results from their use. Medical literature writes about all these so-called miracles that are supposed to happen in peoples' bodies when they take adult herbs, but I think that such miracles don't happen because the phytochemicals in adult plants can be completely gone or highly reduced—by up to 60-75%. However, such phytochemicals are known to be present in high concentrations in embryonic plants.

Plant stem cell extracts serve to repair, rejuvenate and regenerate tissue in the human body. They also have the ability to differentiate into specialized cells once in the body, which means that they are able to treat a wide range of problems. What's more, the phyto-chemicals in embryonic plants have a wide range of physiologic effects upon the body, so they are very broad spectrum in their use, which means that one type of plant stem cell can be used to treat a multitude of problems. For instance, all extracts made from embryonic tissue have high amounts of quercetin and/or other anti-inflammatory agents built into them, which means that a single remedy can be anti-spirochetal, anti-fungal, anti-bacterial, and anti-viral, as well as anti-inflammatory. This is advantageous, because it means that as microbes are being killed, inflammation is being reduced in the body because of the built-in anti-inflammatory properties of the plant. At the same time, other aspects of the immune system are being repaired and supported, as well. Additionally, the more heavy-duty stem cell products can address all types of infections. While some remedies are specifically antiviral or antibacterial, others have properties of the "big four" built into them; meaning, they are anti-viral, anti-bacterial, anti-fungal and anti-parasitic.

Plant stem cells have many uses, and I recommend them to my patients for a variety of different symptoms and problems. One of the really spectacular remedies that I use in my practice is called

Maize, which is one of the strongest anti-bacterial products in the herbal family of stem cells. It has over 200 phytochemicals, thirty-some of which are anti-inflammatory. This is very advantageous because bug killing and detoxification create inflammation in the body, so when practitioners give their patients a product that is anti-bacterial as well as anti-inflammatory, they are addressing multiple pieces of their healing puzzle.

Another example of a multi-purpose plant stem cell product is Grapevine. In its embryonic form, Grapevine is anti-viral, anti-bacterial and anti-inflammatory, as well as an immune system booster and heavy metal chelator. So it's one product, with five very different actions upon the body.

Another great thing about the plant stem cell extracts is that the recommended daily doses are so low, most people usually only need nine drops per day of a single remedy. Also, due to their biochemical constituents, and to the smaller dose sizes, the remedies have better osmotic potential, which results in better absorption and action in the body. Finally, because they are so multi-faceted, fewer adjunct supplements are needed for healing, which makes them cost-effective.

The number of embryonic extracts that people with chronic Lyme disease need depends upon the person, his or her constitution, laboratory findings, and specific problems. People who are super sensitive, asymptomatic or in remission may only need one or two remedies. Those who are really sick and need a lot of extra support; for example, those with cancer or severe immune dysfunction, might need up to thirteen different remedies. Practitioners who support cancer patients, for example, must do many things with their patients; induce apoptosis (programmed cell death), re-regulate and change their immune system responses, regulate their detoxification processes, restore their nutrient deficiencies and then provide them with remedies for specific symptoms. But amazingly, plant stem cells can do all of these things.

Another great thing about the plant stem cell extracts is that because they are derived from plants, not humans, there isn't the same kind of moral controversy over their use as with human stem cells.

The Difference between Herbal Gem and PSC Plant Stem Cells

According to my understanding, Plant Stem Cell Nutrition (PSC) produces its products somewhat differently from Herbal Gem. For instance, PSC takes the time to pick off the paper casing around its buds with tweezers, whereas Herbal Gem doesn't. This makes the levels of undesirable tannins in PSC's products lower than those of Herbal Gem's. Also, PSC uses a 60% alcohol extraction process, whereas Herbal Gem uses only a 30% extraction process. Some medical literature states that maximum extraction of the plant's beneficial properties is achieved by using 60% alcohol. I prefer PSC's products over those of Herbal Gem's for these reasons, and also because PSC's products contain organic grape alcohol, which means that they have high amounts of antioxidants, like resveratrol. Grape alcohol is also less allergenic than grain alcohol.

Finally, it's important to note that the plant stem cell extracts from both companies are full extracts, not dilutions, which makes them very potent.

*Please note: These paragraphs contain my unofficial assessment of these products only.

Buhner's Herbs as Stem Cells

I have found that the herbs described in Stephen Buhner's book (*Healing Lyme*, Raven Press) are extremely beneficial in the management of Lyme disease, and for that reason, I have requested that PSC Distribution make the herbs that he recommends for Lyme disease, but in embryonic form, and especially andrographis, boneset, cat's claw, and artemisia. The stem cell form of these herbs should have a much stronger and better action upon the body than the adult plants, as well as a broader range of uses at smaller doses. I was particularly insistent that PSC develop plant stem cell remedies from andrographis, because this herb has phytochemicals that are specific for Borrelia, as well as a high affinity for the nervous system. As a result of my request, the andrographis product will be available in the near future, and it will be interesting to see how it works. My Lyme patients have benefited tremendously from using Buhner's herbal protocol, so using the embryonic form of these herbs should provide even better results for them. Finally, and as I mentioned earlier, all of PSC's products are made in grape alcohol, so there is a high content of resveratrol in all of their extractions.

Other Herbs That Are Being Used as Stem Cells

Some of the other herbs that will soon be available in embryonic form include pau d' arco, devil's claw, (which should be really effective for treating symptoms of pain and inflammation), nigella, wheat, dandelion, eyebright, yarrow and arnica (again, in the herbal, not homeopathic form). These are herbs that are supposed to have great effects upon the body, but which disappoint when used clinically, due to their low phytochemical content. So I think that practitioners will start to see how powerful these herbs can be when used in plant stem cell extract form, and start getting the results that they are supposed to be getting with the adult herbs. PSC Plant Stem Cells is also making stem cell remedies that can be administered as intramuscular injections, which will be beneficial for people with neuro-degenerative conditions such as MS and Lou Gehrig's, as well as for those with intense, unmanageable pain.

Detoxification

Using Plant Stem Cell Extracts for Detoxification

Interestingly enough, plant stem cells can also be used for detoxification, because they have constituents such as phytochelatin synthase, metallothioneins, oligoelements and phytochemicals built into them which aid in the chelation, binding, excretion, and mobilization of metals. All plant stem cells function as drainage remedies, but the ones that are most useful for overall purposes of detoxification include Grapevine, European Alder, White Willow, Hazel, Cedar of Lebanon, Mountain Pine, Black Poplar, Bilberry, Linden Tree, Rosemary and Juniper. Dr. Richard believes that plant stem cells are superior chelating agents to DMSA and DMPS, as well as others, stating that they are a much more effective, as well as safer, way to rid the body of heavy metals. Also, with plant stem cell extracts, practitioners don't have to worry about problems such as patient sulfation pathway sensitivity, kidney dysfunction, yeast flares and other issues that can arise as a result of using the former chelation agents. In my practice, I use the embryonic remedies in addition to other detoxification agents such as cilantro, chlorella, pectins (apple, citrus, and grapefruit) alginates, clays and charcoal.

Other Detoxification Strategies

In addition to plant stem cells, I recommend ionic cleanse foot baths, detoxification diets (usually food elimination diets and those that follow food combining rules), juicing, green water, saunas, colonics, coffee enemas, electrolytes and minerals, and alkaline water that has a Ph of 9.5, to detoxify the body of Lyme-related toxins. Between the environmental toxins, infections, and stresses of everyday life, most people are "burning the candle at both ends" and "running acidic", and it's important that they keep their bodies alkaline in order to heal from chronic illness. As much as we would like to think that it's possible to correct the body's pH by just having a green drink, I have found that normalizing this particular imbalance is difficult to do. One of the more effective ways of accomplishing this is by drinking alkaline water. One Internet site with great information on ionizers that alkalinize water can be found at: www.waterionizerauthority.com. Tyent and Jupiter are two high quality brands.

It's also a good idea for those with Lyme to keep a quality air filter in the house, to help mop up indoor mold spores, viruses and air pollution. I recommend products made by Austin Air for this purpose.

Even though plant stem cells are quite effective for detoxifying a number of substances from the body, people sometimes require additional toxin binders, especially if they are doing biofilm removal protocol. That said, I have observed that those who use stem cell extracts need to take fewer of the traditional toxin binders, such as chlorella, charcoal and pectin, and/or are able to reduce their usage by anywhere from 25-75%.

Finally, it's important that people with Lyme eliminate all possible sources of toxicity from their environment, including household solvents, pesticides, insecticides, vaccines, phthalates, plastics, genetically modified foods, and chemicals. It's common to cite heavy metals or mercury as the principal source of toxicity in the body, but there are so many other things that contribute to its overall toxic burden, as well.

Treating Detoxification Problems

I'm not an expert in the subject of genetic profiling to identify genetic defects that affect the body's ability to detoxify. I know a little about sulfation, NOS and methylation pathway problems, and that these can be corrected somewhat by taking nutritional supplements and plant stem cell remedies. I believe, in any case, that genetic defects can be overcome, and this belief is supported by studies in epigenetics, which is proving to be an exciting field of study. Bruce Lipton, PhD, has done great work in this area and I highly recommend his book, *The Biology of Belief* to anyone who wants to learn more about epigenetics.

In addition, I think that it can be helpful for those with compromised detoxification mechanisms to offload toxins from their bodies by using detoxification methods that make use of organs besides the liver. Clay baths, castor oil packs, foot baths, saunas and lymphatic drainage, for example, make use of the skin for detoxification. Detoxification can also be facilitated by laser and light therapy. Quantum Neurology is one type of therapy that practitioners use to balance organ and neurological function in their patients. If my Lyme patients can afford their own light therapy device (there are several available—one I recommend is the Sota Lightworks, from www.braintuner.com) then I can teach them how to use it for detoxification, as well as for liver and kidney support. This light device costs $280, but patients can use it forever. It helps patients financially when their practitioners find healing strategies that they can do on their own, so that they don't have to be so dependent upon their practitioners for all of their treatments.

Diet

Maintaining a healthy diet is important for complete recovery from Lyme disease. I believe, in fact, that it is at least 50% of the equation. First, paying attention to, and altering (when necessary) food proportions can be helpful. Some patients might benefit from increasing their vegetable or protein intake, for example, or from decreasing the amount of a particular type of food that they consume. Combining and eating similar types of foods at mealtimes can be beneficial for those with digestive problems. For instance, consuming only vegetables and other complex carbohydrates during a meal while avoiding proteins, or vice versa (eating protein but not complex carbohydrates in the same meal) may be a good idea. In general, I try to steer my Lyme disease patients away from eating grains and refined carbohydrates. Those with compromised immune systems tend to eat too many sugars, which feed the body's infections, suppress the immune system, cause inflammation and stress the endocrine system. Eating foods that are gluten and casein free also tends to be important for those with Lyme. If biofilms are a factor in healing, (which they almost always seem to be in anyone with a chronic infection) cutting out foods that contribute to its formation, (such as those containing gluten and casein), is likewise a good idea.

I think it's also crucial to avoid genetically modified food, as it creates a whole host of problems in the body, including dysbiosis and Leaky Gut Syndrome. Establishing a proper diet for Lyme disease patients can be tricky, however, since it tends to be difficult for them to get enough vegetables into their diets. Also, too much protein can cause acidity, and if patients aren't allowed to have grains or dairy, then it can be hard for them to find enough satisfying foods to eat. Drinking alkaline water can offset the acidity that results from eating protein, but in any case, most people with Lyme should maintain a diet that is at least fifty percent vegetables.

Consuming organic food is also important. At minimum, patients should consume meat and dairy only from organic sources, due to the high antibiotic and growth hormone content of non-organic meat and dairy. I encourage my patients with Lyme to visit the Internet site: www.ewg.org, and look up the "Dirty Dozen", which contains a list of the non-organic fruits and vegetables with the highest levels of toxins. As well, the site mentions which fruits and vegetables are OK to purchase non-organic.

Treatments for Symptomatic Relief

Pain

Pain can be a difficult symptom to treat. Patients who have taken plant stem cell extracts for their pain have experienced relief, but high doses of these remedies are sometimes needed to treat this symptom, unlike other symptoms, which require lower doses. And if it takes 90 drops of a remedy to treat a person's pain, then that treatment becomes quite expensive. For that reason, for some people, using plant stem cells to treat pain may not be as cost-effective as using them for the treatment of other problems, at least until an injectable form of such remedies becomes available.

Besides plant stem cell extracts, the other big intervention that I advocate for treating pain is cold laser or light therapy, and especially Quantum Neurology Rehabilitation (mentioned earlier), which is a technique developed by Dr. George Gonzalez, D.C., Q.N., that rehabilitates the nervous system. Dr. Gonzalez developed Quantum Neurology Rehabilitation (www.quantumneurology.com) after a massage therapist left his wife paralyzed. His wife couldn't walk and had lost all bowel and bladder function, and had developed other severe neurological problems. While in chiropractic school, he took her to many of the best chiropractors in the country.

At some point, he stumbled upon a study about cold laser, and over the next several years used what he learned to develop a technique that he eventually used to completely rehabilitate his wife. She is a neurological miracle, really, because most people don't recover from an injury of that magnitude. In fact, most neurologists believe that if people with neurological conditions don't heal after six months of treatment, then it's likely that they won't ever get better. However, the Quantum Neurology Rehabilitation techniques have been able to restore neurological function to people ten, twenty, even thirty years after their neurological injuries. That is unheard of; a real miracle.

Quantum Neurology is a non-invasive procedure that allows practitioners to check the functioning of all of their patients' nerves as they rehabilitate them. Functional tests can be performed for the motor, sensory and cranial nerves, as well as for the nerves that innervate the body's viscera or organs. 80% of the body's nerves are sensory, and are responsible for a multitude of functions, including the processing of light and deep touch, pain, pressure, hot and cold perception, vibratory sense, proprioception, and form recognition. Practitioners can restore their patients' nerve pathways with this type of light therapy. It's a very effective, non-invasive procedure that has provided those with Lyme with significant relief from their pain, neuropathy, motor and cognitive dysfunction. What's more, it may be one of the most effective treatments for people with reflex sympathetic dystrophy, fibromyalgia, neuropathy, joint pain, bursitis, and ailments of the like. Light therapy can be used for any type of pain, whether nerve or muscle. In addition, it has many other positive effects upon the body: it increases ATP production in the cell, helps the body to make more of its natural pain-relieving substances (its natural anti-inflammatories), promotes collagen production, increases oxygenation, detoxifies the cells, and promotes greater lymphatic system movement. Basically, it causes the body to heal faster, by up to about 30%. Since nerves heal more slowly than any other part of the body, any technique that increases their rate of healing by 30% is significant.

Furthermore, it's non-invasive and patients know fairly quickly whether it's going to work for them. For a long-standing sciatica problem, for instance, patients may need at least ten treatments, but their practitioners can muscle test them to discover how many treatments are needed and whether the therapy will be beneficial for them. Positive changes can result fairly quickly, although pain can be difficult to treat if it's a direct result of patients' infections.

I have one Lyme patient who had horrible neuropathy, and prior to her first QN session, she had been using a walker. She had all kinds of pain, as well as RSD (Reflex Sympathetic Dystrophy), which is a serious pain syndrome that made her feel as though she was being crushed to death. After several months of treatment with the laser, this woman's pain diminished significantly. Every patient responds differently to the therapy, but I believe that the technique is important and extremely beneficial for many with Lyme disease. Again, many health care practitioners have assumed that if they just kill the Lyme bugs, then their patients will get better, but that isn't true in all cases.

Anxiety and Depression

Testing for and managing my patients' neurotransmitter deficiencies and dysfunction is an integral component to helping them to heal from Lyme disease and chronic illness. NeuroScience is one lab that performs a complete neurotransmitter panel, using urinary and/or saliva tests. The lab checks things like patients' levels of histidine, GABA, epinephrine, dopamine and serotonin, and then recommends supplements for them to take, based on their test results.

One neurological balancing product that I have observed to be beneficial for many people is TravaCor, which balances a wide range of neurotransmitters. Another is Kavinase, which is a special type of GABA that has a positive effect upon GABA receptor sites, more so than other types of GABA, and is especially beneficial for people with insomnia or for those who are anxious and feel wired.

I also often recommend Linden Tree, which is a plant stem cell product that detoxifies the nervous system, helps to raise serotonin levels and relieves anxiety and insomnia. So a typical protocol for managing my patients' anxiety and depression might include stem cells, along with NeuroScience products or other supplements that positively affect neurotransmitter levels. It might also include homeopathic remedies, such as flowers or gemstones, which can be beneficial for some people.

Insomnia

Insomnia can be a very difficult symptom to treat. Often, by the time Lyme patients with insomnia come into my office, they have already tried all of the "basic" natural remedies, such as magnesium, chamomile, valerian, and hops. Plant stem cell extracts can help to restore sleep in some of these patients, although there are currently only a couple of remedies that are made specifically for sleep dysfunction; Fig, Linden Tree, Silver Birch Seeds and Cedar of Lebanon. The latter remedy contains high levels of sesquiterpene, which increases oxygen around the pineal gland's receptor sites, and stimulates the release of melatonin. California Poppy can also be beneficial for the treatment of insomnia. If my patients don't respond well to any of these products, I recommend that they get their neurotransmitters tested, and if their levels are really low, then I might recommend that they take melatonin, in addition to other neurotransmitter precursors. I don't think that it's good for people to get dependent upon melatonin, but at the same time, it's a relatively safe hormone to take, and has good antioxidant effects upon the body. If my patients' neurotransmitters are out of whack, then I will try to get those back into balance before prescribing them a sleep remedy.

Practicing good sleep hygiene is likewise important. Some people's circadian rhythms are so messed up that they don't even try to get to bed until after eleven o'clock. Practicing some rituals, such as turning off electromagnetic devices and not watching TV in the bedroom right before bedtime can be helpful, as can trying to get to bed at the same time every night.

Treating Hormonal Dysfunction

Assessing and managing patients' hormonal dysfunction is a key piece to solving their Lyme puzzle. Hormones are especially important for managing energy and for the ability to cope with stress. They also play an important role in immune system function. Most people with Lyme have widespread hormonal dysregulation.

I use ART testing, as well as labs (blood, saliva and urine) to look for hormonal imbalances in my patients. For those that are already on a protocol to help manage their hormones, and who still have fatigue, I'll run an organic acid urine test which reveals whether the cells' mitochondria are dysfunctional. (The mitochondria are the powerhouse of the cell). By doing targeted nutritional therapy, I can heal their mitochondria, and get their cells to start producing energy again.

Amazingly, stem cells can modulate hormonal imbalances. If the amount or functioning of a certain hormone is too high, then the stem cells can bring it down. If it is too low, then the stem cells can raise it.

Additionally, stem cells have a regenerative effect upon the body. For example, one stem cell remedy called Black Currant functions as a natural type of cortisone but doesn't have the same side effects upon the body as synthetic cortisone, or even so-called natural cortisone. Instead, it has a regulatory effect upon the immune system, so those who take it get the anti-inflammatory effects of the hormone without the devastating effects of synthetic cortisol. At the same time, it regenerates the adrenal glands, so that they eventually produce balanced amounts of their own cortisol.

Sometimes practitioners get stuck into the trap of thinking that whenever their patients' cortisol or other hormone levels are low, that it's necessary to give them synthetic cortisol or another hormone. This isn't always beneficial, though, because the body can become dependent upon such hormones, instead of learning how to re-make its own. The other problem is that some people may not even have hormone deficiencies; they may simply have imbalances. Dealing with hormonal dysfunction in Lyme disease is so complex, though. The stress of Lyme infections contributes to hormonal dysfunction and hormonal dysfunction contributes to immune system suppression, so practitioners must address all of these little pieces of the puzzle at the same time.

If patients are on a good Lyme protocol and immune boosting program, ideally, their bodies should eventually heal from hormonal dysfunction all by themselves. This doesn't always happen, but if patients have to be on one milligram of DHEA for the rest of their lives, because their bodies have been so damaged and stressed by Lyme, then that would still be better than them taking ten milligrams of DHEA. Also, their hormone levels can be abnormal because their neurotransmitter problems aren't being properly managed, or because there is some type of stress in their lives that isn't being dealt with, such as psychological or emotional stress, or a food allergy. So dealing with these problems may be more important for them than simply supplementing their bodies with a hormone.

Lifestyle Recommendations for Healing

One problem that I often notice in my patients is that as they start to feel good, they tend to go out and injure themselves. It's as if they say to themselves, "Wow, I was able to sit on the floor for five hours for the first time in seven years!" And I must tell them, "Well your body didn't like that!" So they need to be mindful of overdoing it. It's hard, though, when they have been feeling so sick for so long. When they get a ray of sunshine—that is, an improvement in symptoms, then they really want to take advantage of it, because in the back of their mind, they are wondering, "Okay, so how long is this good feeling going to last? How long before I feel like crap again?" While I understand their thinking, it's also important for them to not undo all of the hard work that they did to get better. I see this sort of thing happen often when my patients do Quantum Neurology. They get some neurological functions turned back on again, they feel good and so go out and take a hike but soon feel awful again, because they did too much, too fast.

Also, it's vital for people with Lyme to minimize stress as much as possible. I find that my patients can become easily overwhelmed by life, because they don't feel well, and that feeling completely paralyzes them. They have so much to do and they can't even bear to start, so I advise them to simplify their lives as much as possible; to get rid of stuff and unclutter their homes, for instance. I also tell them to set routines, in the morning, afternoon and evening, and then stick to those. I might also tell them to make a meal menu for the week and then shop off of that menu so that they know what they are going to eat every day. Doing little things like this can help them to deal with the feeling of being overwhelmed.

Also, I think that it's important for them to take baby steps when attempting to de-clutter their lives. Marla Cilley, the woman who runs the website: www.flylady.net inspired my thinking on this. Flylady has a completely free, on-line mentoring program that was originally designed for stay-at-home moms, but which has evolved into advice for the chronically ill, as well. She tells her readers things like, "Your house didn't get this way overnight, so you aren't going to de-clutter it overnight" and then provides them with manageable suggestions for de-cluttering their lives. As one example, she will tell readers to set a timer for fifteen minutes, and do only one task during those fifteen minutes. Once those fifteen minutes are over, they can decide whether they want to spend another fifteen minutes on that same task, or on something else. It's a psychological game that works, because, for example, if people tell themselves that they have to do their taxes, and they know that this task is going to take forever, then they might not do it. If they know that they only have to spend fifteen minutes working on it, however, then they might find that they are better able to do it, and as a result, actually end up getting more done than if they had tried to do the entire task upfront.

So I encourage routines for my patients, because it takes a lot of the thinking and decision-making out of life. The more routines that they have, the less thinking they have to do. At the same time, they must be forgiving and loving towards themselves when they fail in their tasks.

Finally, people with Lyme disease must listen and tune in to their bodies, and not turn a blind eye to its needs. Sometimes it takes getting hit by a Mack truck before people start paying attention to what they need, though, especially Type A people, who are not very good at listening to their bodies. It's important to honor the body's need for rest, nourishment, play, creativity, prayer and rejuvenation, and to learn to let go and prioritize what's important in life.

Therapies for Healing the Emotions and Spirit

It's important for Lyme disease sufferers to address unhealed emotional trauma as part of their healing process. For this, I recommend the Advanced Cell Training (formerly IRT, Immune Response Training) program. More information on ACT can be found at: www.advancedcelltraining.com. This is a powerful healing modality that addresses symptoms caused by emotional trauma as well as those caused by Lyme. The founder of the therapy, Gary Blier, allows participants to complete three sessions with a money-back guarantee (at the time this book was published). So if they don't notice a change in their symptoms after three sessions, then they don't have to pay for those sessions. I tell my patients that it's worth trying, because they have nothing to lose financially from doing it.

I also recommend energetic tapping techniques such as EFT (Emotional Freedom Technique), for healing conscious trauma, or the problems that Lyme sufferers are aware that they have, such as depression over not being able to do the same daily activities that they could do prior to illness. This is an inexpensive, effective and easy-to-learn technique that can be done anytime or anywhere. Patients can learn to do this technique on their own; there are lots of websites that demonstrate how to do it. Or they can first go to an

EFT practitioner to learn how to do it, and then practice the techniques at home. When a problem comes up during the technique that they themselves can't resolve, then they can always go back to the practitioner to work through it.

For a great technique that taps into subconscious beliefs or traumas, I recommend Psych-K. It's great at accessing buried trauma, re-programming the brain and removing the subconscious beliefs that are sabotaging patients' healing and keeping them from reaching their goals. Psych-K is also nice because it is a technique that can be combined with muscle testing, which enables patient and practitioner to discern exactly which emotional issues need healing. Patients can then take that information and re-train their brains to re-create healthier beliefs.

I also like therapies that require active participation from patients, unlike traditional talk therapy, which is focused mostly on patients sharing their past issues and then receiving advice for healing those. Not that there's anything wrong with this type of therapy, but I worry that it can get people stuck in the "story of their illness", because they keep recycling and repeating it to a counselor, and by doing so, reinforce it deeper and deeper into their belief system. This same problem also occurs with some of the on-line Lyme disease chat groups. I think there is a time and place for these, but they can also get people stuck into this energetic vortex of Lyme and illness that becomes difficult to climb out of.

In any case, it's important to reach the subconscious mind when healing emotional trauma, and talk therapy doesn't always do that. And while EFT, for example, starts out as a conscious therapy, subconscious wounds can get healed in the process, because EFT taps into the subconscious, or unconscious, mind, as well as the conscious. I think that books like *The Secret* have a place and a value for some, but if a person has an underlying subconscious belief, such as, "I don't deserve to be well," all of the conscious affirmations in the world aren't going to shift that belief. Since 80%

of our mind is run by the subconscious, it's important to do therapies that reach the subconscious mind.

So, while I believe that it's important for people to be mindful of their thoughts, they must go deeper and access the subconscious mind to discover what harmful beliefs are stuck there and which are driving them and their decisions. Besides Pysch-K, APN (Applied Psycho-Neurobiology) and PK (Psycho-Kinesiology) are other modalities that get to the root of emotional problems. Lyme-literate physician Dr. Klinghardt's therapies are of this sort.

RET, Rapid Eye Therapy, is another good healing intervention that reaches the subconscious mind. This therapy is gentler than EMDR (Eye Movement Desensitization and Reprocessing), which forces people to re-live their traumas. Practitioners must be careful of therapies that cause this to happen. There are ways of making patients aware of their traumas without forcing them re-live them. Besides, when people re-live their traumas, those memories can get pushed even further into their cellular memory.

Dr. Cowden, in his healing seminars, states that practitioners should muscle-test three statements on their patients to help them to discern what their emotional blocks to healing are. Those statements are: "I am well," "I want to be well," and "I deserve to be well." He finds that most people "blow out" on at least one of the statements. After muscle testing the questions, different interventions can then be applied to reverse the unhealthy beliefs. One of Dr. Cowden's interventions is prayer, which I think works for some people but not others. Some will need to apply energetic and cognitive approaches, such as those that I mention above. Also, the majority of people that I know with Lyme disease have a strong spiritual background and may pray often, but that doesn't mean that they have necessarily dealt with the past emotional trauma that is contributing to their illness.

Another technique that I recommend is called the Healing Way Method, which involves no harsh re-experiencing or re-living of past traumatic experiences. The Healing Way Method is an advanced healing system designed to serve the spiritual evolution and healing of human kind, by healing distorted beliefs, unconscious attitudes and automatic emotional responses and by enhancing people's awareness of who they really are and their connection with the Divine. It is an intention-based therapy, meaning, patients decide what they want to change about their lives. They verbally state and write out their intentions, which then serve as a springboard for everything else that follows in the healing process. Through this therapy, patients are able to transform their life situation and reach their intended goals for personal change and development. More about this therapy can be found on the Internet at: www.healingwaymethod.com.

Finally, homeopathy, color therapy, and neurotransmitter modulation can be beneficial for processing and healing emotional trauma. I also recommend the book, *Feelings Buried Alive Never Die,* by Karol Truman.

Profiling the Person That Heals Fully from Lyme Disease

In general, it's easy to get sick people to take their supplements. Getting them to change their diets and deal with emotional trauma, however, is much more difficult. Also, sicker patients have more emotional baggage that they must deal with, and consequently, their healing is more complicated, unless they are able to do the difficult work of healing this emotional trauma. People who maintain unhealthy diets and fail to deal with their emotional challenges struggle to get well.

That said, it seems that practitioners have been taught that if their patients just deal with their emotional stuff, then that will fix everything. But I knew one lady who did some emotional healing work and as a result, had such a bad Herxheimer reaction that she ended up in the hospital for three days. Dealing with the emotional stuff had almost killed her! I was dumbfounded, and thought, *What in the heck is this? People are supposed to get better when they deal with their emotional stuff, not worse!* So as a practitioner, you can think that you have it all figured out, but then you find that you don't and it turns out that there is still a lot of mystery involved in the healing process. So when my patients don't get well when I expect them to, I now think, *Well, this may be the path that they are meant to be on. This (business of healing) has nothing to do with me, after all. It really doesn't.* I put my heart into my work and I make recommendations to Lyme disease sufferers, but in the end, their healing journeys have nothing to do with me. I mean, I want to help them so badly, but their path in this world and God's plan for them are really out of my hands.

I was disappointed by what happened with the woman who got worse when she healed her emotional trauma, though, because I had encouraged her for so long to deal with her emotional problems, assuring her that once she did, she would get better. Fortunately, her perspective has been that her healing crisis was just another step in the healing process, but part of me kept thinking, *Why did this have to happen? Dealing with her emotional issues was supposed to be the last piece of her healing puzzle! Why didn't she get better?* But this kind of thing can happen. With all the tools and techniques that I use in my practice, patients' healing happens in layers. We peel off one layer of illness, and then another comes up, and sometimes, the new layer involves the manifestation of new symptoms. It's as if the subconscious mind and/or the body says, "Great, thanks for finally paying attention to me, now deal with this!" As a result, patients will get symptoms that they never had before, and these become the next piece of the puzzle that they have to work on.

Is Lyme Disease Always the Primary Reason for Symptoms?

Lyme disease is called the great mimicker, because it mimics over 300 other diseases. Some doctors say that Lyme disease is always the primary cause for symptoms in the chronically ill who have Borrelia and co-infections, whereas others believe that Lyme is only part of the problem. Both perspectives are probably valid and whether Lyme is primary or secondary in the overall symptom picture depends upon the person. For example, some people might have viruses that have been in their bodies forever and which have finally brought their immune systems down, and then their Lyme "wakes up" and decides to have a party with their collagen! Then there are others who, prior to getting infected by Borrelia, were totally healthy people, but after a walk through the woods, developed Lyme disease. I try not to get hung up in figuring out what was the first cause of my patients' symptoms, though. I simply try to make recommendations for their healing based on their symptoms and tests and where they are currently in their healing journey.

In any case, whether or not their symptoms are caused mostly by Lyme disease, it's beneficial for them to not look at their illness through "Lyme lenses." For instance, when a patient gets a little bump on his or her skin and says, "I'm sure that it's Bartonella," I respond, "It could be, or perhaps you were wearing a shirt that was chafing you." Not every symptom is related to Lyme disease. Also, while it's important to be educated about Lyme disease, I don't think it's beneficial for people to get caught up in a "Lyme disease" mindset. Sometimes a cold is just a cold, and an eye twitch is just an eye twitch. It's good to notice symptoms, but not become obsessive about them.

Patient and Practitioner Challenges in Treating Lyme Disease

One great challenge that practitioners have in treating Lyme patients is getting them to believe that emotional strategies can be helpful for their healing, even when patients claim that they have "already done them all."

Another challenge is when "the cure becomes worse than the disease". Sometimes the way out of illness is extremely difficult. As patients respond to treatment, they can become more symptomatic. And although practitioners may try to support them as much as possible during this process, for some, this support just isn't enough. Compliance is challenging for patients when they feel sicker while on a treatment regimen, especially when they don't seem to be making much progress in their healing.

Dealing with patients' financial limitations is another great challenge for both practitioners and patients. Many Lyme sufferers have been financially devastated by disease because they aren't working and have lost a lot of income as a result. Many don't have much of a support system, either, but they need a lot of treatments to get back on track, and it's financially impossible for them to pay for these treatments.

Not everyone can afford saunas, Quantum Neurology or footbaths, let alone supplements and organic food. If patients are on a limited budget, they probably can't afford organic food, and to me, that is a stumbling block in their recovery.

Then again, this may not be true if you believe in the philosophy that what's happening in a person's life is what is supposed to be happening. Part of me resists this philosophy though, and thinks, *If only this patient could buy this ... if only she could afford that, she would be okay.*

Unfortunately, in the end, I think that generally, those who have adequate financial resources have a greater chance at healing than those who don't.

On the other hand, I know some Lyme disease sufferers who have adequate financial resources because they work, and while they are functional enough to have a job, they can't seem to fully heal because they have to push themselves all of the time. The symptoms of such people improve dramatically when they go on vacation! So despite the fact that they might have more financial resources than others because they are working, they don't heal because they have to deal with the stress of work. This is another challenge of treating Lyme patients.

How Friends and Family Can Help the Sick

Friends and family can better support their loved ones with Lyme disease by giving them more money to pay for treatments! Helping them to do the little things is important, too. Cooking meals, shopping and cleaning the house, for example, can make a huge difference, as can getting them organized so that their houses are less cluttered, offering to take them to appointments, or organizing their supplements for the week. Such tasks can be really challenging for the sick. People with Lyme get overwhelmed by what they have to do, so sometimes they don't do anything. It's as if they become paralyzed. For that reason, helping out with such tasks is important. I mean, I'm not even sick, and I know that it would be a big deal to me if someone came over once a week to cook for me!

Honoring the sick person's experience is also helpful. Friends and family members should become educated about the disease and believe their loved ones when they tell them about their symptoms. They are not making them up! They also need to acknowledge and encourage them.

Exercise

The type of exercise that people with Lyme disease should do depends upon the person and his or her condition. Some people respond well to aerobic exercise, working out with weights and really sweating three times a week. For others, such exercise is impossible, and they need to do things like stretching or yoga. I encourage my patients to do whatever works for them. There are many ways to get the heart rate up without going out and doing aerobic exercise. Ideally, people should find activities that they enjoy doing and which involve some kind of movement and attention to the physical body, but which are within their physical limitations. They should make sure that whatever activity they do is fun, so that it keeps them interested and motivated. And they shouldn't forget to take baby steps when starting an exercise program!

Less-than-Beneficial Lyme Disease Treatments

When patients take too many prescription medications, this is detrimental to their healing. I often see this problem with autistic kids who have Lyme disease; they are on Valtrex, anti-psychotic medications, and all kinds of antibiotics. While I understand that medications are sometimes necessary, I worry about the long-term effects that such medications have on the immune system and gut. I am also concerned that we are overusing antibiotic therapies, and creating more "super bugs" as a result. Killing bugs is just one piece of the puzzle, anyway. Supporting patients' immune systems, balancing their hormones, and regenerating their tissues and organs are just as important.

Treating Structural Problems

Treating Lyme disease is such a multi-factorial process. Rarely is it as cut and dry as treating infections, and for that reason, it's important for practitioners to address as many factors as possible that are contributing to their patients' diseases. Besides physical toxins and the issues that I mentioned in earlier parts of this chapter, such factors include geopathic and electromagnetic stress, allergies and structural problems.

A lot of practitioners don't address and treat their patients' structural problems, but so much of the body's energy is geared towards maintaining structure, so if practitioners and patients aren't addressing this piece of the Lyme puzzle, then patients will have less energy available for healing. When the body's structure is misaligned, the nervous system can't deliver the proper signals to the organs and tissues. There is static on the line. For example, when a misaligned bone irritates the nerve that goes to the liver, the result is a malfunctioning liver.

People with Lyme disease tend to have horrible posture as well as difficulty holding chiropractic adjustments. This happens for several reasons. First, the Lyme bugs attack collagen, and this then breaks down the body's structural support system. Secondly, when the adrenal glands are weak, this creates ligament laxity (ligaments also aid in maintaining the body's structure). Fortunately, plant stem cells can support the body's soft tissues and promote new collagen production.

If people with Lyme don't attempt to fix their structural problems, then they will get worse symptomatically, and develop more arthritis, joint and muscle pain down the road, and not because of Lyme, but because of structural problems. People underestimate the importance of structure in human health. Chiropractors understand it, but chiropractors tend to know little about Lyme disease, so it's important that they learn about Lyme, too. It's also important that Lyme-literate health care practitioners understand the importance of fixing structural problems when helping their patients to heal from Lyme.

One of the techniques in Quantum Neurology involves adjusting the body's spine and extremities with a tool called the Arthrostim. The Arthrostim is a device that looks like a gun and sounds like a jackhammer. This tool taps bones back into place, but it can also be used for releasing trigger points and doing visceral release, or for freeing up restricted organs. So it's a multi-purpose tool which can be extremely helpful for fixing structural problems in those with Lyme. What's more, since Quantum Neurology also rehabilitates the nervous system, practitioners can functionally heal their patients' nervous systems at the same time that they address their structural problems. Finally, the therapy can also remedy ligament laxity to some extent, but since we are talking about a population that can't hold its adjustments well, more importantly, the device frees up energy in the body for healing as it alleviates symptoms.

People with Lyme disease have vertebral segments and ligaments that are hypermobile due to laxity, but the vertebra and ligaments that surround these may be hypomobile, and, when left unmanaged, may cause degeneration. Getting chiropractic adjustments and doing treatments such as those found in Quantum Neurology can help to correct and prevent degeneration. When patients are on a good Lyme treatment plan that involves killing bugs, supporting the immune and musculoskeletal systems and regenerating collagen, then their structural problems become easier to address.

Finally, I believe that a multifaceted approach to treating the spine is best. Some of the plant stem cell extracts are good at regenerating collagen and supporting soft tissue health, as are other supplements on the market. Therefore, doing a combination of hands-on techniques, working on the nervous system via cold laser, and taking supplements comprise the best comprehensive strategy for addressing structural problems. Whatever can be done to support the body's structure, to free up as much healing energy as possible, will aid significantly in patients' healing.

For collagen supplementation, I recommend PCHF(S) Collagen Complex, which is a mix of vitamins and minerals that support collagen production. I also recommend an amino acid product called MAP that is low nitrogen wasting, which means that it's highly absorbable. This product was originally developed for elite athletes, but was found to significantly help cancer patients whose muscles were wasting away. Some Lyme disease patients who have used this product notice positive change within two weeks of starting it. Many of the plant stem cells are excellent for rejuvenating and restoring soft tissue. Cedar of Lebanon is a plant stem cell remedy that also helps to promote collagen production. It's called the natural Botox, because after several months, it's supposed to fill in one's wrinkles! Finally, laser (or light) therapy is also beneficial, because, in addition to stimulating collagen production, it reduces inflammation and stimulates mitochondria to produce energy.

Last Words

People with Lyme disease should always remember that healing this type of illness is a marathon, not a sprint. They should stay vigilant and work on as many pieces of their healing puzzle they can. We practitioners out here in the field are constantly looking for better, quicker and easier ways to deal with this illness. To those with Lyme disease, I would just like to say: You can overcome! Don't be afraid to try different treatments, and "to go out-side of the box." If you have a great kinesiologist, you can better guide your treatment options. And please remember that you are NOT your illness!

How to Contact Elizabeth Hesse-Sheehan, DC, CCN

Experience Health, Inc.
Dr. Elizabeth Hesse Sheehan DC QN
12121 100th NE
Kirkland, WA 98034
www.experiencehealth.info

• CHAPTER 13 •

Jeffrey Morrison, M.D.
NEW YORK, NY

Biography

Dr. Jeffrey Morrison is a medical doctor who champions a nutritional approach to healthcare as well as preventing and reversing degenerative diseases. Dr. Morrison's treatments are aimed at enhancing the body's ability to heal and detoxify itself. Safe, non-toxic and non-invasive treatments are proving to be more powerful than conventional treatments, which involve drugs and surgeries that are often dangerous.

Dr. Morrison completed his undergraduate degree in psychology at the University of Rochester and received his medical doctorate from Jefferson Medical College in Philadelphia. He is trained and board certified in Family Practice and has completed additional training in environmental medicine.

In 2001, Dr. Morrison was on the medical staff at the Atkins Center for Complementary and Alternative Medicine in New York City, where he worked under Dr. Robert Atkins, the developer of the famous low carbohydrate diet, the Atkins Nutritional Approach (or

Atkins diet, as it is commonly referred to). He then went on to become the medical director of the Wellness Medical Center of Integrative Medicine in New York City.

In 2002, Dr. Morrison opened The Morrison Center on Fifth Avenue, just steps away from Manhattan's Union Square. Since then, Dr. Morrison has used his successful integrative medicine and nutritional approach for both health optimization and the treatment and prevention of degenerative diseases, such as arthritis, Lyme disease, high blood pressure, hormone imbalance, obesity, diabetes, chronic fatigue, anxiety, depression, heavy metal poisoning and many other ailments.

Dr. Morrison is a member of the American Academy of Environmental Medicine (AAEM) as well as a lecturer and board member for the American College for the Advancement in Medicine (ACAM). He has appeared on television, written journal articles and chapters for textbooks, and lectured throughout the country in the field of integrative and complementary medicine.

Dr. Morrison has been featured as a health specialist on The Discovery Channel, Next Top Model, and in several documentaries related to anti-aging. He has also contributed to articles in publications such as Cosmopolitan, Men's Journal, Shape, Fitness and New York Magazine, as well as to other health related resources around the United States.

Healing Philosophy/Treatment Approach

I became involved in the treatment of Lyme disease when patients started coming in to my practice with symptoms of Lyme and I realized that I didn't know how to treat them. So in 2005, I received six months of advanced training in the treatment of tick-borne infections from Lyme-literate physician Dr. Burrascano, and that helped to shape what I do today.

When treating Lyme disease, my goal is to make sure that I have identified what infections my patients have, which I do through blood work and by taking a thorough history of their symptoms. It isn't always clear to me why some patients don't get better, even after being treated for Lyme disease. Accordingly, when treating them, it's important for practitioners to make sure that all of the common Lyme co-infections have been considered, including Babesia, Bartonella, and Ehrlichia, as well as the opportunistic infections such as Chlamydia pneumoniae and Mycoplasma, and viruses such as HHV-6 and Epstein-Barr.

Often, one person who gets a tick bite will get symptoms, while another won't, which means that genetics and environmental factors probably also determine whether a person will develop chronic Lyme disease. For this reason, in addition to treating the infections, I also treat the immune system and correct for any nutritional deficiencies. Checking quantitative immunoglobulin levels, IgG subtypes, B-12 and folic acid levels, 25-hydroxy Vitamin D, ferritin, and red blood cell levels of magnesium are an important part of this assessment.

I also find that my patients tend to have a hard time getting over infections if they have high levels of environmental toxins in their bodies, such as accumulations of mercury and lead. So I will also establish protocol for removing these toxins, when necessary.

Two other common problems which Lyme patients have and which impact their healing are yeast overgrowth or parasitic infections in their digestive tract. Sometimes, their symptoms are more related to one or both of these issues than to the Lyme infections, so I perform stool testing to clarify whether they are a problem and then treat as necessary.

Finally, I check hormones, including cortisol, DHEA-S, testosterone and growth hormone, as well as others, and if there are imbalances, I correct those, as well.

Treatment Protocol for Borrelia and Co-Infections

Borrelia

If my patients have chronic Lyme disease involving just Borrelia (and no co-infections), then I will give them whatever medication is needed to get them better. That could be oral doxycycline, or another medication. In my practice, we sometimes use a combination of antibiotics to treat Borrelia but I find that it isn't always necessary to give patients multiple antibiotics. When it is necessary, Ceftin (cefuroxime) and azithromycin are one combination of medications that I often use. Omnicef (cefdinir) and Biaxin (clarithromycin) is another good combination. I never know which combination is going to work best, however, because every patient is different. Sometimes, the best way to know is by looking at what medications have or have not worked for them in the past, as well as which treatments they still haven't tried.

In addition to the above oral medications, I might also give Flagyl (metronidazole) to my patients, which I prescribe in-between courses of bactericidal antibiotics. For instance, I might have a patient take Ceftin with azithromycin, and then rotate these two drugs with Flagyl. If oral antibiotics are insufficient, I may then use intramuscular Bicillin (penicillin) injections. The next level of treatment, if patients don't respond well to oral medications and/or injections, would involve giving them intravenous antibiotics. In my practice, we try to avoid IV antibiotics, because there are a lot of risks with these, even though they provide a lot of benefits. Intravenous therapy requires a PICC line, (peripherally inserted central catheter) which is left in the patient's body anywhere from four to twelve weeks at a time. PICC lines create susceptibility to skin infection and can irritate blood vessels. The catheter is placed close to the heart, which could also cause irritation in the body if it's placed incorrectly. So there are risks with IV therapy and I tend to administer it only to patients that don't respond well to oral or intra-muscular antibiotics.

Babesia and Bartonella

For the treatment of patients with Babesia, I use Mepron (atovaquone) and azithromycin, or Malarone (atovaquone plus proguanil). I also usually use artemisia, which is an anti-parasitic herb. It's not always obvious when the infection is gone after treatment, so I usually allow one to three months' time to asses patient response to these treatments. Also, it's important to note that the medications themselves can debilitate patients and sometimes it's difficult to know whether they are still having symptoms as a result of their infections or are having side effects from their treatments.

For the treatment of Bartonella, I prescribe Levaquin (levofloxacin), Bactrim, or rifampin, for one to three months.

Treating Opportunistic Infections

While it can be important to discover whether patients have opportunistic infections (which are not the same as common Lyme co-infections), I don't necessarily treat these, because I think that they are not usually the cause of symptoms. They only tend to cause problems if patients have other major issues in addition to Lyme, such as an overgrowth of yeast, heavy metal toxicity or nutritional deficiencies, and tend to go away once these other problems are addressed. For example, I have used antiviral medications for opportunistic infections in the past, but have inevitably been frustrated because they usually didn't make the patient feel better and didn't get rid of the infection.

Are Lyme and Co-Infections Always the Primary Cause of Symptoms?

Lyme and co-infections are not always the first, or primary, cause of symptoms in my patients that have chronic illnesses involving Lyme. That's why I do other things in my practice in addition to treating Lyme and co-infections, such as detoxification protocol and addressing nutritional deficiencies, yeast overgrowth, and hormone imbalances. For some people, one or more of the above problems is more pronounced in their overall symptom picture than the Lyme infections. So the question is always, what is the underlying cause of patients' symptoms? Sometimes this is easy to figure out, but at other times, it's more complicated.

Treating Yeast Infections

If patients have yeast overgrowth, then this can cause inflammation in their bodies, as well as Herxheimer reactions when the infection is killed off by treatment.

Dietary modification is the single most important treatment for yeast. It's important for patients to maintain a low yeast and carbohydrate diet. Sugar, bread, hard cheese, vinegar, and baked goods are among the foods that they should avoid. I also prescribe certain herbs, such as caprylic acid, berberine and grapefruit seed extract, or drugs such as Nystatin powder, Nizoral, and Diflucan, to help get rid of the yeast.

Heavy Metal Detoxification

If patients have significant heavy metal toxicity, then it's important to rid their bodies of these metals, because they have a negative impact upon the immune system. They lower natural killer (NK) cell activity and create susceptibility to autoimmune disease. Also, patients have much more difficulty healing from chronic Lyme disease if they have high levels of heavy metals, so it is necessary to address these, along with infections.

The symptoms of heavy metal toxicity are sometimes similar to those of Lyme, and may include poor concentration, memory changes, tremors and brain fog, so I must take this fact into account when diagnosing patients. After a preliminary clinical diagnosis, I perform blood tests for mercury, lead or the metal in question, as well as a provoked heavy metal urine test. The urine test involves giving patients a chelating agent such as DMSA, or calcium EDTA, and then asking them to collect their urine for six hours to see if any metals come out in the urine. If they have high levels of metals, then I also make sure that it isn't due to a current exposure and then perform some type of detoxification protocol. This might include saunas and taking certain nutrients that improve the elimination of metals, such as sulfur-containing amino acids like MSM and alpha-lipoic acid. I may also recommend agents such as DMSA or calcium EDTA. Ionic footbaths or colonic therapy can be helpful, too.

Treating Hormonal Dysfunction

Balancing patients' hormones is an important component of any successful Lyme disease protocol. The hormones of the body function like an orchestra, and when one group of hormones is off balance, then the others get sent off balance, as well. In my practice, we check the functioning of a variety of hormones, including the sex hormones such as estradiol, progesterone, testosterone and DHEA-S. We also check pituitary hormones such as LH (luteinizing hormone), FSH (follicle-stimulating hormone), prolactin, and HGH, or growth hormone. We check adrenal hormones such as cortisol and pregnenolone, as well as thyroid hormones, including TSH, Free T3, and Free T4. Blood tests are a very accurate way to measure the hormones. Depending upon our level of suspicion about which hormones might be off-balance in our patients, we may perform follow-up tests to better clarify where and/or what their specific problems are. So for instance, if patients have low cortisol levels, then this would suggest that they have an adrenal problem, and we would follow up with a Cortrosyn stimulation test to confirm this. This test determines whether the body can create cortisol in response to stress, and if it reveals that patients' cortisol levels are low, then we support their adrenals with cortisol replacement therapy or supportive herbs.

In my practice, we use bioidentical hormone replacement (BHRT) for most hormone problems. BHRT refers to replacing hormones with the same type of hormones that the human body produces. These are made at compounding pharmacies.

For treating thyroid problems, I may recommend a product called Armour thyroid, which is considered to be bioidentical, but not everyone has good results with it. For example, patients with autoimmune thyroid conditions might fare better with non-bioidentical thyroid replacement, such as Synthroid.

Response to bioidentical hormones can vary. For example, if patients respond well to bioidentical cortisol, they tend to respond very well. If they don't respond well, I tend to know very quickly by their symptoms. Sometimes, using alternatives to bioidentical cortisol, such as ginseng or licorice, or nutrients that support the adrenals, such as fish oil, and Vitamins B-5 and C, can be beneficial.

Hormonal dysfunction can sometimes be the primary cause of symptoms in those with Lyme disease. Too often, people get stuck into thinking about chronic illness in terms of categories, such as "Lyme", and they don't stop to consider whether there might be another problem in the body that is allowing the Borrelia infection to thrive.

Treating Nutritional Deficiencies

Basic nutrients that I recommend to my patients include a good multi-vitamin, fish oil, (at least 1000 mg, 2x/day), magnesium glycinate, (200 mg/day), Vitamin C, (1000 mg, 2x/day), probiotics (Essential Formulas makes a good product), and digestive enzymes (like Benezyme). Also, I often recommend Cordyceps mushroom (200mg/day) because it increases Natural Killer cell counts and improves patients' energy. Vitamin B-12 (1000mcg/day), as an injection or sublingual liquid can aid in energy, memory and mood. Iron supplements, in the form of iron glycinate, are sometimes necessary if patients have anemia. Ferrasorb by Thorne Research, Inc. is one good iron product that I use. Finally, I also use intravenous Vitamin C and trace nutrients in my practice, since these seem to be beneficial for strengthening patients' immune systems. Sometimes, I will add magnesium to the Vitamin C IV, and I find that people have absolutely fantastic results with this combination.

The nutritional supplementation protocol that I recommend for my patients also depends upon their symptoms. Most of them have vitamin B-12 deficiencies, partly because it's one of the most difficult nutrients for the body to absorb. Also, if they have been on antibiotics, then they are likely to have a loss of beneficial bacteria in their guts, which is needed to help absorb the B-12.

Most of my patients are also deficient in Vitamin D. Women tend to have low iron levels. If patients have been on Mepron, then they have low levels of Co-Q10, because Mepron depletes Co-Q10. Magnesium deficiencies are probably also as common as B-12 deficiencies. Magnesium levels get depleted whenever a person is under stress, which is basically anyone being treated for Lyme disease, and once intracellular magnesium levels get low, they are hard to replenish, because the cellular mechanism that is responsible for pumping magnesium into the cell becomes dysfunctional. A person with a magnesium deficiency might have chronic muscle cramping or twitches. Magnesium deficiencies also add to the problem of chronic fatigue, because magnesium is needed to stabilize ATP, the energy currency of the cell.

I believe that nutritional deficiencies can also sometimes be the first, or primary, cause of patients' symptoms, and can be present whether or not they have taken antibiotics for Lyme disease. People in the United States don't eat an optimal diet. They tend to eat junk food, or if they eat their veggies, those veggies are often depleted in nutrients because of the prevalence of non-organic farming practices and nutrient-depleted soil. So they may be consuming inferior food products, even though they might be trying to eat the "right" types of food. Then there are the chronically ill, who require higher levels of nutrients in order to heal. This popular concept that people have similar nutrient needs is rubbish. Nobody would expect an Olympic athlete to have the same nutritional needs as someone who sits on the couch all day. And in the chronically ill, the immune system is running an Olympic marathon, and therefore, the bodies of such people require more nutrition than the bodies of those who aren't ill. Our bodies are machines, (with the difference that, unlike a machine, the body can heal itself) and will run properly if we give them the proper nutrition, but we have to make sure that the building blocks are there so that they can heal themselves. This sometimes means giving IV vitamin or intramuscular vitamin shots to my patients, in addition to recommending a proper diet and supplements for them.

Magnesium

In my practice, we are also known for giving a lot of magnesium injections to our patients. As mentioned earlier, this is important because once magnesium levels are low inside of the cell, the only effective way to raise them is by ensuring that the magnesium gets to where it needs to go inside the body. The body's magnesium levels are ordinarily higher inside of the cell than outside of the cell, while calcium levels are higher outside of the cell, but when cells become dysfunctional, the cell's magnesium pump gets damaged and the result is that magnesium cannot build up inside of the cells properly. So in order to overcome the barrier to entry, there must be higher concentrations of magnesium outside of the cell. This can be achieved through the administration of magnesium injections, which restore the calcium/magnesium pump back to normal.

The body has an efficient way of regulating magnesium, and its ability to achieve a high concentration in the cells via oral administration is limited. Hence, I find it necessary to give my patients magnesium intramuscularly or intravenously in order to get a high peak concentration of the mineral in their blood. Administering magnesium in these ways has to be done under a doctor's supervision, because there are risks to the procedure. For instance, if someone has kidney damage or low blood pressure, then that could create problems.

Dietary Recommendations

In general, if yeast isn't a primary problem for my patients, I recommend that they follow a diet that we in my practice call the Balanced Approach meal plan. This plan allows for the consumption of the following protein sources: free range chicken, grass-fed beef, turkey, duck and fish that is low in mercury. Tuna fish, for example, should be avoided. Most vegetables are also allowed on this plan, but I advise patients with joint symptoms to avoid night-shade veggies, such as white potatoes, tomatoes, eggplant and peppers. Seaweed is OK, as are low glycemic index fruits, when eaten only seasonally. So in the spring, for example, citrus fruit, summer berries and cherries are fine to eat; in the fall, melons, apples and pears are best. The reason that I recommend eating fruits seasonally is because they are not as likely to be picked too early or sprayed with pesticides or preservatives when grown in season. Also, getting food locally is best because it supports local farms and the food doesn't have to be picked early and shipped. When fruit is picked too early, its level of nutrients is lower than in fruit that has been allowed to fully ripen. In addition to the above foods, I also recommend whole grains, such as brown rice, buck-wheat, millet, quinoa, and oatmeal. I find that if whole grains are unprocessed, they tend to be OK for most people, but it also de-pends upon the person. Beans are OK, as are healthy oils, such as olive, coconut and grapeseed. Finally, avoiding white foods is important, including white rice, bread, potatoes and dairy products (except yogurt, for some people).

Detoxification

I strongly believe that most patients with chronic Lyme disease should do some type of bowel, liver and colon detoxification and cleansing protocol. I sometimes recommend a specific detoxifica-tion diet to my patients, which basically involves using a rice-based protein shake as a meal replacement, while eliminating certain types of food from the diet. Information on this detoxification diet can be found on my web site, www.TheMorrisonCenter.com.

In addition, I recommend homeopathic remedies to improve liver, kidney and lymphatic drainage. One brand of remedies that I use is Pekana from Germany. The Pekana detoxification kit includes three different remedies, one for each of the above organs/systems. Also, I make sure that my patients take a soluble fiber, such as psyllium husks or flaxseed, to ensure regular bowel movements—at least one to three per day. This guarantees that the body's exhaust system is working properly. I believe that if patients take a soluble fiber, along with bentonite clay, then it's not usually necessary for them to take other toxin binders.

Lifestyle Recommendations

I tell my patients to stick with a routine during the course of each day. Going to sleep before 10:30 PM and getting at least eight hours of sleep or whatever the body needs, is important, as is waking up at the same time every day. Having breakfast, lunch and dinner, and exercising at the same time every day is likewise beneficial. Routines can really take stress off the body.

Treatments for Symptomatic Relief

Insomnia

I tell my patients to sleep in a completely dark room. If they don't, they should get blackout shades or some kind of mask to wear over their eyes at bedtime. They should absolutely not watch television in the bedroom, nor read in bed. The bed is for two things; sleep and you know what else! I also tell them to go to sleep before 10:30 PM, because after that time, the adrenal glands start to wake up and give them a second wind, so that it becomes difficult for them to fall asleep.

The supplements that I recommend for sleep include melatonin, in doses of .5 mg on up; GABA, (500-1500 mg), 5-HTP (100-200 mg), and valerian root (500-1,000 mg). Also, sometimes just drinking chamomile tea can help. I do find that pharmaceutical medications are necessary for some patients, but again, it depends upon the person. The medications that I might recommend include Ambien, Sonata, Rozerem, or even Xyrem.

Pain

Proper treatment for pain depends upon its cause. Sometimes, it's a result of low magnesium levels in the body, and if this is the case, then I administer magnesium injections to my patients. I might treat nerve pain with Neural Therapy, which is an injection technique that helps to re-set the nervous system and re-polarize nerve fibers. For pain in a specific joint, I may inject procaine, and/or DMSO, which are anti-inflammatory substances, in and around the affected area. I also recommend fish oil, MSM and boswellia, as well as bitter spices like curcumin and turmeric. For some people, I will use low dose Naltrexone, or plaquenil, but I don't like to use Neurontin or other narcotics in my practice.

Depression/Anxiety

For the treatment of depression, I may recommend SAM-e (1200mg daily) or rhodiola and 5-HTP (100mg 2x/day). For anxiety, I recommend the amino acid L-theanine (200/mg, 2-6 capsules per day), GABA (500 mg, 1-2 capsules, 2x/day) and/or ashwagandha, which is an adrenal tonic (500 mg, 2x/day). As well, fish oil and a product called Pro DHA can be beneficial, as can homeopathic remedies, such as Rescue Remedy.

If patients have Post-Traumatic Stress Disorder, I recommend that they do a therapy called Somatic Experiencing, which significantly relieves the anxiety associated with this condition by helping to bring the body out of the fight-or-flight response.

I may also refer some of my patients with emotional problems to a holistic psychiatrist, who can prescribe them pharmaceutical anti-depressants, if necessary.

Emotional trauma can play a big role in patients' symptoms, and, like nutritional or hormonal deficiencies, can also be a main cause of symptoms. In my experience, I have observed that there is always a physical and emotional component to illness and both must be addressed in order for patients to feel well again.

Another practice that I recommend for healing depression and anxiety is meditation, but I advise my patients to work with a practitioner to learn how to do this properly. Exercise is likewise important, and I recommend practices such as yoga, Pilates, or even weight training, depending upon on one's physical ability. The most important thing is that patients do something to move their muscles and improve circulation, because this will help their minds and bodies to recover.

Mistakes in Treating Lyme Disease and Less-Than-Beneficial Treatments

If patients are being treated for just Lyme disease and not improving, then they should ask the doctors who are treating them if it's possible that they have some other infection or reason for their symptoms. By doing so, they are breaking the mindset (among practitioners and patients alike) that the only problem that those with Lyme disease have is Lyme disease! I mean, Lyme is a terrible disease, and it affects people in a chronic way, but not everyone has *just* Lyme disease. Patients and practitioners must therefore comb through the options to determine what is going on. For instance, in addition to ongoing antibiotics for Lyme, sometimes patients need rehabilitation from the negative effects that Lyme has had upon their bodies.

Also, just as underlying deficiencies and imbalances in the body can contribute to chronic Lyme disease, Lyme disease itself can likewise trigger or worsen underlying problems in the body. For example, gluten sensitivity can emerge in people with Lyme. Prior to Lyme disease, the gluten sensitivity may have been latent or sub-clinical, but it can surface when the body gets hit with Lyme disease and related co-infections, and can then take more of a center-stage role in the overall symptom picture.

Roadblocks and Challenges to Healing

There are several reasons why people don't heal from Lyme disease, or why their healing becomes complicated.

The first is genetics. Some people are genetically predisposed to illness and just don't have the immune system to handle infections properly. For instance, Ritchie Shoemaker, M.D., in his book, *Mold Warriors,* writes about genetic defects that hamper people's ability to detoxify biologic toxins that are produced from infectious agents.

Also, emotional problems can complicate or block healing. Some people, for instance, internalize their illness, and believe that it's a result of something they did wrong, or that they deserve to be sick. Yet others get discouraged because the road to recovery is long, but it's important for them to stay positive and hopeful, and to continue searching for a cure.

The healing process is sometimes quick, but more often, it takes a long time, and patients need to be prepared to go through this process with realistic expectations. It's beneficial when their treating doctors can be available, not only to give them treatment information, but also to be emotionally supportive towards them. In my practice, I try to give my patients as much emotional support as they need. I may also refer them to a therapist for additional emotional support. I find that this helps immensely with their recovery.

Another roadblock to patients' healing is not finding the underlying cause(s) of their symptoms. This might be the single most difficult challenge in treating Lyme disease. Healing requires digging and searching and sometimes re-evaluating patients and their protocol from beginning to end. For instance, when they have been on a protocol for a year, or year and a half, and they just can't break through a healing plateau, I must tell them, "You know what, we are not getting the progress that I expect, so let's re-evaluate everything from the beginning." And then I do another work-up on them, which involves running more blood tests, taking another history and doing a physical exam. Inevitably, I end up finding a problem that we didn't initially consider.

Just this week, for example, I discovered that someone that we had been treating for chronic Lyme disease really had a yeast issue as the overriding cause of her symptoms. The patient had thought it was Lyme, but after a complete re-evaluation, I decided that it was a yeast issue, so we started treating her with antifungals, and then she got much better. As physicians, we would like to hope that we get it right the first time, all of the time, but this doesn't always happen.

If people with Lyme are getting well on a particular protocol, then they should continue with whatever it is that they are doing. The most important thing is that they are getting well. I find that if patients aren't improving on their current protocol, but want to get well, then they will seek out whatever treatments are necessary to accomplish that. A person that is motivated will do whatever it takes to get well, and money is not usually a factor in the process.

Friends, Family and Final Words

Family members should take the time to listen to what their loved ones with Lyme disease are going through and participate in their healing journey to the degree that their loved ones allow. In doing so, family members can learn about the healing process and the type of disease that Lyme is, so that they can be supportive, both emotionally and in making sure that their loved ones are doing everything that needs to be done in order for them to get well.

Finally, people with Lyme disease should maintain hope. There are solutions out there; they just need to be discovered.

How to Contact Jeffrey Morrison, M.D.

The Morrison Center
103 Fifth Avenue, 6th Floor
(Between 17th and 18th Street)
New York, NY 10003
Phone / Fax Numbers:
Office: 212-989-9828
Fax: 212-989-9827
Website: www.TheMorrisonCenter.com
Email: staff@themorrisoncenter.com

• A P P E N D I C E S •

Why Lyme Treatments Fail
By James Schaller, M.D., M.A.R.

My average patient has been to 10-50 physicians before me. Such patients have not been healed of their Lyme disease. Below are some common reasons for their treatment failure:

1. ***Many patients and practitioners are profoundly ignorant about how to interpret a Western Blot Test.*** They say it is either "negative" or "positive." Wrong. If a person has one "fingerprint band", they have Lyme disease. These highly specific bands, widely accepted in the world literature, are 13, 14, 17, 21, 23, 24, 25, 28, 31, 34, 35, 37, 39, 47, 50, 54, 83, 84, 93 and 94. The lab can be a junk lab that invests nothing to optimize their testing kit, but if one of these bands is positive—Lyme is present. IGeneX has the best Western Blot in the world. No other lab has invested so much, for so long, to create the best test. If your clinician wants to first use an ELISA, simply run. To put it bluntly, the ELISA test as a screening tool is useless, missing even the most obvious PCR positive patients with clear past histories of massive Bull's Eye rashes, which, while not the norm, provide evidence of spirochetes.

2. ***Practitioners are not aware of current treatment approaches***. Practitioners who follow a year-after-year IV treatment approach are not "up-to-date" in their knowledge of Lyme. Ten years of Lyme disease treatment is not acceptable. These so called "cure" treatments often merely lower the body's pathogen load or decrease symptoms without fully eradicating all the different types of infectious agents.

3. ***Some treatments are simply useless. For example, the use of hyperbaric oxygen (HBOT), for the treatment of tick-borne infections fails***. The use of HBOT in mice studies is not applicable to humans. To prove that HBOT is useless for the treatment of tick-borne infections, I decided to perform a self-funded study to examine its benefits for the treatment of Lyme (Borrelia), Babesia, Ehrlichia and Bartonella. After receiving 120 treatments at 2.4 atmospheres for 90 minutes each, all participants still had clear positive findings for all four infections. Therefore, there is no validity to the claim that HBOT "kills" Lyme disease. I have talked to the late Dr. Fife in detail and carefully evaluated the HBOT research of Dr. Robert Lombard, which has further confirmed this finding. I love this treatment for many medical problems, but it is not a cure for tick-borne infections. It may help other aspects of patients' suffering.

4. ***Ignoring new data leads to treatment failures***. All medical groups have founders who represent the core of their organization. These founders are closed-minded about receiving new information. This is simply human nature. For example, I have published many new books on advanced tick-borne infections, all showing new critical information. For some "Lyme-literate" physicians, it took educated patients throwing a copy at them before they read this new information, and by then, years had already passed. Some health care workers believe in a Lyme literate Pope or President, but no such expert exists. Sure, some offer useful information from past investigations. However, no one has

mastered modern tick-borne medicine and all the newest co-infection information.

5. ***Sick physicians are trying to treat sick patients.*** I have been asked by a number of physicians to share my various findings, because they have become ill themselves and need treatment help. I have asked them to stop treating themselves, and to do an hour consultation with very extensive labs. Most have refused. Tragically, what they could have learned by fixing themselves would have translated into real help for their patients.

6. ***Current treatment recommendations are profoundly flawed.*** IV treatments are often used without herbal or synthetic antibiotic cyst busters. The most common treatment for Babesia is 750 mg/teaspoon of Mepron, taken twice a day. The most commonly used herbal Babesia cures are artemisinin, dihydroartemisinin, or artesunate (for example, Zhang Artemisia from Heprapro.com). The latter involves a standard dose of one capsule three times a day—yet all four of the approaches listed above fail at published and recommended doses, even after long trials of treatment.

7. ***A lack of two-year blind studies leads to treatment failures for Bartonella.*** For example, I have found that high doses of Levaquin, Rifampin, Zithromax, doxycycline, Mycobutin, Ceftin, Omnicef, Cumanda and Banderol, all fail to cure Bartonella. These antibiotics, along with Rife machines that are used at various frequencies and power, may lower the body's pathogen load and lead to initial and convincing feelings of improvement, but none of these treatments leads to a cure for Bartonella.

8. ***The current tests for Babesia, Bartonella and Ehrlichia are markedly flawed.*** Some DNA or PCR tests that are processed by a popular East Coast lab, often miss a positive infection up to ten times. If a lab needs to produce ten urine or blood samples to show a positive result, it is not

functional. Some labs are only fair at tissue PCR testing, when the tissue has clear Lyme, Babesia and Bartonella that can be observed microscopically. This is a diagnostic disaster. Amazingly, some rely upon large national labs to do manual examinations of red blood cells to look for Babesia and Bartonella. I have never seen a large national lab detect Babesia or Bartonella in over 600 manual smears. No national lab has been able to capture these infections even once in patients with certain strains of Babesia and Bartonella. I have repeatedly offered to assist them in improving their technology by linking them with hematology experts in tick-borne infections. They did not care that their manual smears were worthless, and I was repeatedly ignored.

9. ***The knowledge base about both Bartonella testing and treatment borders on the catastrophic.*** Bartonella is one of the most common infections in the world. Calling it a "co-infection" may be an error. If anything, Lyme (Borrelia) might be the "co-infection." Bartonella is found in vast numbers of common vectors including dust mites, fleas, flea feces, pet saliva, ticks, etc. Amazingly, it can turn off or lower antibodies to Lyme disease, Babesia, Ehrlichia, Anaplasma and even itself. Bartonella floats in blood and also enters all blood vessel walls without causing a fatal fever, and indeed, actually lowers fevers. It is the ultimate stealth infection. It turns off antibodies, fevers and immune function defense chemicals as it damages organs in anywhere from 20-60 different ways.

10. ***The use of fixed "protocols" or "procedures" in the treatment of tick-borne infections is sadistic "machine mill" medicine.*** Why? It treats each ill human person as a machine that is built the same and has the exact same problems, which in turn objectifies the patient and flirts with the sociopathic. We see this mindset in serious criminals, who mold people into objects in an effort to fit their skewed perceptions of the world. It is junk medicine to apply a blanket protocol to a unique human body, with a complex and multi-faceted infection

cluster and unique biochemical response. Doing so is useless "mill medicine," plain and simple.

11. ***Since Bartonella turns off the production of antibodies to infections like Babesia microti or Babesia duncani and Lyme disease, this infection must be considered in all initial consults, but it often isn't.*** I would suggest that practitioners learn the 60 different skin patterns that can be created by Bartonella or a mix of Bartonella/Lyme infections. It would also be useful for them to become familiar with the indirect lab markers that are associated with Bartonella infections, as well as those that are associated with mixed Bartonella/Babesia infections, such as IL-6, IL-1B, TNF-a, ECP, and VEGF. We discuss clinical patterns that are seen as a result of these lab results in the *Babesia 2009 Update* book and *The Diagnosis and Treatment of Bartonella* book (available from www.lymebook.com).

12. ***Some patients have very few Babesia protozoa parasites, but they are causing serious trouble in their bodies. Practitioners don't recognize them to be a problem, however.*** Their small numbers cause them to be missed in visual FISH exams, PCR and antibody tests.

13. ***Most labs don't test for new species of Babesia and Bartonella, such as Babesia duncani or the many other documented species of Babesia (15) or Bartonella (10) that infect humans, but practitioners cannot rule out the presence of these infections just because patients test negative for them.*** One way to reduce treatment failures is to use new medical tricks to detect stealth Babesia. (Babesia can cause symptoms of ongoing fatigue, headaches and weight gain, as well as others, while hindering the treatment of Lyme disease).

   a. The "trick" is simple: A patient is given at least two Babesia killing medications such as Mepron and artesunate or Malarone (given for the proguanil).

These medications are used for ten days at a dose that both patient and physician feel is worth the risk. Usually, at least one of the medications will kill a few Babesia parasites. Approximately ten to fourteen days later, a follow up lab test is performed, in which blood is drawn and special attention to ECP levels (which are produced to kill parasites) is given. The new ECP level is compared to the baseline. If the ECP rises significantly, it is usually a sign of Babesia "die-off". (Eosinophils release ECP and possibly inject Babesia debris). Changes in IL-6, IL-1B, TNF-a and VEGF as a result of this test are also indicative of Babesia die-off.

b. An added option is to wait six weeks after doing this "trick" and have the patient tested for antibodies to Babesia microti or duncani. One youth patient with profound illness was finally diagnosed in this manner, and after three weeks of triple Babesia treatment had significant clinical improvement for the first time in six years. Not being able to detect stealthy, low-volume Babesia is a common problem when treating tick and flea-borne infections. Talented health care workers commonly miss these red blood cell parasites, but this trick usually causes the parasites to show up and can save patients from years of failed treatment.

14. ***The Bartonella testing of most national labs is useless. It is stunning to read about so-called "sages" who report that patients don't have Bartonella just because a large lab didn't find antibodies to the infection in their blood.*** First, these "sages" do not understand that Bartonella turns off its own antibodies, and that the large labs only check for one (or two) species that infect humans, and their cut-off titers are unrealistically high. Thankfully, IGeneX Bartonella FISH testing will be available soon nationwide (except in New York State).

15. *Infections and inflammation decrease insight.* Tick-borne infections routinely destroy patients' ability to have insight into treatments and lead to personality changes and/or rigid resistance to testing. This is largely due to an impaired frontal lobe (the part of the brain involved in self-awareness). Examples of decreased insight are demonstrated by the following situations:

    a. Patients feeling like they are cured when they have only experienced improvement in their symptoms

    b. Patients intentionally going to practitioners who use inferior labs.

    c. Patients refusing, with eccentric resistance, to be tested for tick-borne infections.

    d. Patients dismissing positive test results with a wave of the hand.

16. *Some patients insist that their problem is mold and not tick-borne infections. They cannot believe both are important and either one could be "the last straw" for them.* Some patients get ill after a flood, large leak or some other water intrusion problem. They feel they are ill only because of mold mycotoxins in their home that have formed 36-48 hours after water intrusion into drywall, insulation, carpeting and other dust or cellulose-filled materials. The EPA reports that 30% of US structures have indoor mold. Some of these indoor molds have war-grade chemicals on their surfaces. When the tomb room of the last King of Poland, Casimir IV was opened in Paris in 1973, ten of the twelve scientists who were present died. One survivor had expertise in mold and subsequently found three toxic mold species.

17. *Residing in a moldy location prevents people from being cured from tick and flea-borne infections.*

This significant factor was the catalyst for my decision to write two mold remediation books. We have also known since the 1880's that dust and high humidity leads to mold and bacteria growth indoors. Their presence makes Lyme disease much more difficult to cure.

18. ***Lyme has at least one surface biotoxin, the patented BbTox1, and some people cannot detoxify this biotoxin.*** Patients with 15/16--6/5--51 HLA patterns are probably unable to remove Lyme biotoxins (R. Shoemaker) and must take a binder, like Cholestyramine, which has been used to bind biotoxins since the 1970's. Other HLA patterns have been identified in 2009 that may be responsible for the body slowly releasing Lyme biotoxins.

19. ***Many patients who have had tick-borne infections have very high levels of inflammation. High starting doses of antibiotics exacerbate this problem and complicate healing.*** Therefore, all starting doses of medications or herbs should be very low and gradually raised to higher levels. Additionally, liver-protecting substances should be given in conjunction with these remedies. Starting at full dosing in a "medically sensitive" patient is akin to committing chemical battery. Massive die-off reactions may be confused with allergic reactions and can cause panic attacks, shortness of breath, chest pain and severe migraines. This sloppy, one-size-fits all approach, is common in large practices in which a few major "protocols" are routine.

20. ***Medical "Band-Aids" are often required to save a job or a marriage and to care for children, but practitioners don't always prescribe these.*** They are often a highly useful component of care, however. Pain, fatigue, severe insomnia, depression and anxiety often increase with die-off reactions or as a result of the presence of the infections. Band-Aid treatments are therefore often useful and helpful for patients. I treat people who run companies,

schools, very large families and professional teams. They want to sleep 13 hours per day. They need stimulants for a period of time. The use of natural or synthetic stimulant options is discussed in *The Diagnosis and Treatment of Babesia* (available from www.LymeBook.com). Patients do not benefit from sleep in excess of 8 hours. It may just serve to get them fired!

21. **Some healthcare practitioners are not comfortable with being aggressive with their patients' diagnoses and treatment of tick and flea-borne infections. This is a problem.** If healthcare practitioners haven't spent 1,000 hours learning about this complex emerging area of medicine that requires a great deal of study, then their patients need to find practitioners that are serious about it, instead of someone who is just "doing them a favor" by simply running a few tests.

22. **Some patients relapse due to "treatment fatigue." Meaning, they have been treated for many years and are fed up.** They have done IV antibiotics or IV nutrients, have taken 40 pills per day, tried a wide range of specialized treatments, and now are tired of it all. They are at the end of their treatment rope. This is what happens when practitioners do not treat them fully and effectively at the beginning of their treatment. They get treatment fatigue. Patients should consider a short treatment break, and discuss this option frankly with their health care providers. They should not confuse cure with improvement.

23. **The treatment dose that "stuns organisms" is not the same dose that leads to a cure.** A cure is not a mere reduction in bacterial load. For example, using Bicillin once a week with no cyst buster will never cure patients of Lyme disease because it does not remove cysts. So years after receiving this treatment, levels of the body's cancer-fighting cells, marked by some as the CD57, may still be under 90, which indicates active infection. This is one good test that is

possibly specific for Lyme disease and other tick-borne infections. (The C3a and C4a tests are definitely not specific for Lyme).

24. ***Cynical relatives, friends or other health care workers defame Lyme experts, and convince patients to drop healthcare workers who are actually helping them.*** They usually use "the money" argument or "the speed of your recovery" argument to dissuade patients from receiving help from those who are sincerely trying to help them. If patients have been battling for years with multiple infections, they will not be cured in four months.

25. ***Last year, the existence of a Lyme biofilm was proposed. Many spirochetes make biofilms so this was not really a surprise, but not addressing these may undermine treatment outcomes.*** Indeed, many spirochetes in the mouth are known to cause biofilms, and they are believed to limit antibiotic effectiveness. Organizations with millions in grants and research money have never addressed this issue.

    I am currently working on a textbook that addresses the many treatment options for attacking biofilms. No article or book exists that explores the twenty-plus ways that I would propose to beat a Lyme biofilm. It is believed by some professionals that highly specific enzymes, drugs, or one mineral can undermine a Lyme biofilm. Yet enzymes are like highly specific keys, and no single enzyme has been a proven "key" to undermining a Lyme biofilm.

26. ***Self-treatment is easy to pursue but does not lead to cures. The best experts are typically expensive even when they use physician extenders, and their level of expertise may be uncertain.*** The Internet seems to offer many effective treatment options but not all of these are, in reality, good. Some health care practitioners

seem too narrow in their approach to treatment, while others are open to virtually everything. So patients get into a medical boat and push themselves out to sea. They read like crazy. They try treatments a, b and c. They read testimonials of hundreds of patients. They try a wide range of non-prescription options. Some days, weeks or months, they feel better. Other weeks, they don't feel so good. They are upset. They ask themselves, "Why do I have to do all the work and learning?" This is not a good place for them to be in. People exist who have already explored virtually all of the things that those with Lyme are going to explore over the next ten years. They need mentors.

27. *In many of my books and many Internet sites, patients can read about preventing flea and tick bites.* They do not need to be re-infected with Bartonella, Lyme, Babesia or any other infection. They can learn about the basic steps to protecting themselves from tick bites by doing about thirty minutes of reading.

28. *Tick and flea-borne infections cause isolation. They ruin relationships due to the sick person's fogginess, poor insight, depression, various addictions, rage, anxiety and extreme hostility, or because he/she refuses to get treatment. They can even sometimes provoke violence in those infected. This hinders recovery.* Bartonella is likely the worst cause of these problems, but Lyme and Babesia and the die-off reactions that they cause can also increase these problems. Isolation leads to decreased treatment options. It can ultimately lead to divorce and the loss of family relationships and friendships. This, in turn, leads to decreased resources and support while ill. Isolated humans, as Mother Teresa often said, are the poorest beings on earth.

OTHER REASONS FOR LYME TREATMENT FAILURE EXIST, BUT IT IS IMPORTANT FOR PATIENTS AND PRACTITIONERS TO AT LEAST KNOW THESE BASIC ONES.

ABOUT DR. SCHALLER: James Schaller, M.D., M.A.R., is the author of 26 books with six on tick-borne infections. He has published more books on tick-borne infections than anyone in print. Dr. Schaller is the author of 27 peer-reviewed journal articles and is one of the most prolific and creative LLMD's in the world. He is a full-time self-funded researcher, with a part-time private practice offering tailored care to patients. You can visit Dr. Schaller's website at: www.personalconsult.com.

The following books by Dr. Schaller are sold through the company that publishes the book you are now holding, BioMed Publishing Group, available from www.lymebook.com:

- *The Diagnosis and Treatment of Babesia*

- *The Use of the Herb Artemisinin for Babesia, Malaria and Cancer* [this book discusses all Artemisia derivatives]

- *Mold Illness and Mold Remediation Made Simple*

- *Bartonella: Diagnosis and Treatment* [2-part set]

- *2009 Babesia Update: A Cause of Excess Weight, Migraines, and Fatigue*

- *The 35 Causes of Lyme Disease Treatment Failure* [Expected release date: December, 2009]

Microbes, Toxins, and Unresolved Conflicts:
A Unifying Theory

Based on an interview with
Dietrich Klinghardt, M.D., Ph.D.

Article Written by Scott Forsgren, Founder and
Editor of www.BetterHealthGuy.com

Throughout my journey with Lyme disease, I have looked for teachers and mentors that could help shape my understanding of the disease process taking place within my body everyday. From the onset, it was not enough to accept that the meltdown I was experiencing was the result of a simple infection. I knew that there was more to the complex puzzle of my illness. I also felt that a treatment approach based solely on attempts to manage infection would not result in the higher level of health that I had set out to once again attain.

After eight years of illness and what at times felt like the end was looming, I was diagnosed with Lyme disease in July 2005. I finally had a name for the disease that had ravaged my body for so many years. I was now better able to direct my research towards finding effective treatment options.

Shortly after, I learned of Dr. Dietrich Klinghardt, M.D., Ph.D. in Seattle, Washington. Dr. Klinghardt is renowned by many as the top expert in the field of Lyme disease.

As I began to learn more about the work of Dr. Klinghardt, a light suddenly turned on. I understood my illness in a completely new and different way. I understood how to approach my recovery in a way that, for the first time, made me feel empowered to get well. Since the day I met Dr. Klinghardt, my journey has been forever positively changed.

The "Klinghardt Axiom" looks at the multiple contributors to illness and serves as a single unifying theory for chronic illness. This axiom has three major components: microbes, toxins, and unresolved emotional conflicts. It looks at the relationships within this triad and explains how most attempts to recover from a chronic illness will not be successful without a treatment program that addresses each of these components simultaneously.

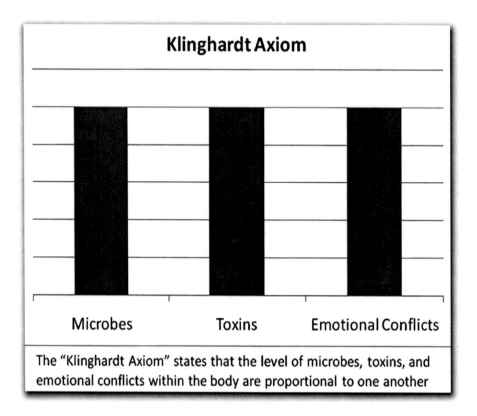

The "Klinghardt Axiom" states that the level of microbes, toxins, and emotional conflicts within the body are proportional to one another

The "Klinghardt Axiom" states that "The body always strives to achieve equilibrium between stored unresolved emotional issues, toxins, and the presence of pathogenic microbes." It is only through a well-planned treatment protocol that considers all of these factors that the patient will return to a state of wellness. Let's look further at some of the relationships described by the axiom.

The level of infection in a body is directly correlated to the level of toxins, or toxic body burden. If the toxic body burden is high, the level of disease-causing microbes will also be high. This leads to a total combined body burden which results in chronic disease. Once this state is reached, there are no easy solutions. One cannot attempt to address the body burden of infection through an anti-microbial protocol alone. It will simply fail. The toxic body burden must be addressed as well if there is to be any chance of success in reducing the infectious load of the patient.

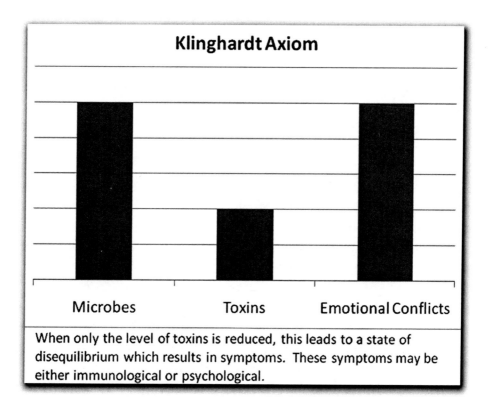

Klinghardt Axiom

| Microbes | Toxins | Emotional Conflicts |

When only the level of toxins is reduced, this leads to a state of disequilibrium which results in symptoms. These symptoms may be either immunological or psychological.

Toxins can come from multiple internal and external sources such as heavy metals, flame retardants, insecticide residues, mycotoxins from mold, Lyme biotoxins, and many more. These toxins lead to a suppression of the immune system in the various body compartments where they reside. Once these toxins contaminate an area of the body and immune surveillance and function is reduced, this body compartment becomes the ideal breeding ground for pathogenic microbes and numerous infections move in. They not only move in, but they are essentially free to further damage the body as a result of the immune system's inability to address these organisms in areas where the concentration of the toxins are highest.

If one attempts to reduce the level of infection without concurrently reducing the toxic body burden, any positive results will be short-lived. Once the anti-microbial agent is stopped, the infections will once again move into their former home where they will thrive in the presence of a toxic environment.

Microbes grow and prosper proportional to the level of stored toxins in the body. A more successful treatment approach is to lower both the level of toxins and the level of infectious organisms in the body simultaneously. In fact, it may be the case that a focus on toxin reduction and immune support and modulation will result in a successful outcome even in the absence of an aggressive anti-microbial program.

If we take the impact of toxins on microbes one level higher, we must consider the impacts of electromagnetic radiation, a very powerful toxin to the human body. Electromagnetic fields (EMFs) from cell phones, cell towers, cordless phones and other sources strongly drive the growth of many microbes within us.

Molds, for example, increase their rate of growth and put out far more virulent mycotoxins in the presence of EMFs. They feel that they are being attacked and respond by fighting back. It is suggested that all levels of the microbiome are influenced by electromagnetic radiation including viruses, spirochetes, Mycoplasma, streptococci, staphylococci, and numerous others. Thus, in looking at the impact of toxins on microorganisms, we must not only consider our internal toxic body burden. We must look at the toxic forces around us and make every effort to minimize the external toxins which also have powerful disease-promoting properties.

Next, we turn to emotional conflicts and how past traumas are a significant factor in healing. In Dr. Klinghardt's teachings in the area of Applied Psycho-Neurobiology (APN), Dr. Klinghardt talks about the relationships between specific emotions that we hold and organs that are impacted by these emotions. For example, anger and frustration are the primary emotions associated with the liver. Likewise, fear and guilt are associated with the kidneys. Being overcritical or controlling impacts the large intestine. The emotions of loneliness or abandonment impact the small intestine.

When these emotions are present and not dealt with, they alter the blood flow in the associated organs. Unresolved conflicts create loops of arousal in the subconscious and are expressed by branches of the sympathetic nervous system which leads to hypoperfusion and vaso-constriction (reduced blood flow) as well as a hypersensitizing of pain receptors. When the blood flow is

"The body always strives to achieve equilibrium between stored unresolved emotional conflicts, toxins, and the presence of pathogenic microbes."

reduced, immune surveillance in those organs is also reduced and oxygen and nutrient delivery is depressed. As a result, the levels of infections and toxins increase as the immune system is no longer able to perform its job in those areas. If the organs which are impaired are organs of detoxification such as the kidneys or liver, there is an overall decrease in the clearance of toxins which results in a redistribution of toxins into the connective tissue and into the matrix.

The matrix is the space between the cells–the area in the body that includes the blood vessels, lymphatic vessels, autonomic nerves, fibroblasts, collagen, elastin, glycosaminoglycans, proteoglycans, cell membranes of neighboring cells, cells of the immune system, and nutrients. The matrix is where nutrients and information-carrying substances move into the cells and toxins move out of the cells.

The matrix as a whole is a significant storage site for toxins in the body. Psychologically the matrix is related to unresolved emotional conflicts with the mother. It is essentially another organ of the body. If the body can detoxify more each day than it takes in, there is no need for a storage organ. If, however, the body cannot detoxify what it encounters on a daily basis, the matrix then becomes a backup storage container and acts like a sponge. Once the matrix is contaminated, the nutrient, water, and oxygen transport into the cells is impaired, the transport of metabolic waste from the cell to the excretory pathways is blocked and chronic illness follows. Borrelia spirochetes live in the matrix and are collagen-eating organisms that feed on connective tissue. One of the key elements of a good detoxification protocol is to ensure that the matrix is no longer serving as a sponge for toxic waste.

It is easy for most people to accept that microbes or infections are a significant factor in a condition such as Lyme disease. It becomes slightly more difficult for some to fully grasp how our toxic body burden promotes the proliferation of the disease-causing microbes. It is often an order of magnitude more challenging for a patient to accept that emotional traumas or conflicts may be a contributor to their illnesses. However, these conflicts very significantly impact our ability to detoxify which results in increased toxin accumulation and a higher level of microbes. It is only through a treatment program which works to address each of these three factors that the patient will find and achieve lasting wellness and a new, optimal state of health.

Resources:

Dietrich Klinghardt, M.D., Ph.D. is a highly-respected pioneer in the field of chronic illness and treatment of Lyme disease. Dr. Klinghardt studied medicine in Freiburg, Germany. He has since created a comprehensive diagnostic system known as ART, or Autonomic Response Testing, which has transformed many medical practices and helped numerous practitioners become gifted healers.

Dr. Klinghardt has recently released a new 5-DVD set geared towards educating patients and practitioners. The set is entitled "Protocols for Patients and Practitioners: Fundamental Teachings of Dietrich Klinghardt, M.D., Ph.D." and is available now at:

www.lymebook.com/dietrich-klinghardt-dvds

The "Klinghardt Protocol 2008" which discusses approaches to treatment of chronic illnesses and Lyme disease can be found on Dr. Klinghardt's web site at:

www.klinghardtneurobiology.com

About the author of this article:

Scott Forsgren, author of this article, is the editor and founder of BetterHealthGuy.com where he shares his twelve year journey through a chronic illness only diagnosed as Lyme disease after eight years of searching for answers. He has attended numerous conferences taught by Dr. Klinghardt as well as having been a patient of Dr. Klinghardt for the past 3 years. Dr. Klinghardt has been a powerful mentor, teacher, and guide as Scott has worked to understand the disease which had previously taken so much of his life and as he moves toward a place of health and wellness.

About Connie Strasheim

Connie Strasheim was born in 1974 and raised in Denver, Colorado. She holds a Bachelor's degree in Spanish for Business and graduated in the top two percent of her class from the University of Colorado at Boulder. In addition to other types of employment, she spent her twenties working as a flight attendant for United Airlines in New York and traveling around the world. In her spare time, she participated in and led humanitarian missions to Latin America and wrote travel narratives and novels. These were inspired by her having lived overseas in Argentina, as well as by her travels to over forty-five countries.

In September 2004, and at the age of 30, she "crashed" from Lyme disease (although some symptoms had started to manifest many years prior, during her university years and perhaps even childhood). Over the following year, she visited over thirteen physicians before she was finally diagnosed with Lyme disease in June, 2005, by Dr. Arlyn LaBair at the Fibromyalgia and Fatigue Center in Denver. During subsequent years, in an attempt to heal herself, she became a full-time medical researcher. No longer able to work as a flight attendant, she worked part-time as a Spanish medical interpreter and private Spanish instructor whenever her health allowed her to.

In November, 2007, Connie traveled to Costa Rica to write her first Lyme book, *The Lyme Disease Survival Guide: Physical, Lifestyle and Emotional Strategies for Healing,* and to temporarily experience what was, in some ways, a healthier, less expensive way of life.

Over the past four years, she has experienced significant healing from Lyme disease, although is not fully cured due, most likely, to the damage that Lyme has done to her body and to the continued presence of toxins and/or low-grade infections. Still, she has come a long way since 2005, and continues to heal more and more with each passing year. This year, she hopes to work full-time again, for the first time in nearly five years. Connie lives in Denver, Colorado, and is available on a limited basis for interviews.

•PRODUCT CATALOG•

Lyme-Related Books & DVDs
FROM BIOMED PUBLISHING GROUP

www.LymeBook.com
Phone: (530) 541-7200

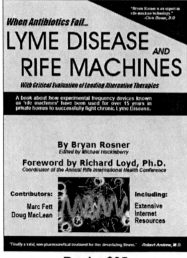

When Antibiotics Fail...

LYME DISEASE AND RIFE MACHINES

With Critical Evaluation of Leading Alternative Therapies

A book about how experimental frequency devices known as 'rife machines' have been used for over 15 years in private homes to successfully fight chronic Lyme Disease.

By Bryan Rosner
Edited by Michael Huckleberry

Foreword by Richard Loyd, Ph.D.
Coordinator of the Annual Rife International Health Conference

Contributors:
Marc Fett
Doug MacLean

Including:
Extensive
Internet
Resources

Book • $35

When Antibiotics Fail: Lyme Disease And Rife Machines, With Critical Evaluation Of Leading Alternative Therapies

By Bryan Rosner
Foreword by Richard Loyd, Ph.D.

There are enough books and websites about what Lyme disease is and which ticks carry it. But there is very little useful information for people who actually have a case of Lyme disease that is not responding to conventional antibiotic treatment. Lyme Disease sufferers need to know their options, not how to identify a tick.

This book describes how electromagnetic frequency devices known as rife machines have been used for over 15 years in private homes to fight Lyme disease. Also included are evaluations of more than 20 conventional and alternative Lyme disease therapies, including:

- Homeopathy
- IV and oral antibiotics
- Mercury detox.
- Hyperthermia / saunas
- Ozone and oxygen
- Samento®
- Colloidal Silver
- Bacterial die-off detox.

- Colostrum
- Magnesium supplementation
- Hyperbaric oxygen chamber (HBOC)
- ICHT Italian treatment
- Non-pharmaceutical antibiotics
- Exercise, diet and candida protocols
- Cyst-targeting antibiotics
- The Marshall Protocol®

Many Lyme disease sufferers have heard of rife machines, some have used them. But until now there has not been a concise and reliable source to explain how and why they work, and how and why other therapies fail. Remember that any medical treatment decision must be made under the care of a licensed physician. Rife machines are not FDA approved and the FDA has not reviewed or approved of this book. The author is a journalist, not a medical doctor.

The Foreword for the book is by Richard Loyd, Ph.D., coordinator of the annual Rife International Health Conference. The book takes a practical, down-to-earth approach which allows you to learn about:

"This book provides life-saving insights for Lyme disease patients."

- Richard Loyd, Ph.D.

- Why rife machines may help after other therapies fail, with analysis of antibiotics.
- Rife machine treatment schedules and sessions.
- The machines with the longest track record: High Power Magnetic Pulser, EMEM Machine, Coil Machine, and AC Contact Machine.
- Explanation of the "herx reaction" and why it may indicate progress.
- Evaluation of popular alternative therapies.
- Antibiotic categories and classifications, and which antibiotics are most efficacious.
- What it feels like to use rife machines.

Paperback book, 8.5 x 11", 203 pages, $35

The Top 10 Lyme Disease Treatments: Defeat Lyme Disease With The Best Of Conventional And Alternative Medicine

By Bryan Rosner
Foreword by James Schaller, M.D.

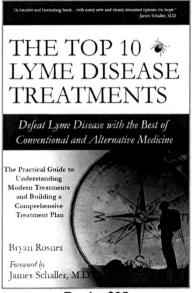

"A creative and fascinating book... with many new and clearly described options for hope."
- James Schaller, M.D.

THE TOP 10
LYME DISEASE
TREATMENTS

Defeat Lyme Disease with the Best of
Conventional and Alternative Medicine

The Practical Guide to
Understanding
Modern Treatments
and Building a
Comprehensive
Treatment Plan

Bryan Rosner

Foreword by
James Schaller, M.D.

Book • $35

This information-packed book identifies ten cutting-edge conventional and alternative Lyme disease treatments and gives practical guidance on integrating them into a comprehensive treatment plan that you and your physician can customize for your individual situation and needs.

This book was not written to replace Bryan Rosner's first book (*Lyme Disease and Rife Machines*). Instead, it was written to complement that book, offering Lyme sufferers many new foundational and supportive treatments to use under the supervision of a physician. New information in this book includes:

- Systemic enzyme therapy, which helps detoxify tissues and blood, reduce inflammation, stimulate the immune system, and kill Lyme disease bacteria.
- Lithium orotate, a powerful yet all-natural mineral (belonging to the same mineral group as sodium and potassium) capable of profound neuroprotective activity.
- Thorough and extensive coverage of a complete Lyme disease detoxification program, including discussion of both liver and skin detoxification pathways. Specific detoxification therapies such as liver cleanses, bowel cleanses, the Shoemaker Neurotoxin Elimination Protocol, sauna therapy, mineral baths, mineral supplementation, milk thistle, and many others. Ideas to reduce and control herx reactions.
- Tips and clinical research from James Schaller, M.D.
- A detailed look at one method for utilizing antibiotics during a rife machine treatment campaign.
- Wide coverage of the Marshall Protocol, including an in-depth description of its mechanism of action in relation to Lyme disease pathology. Also, the author's personal experience with the Marshall Protocol over 3 years.
- An explanation of and new information about the Salt / Vitamin C protocol.
- Hot-off-the-press information on mangosteen fruit (not to be confused with mango) and its many benefits, including antibacterial, anti-inflammatory, and anti-cancer properties.
- New guidelines for combining all the therapies discussed in both of Rosner's books into a complete treatment plan. Brief and articulate for consideration by you and your doctor.
- Also includes updates on rife therapy, cutting-edge supplements, political challenges, an exclusive interview with Willy Burgdorfer, Ph.D. (discoverer of Lyme), and much more!

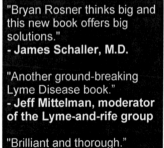

"Bryan Rosner thinks big and this new book offers big solutions."
- James Schaller, M.D.

"Another ground-breaking Lyme Disease book."
- Jeff Mittelman, moderator of the Lyme-and-rife group

"Brilliant and thorough."
- Nenah Sylver, Ph.D.

Do not miss this top Lyme disease resource. Discover new healing tools today!

Paperback book, 7 x 10", 367 pages, $35

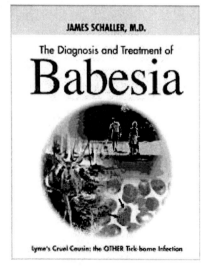

JAMES SCHALLER, M.D.

The Diagnosis and Treatment of

Babesia

Lyme's Cruel Cousin: the OTHER Tick-borne Infection

Book • $55

The Diagnosis and Treatment of Babesia: Lyme's Cruel Cousin – The Other Tick-Borne Infection

By James Schaller, M.D.

Do you or a loved one experience excess fatigue? Have you ever had unusually high fevers, chills, or sweats? You may have Babesia, a very common tick-borne infection. Babesia is often found with Lyme disease and, like all tick-borne infections, is rarely diagnosed and reported accurately.

The deer tick which carries Lyme disease and Babesia may be as small as a poppy seed and injects a painkiller, an antihistamine, and an anticoagulant to avoid detection. As a result, many people have Babesia and do not know it. Numerous forms of Babesia are carried by ticks. This book introduces patients and health care workers to the various species that infect humans and are not routinely tested for by sincere physicians.

Dr. Schaller, who practices medicine in Florida, first became interested in Babesia after one of his own children was infected with it. None of the elite pediatricians or child specialists could help. No one tested for Babesia or considered it a possible diagnosis. His child suffered from just two of these typical Babesia symptoms:

- Significant Fatigue
- Coughing
- Dizziness
- Trouble Thinking
- Fevers
- Memory Loss

- Chills
- Air Hunger
- Headache
- Sweats
- Unresponsiveness to Lyme Treatment

With 374 pages, this book is the most current and comprehensive book on Babesia in the English language. It reviews thousands of articles and presents the results of interviews with world experts on the subject. It offers you top information and broad treatment options, presented in a clear and simple manner. All treatments are explained thoroughly, including their possible side effects, drug interactions, various dosing strategies, pros/cons, and physician experiences.

"Once again Dr. Schaller has provided us with a much-needed and practical resource. This book gave me exactly what I was looking for."

- Thomas W., Patient

Finally, the book also addresses many other aspects of practical medical care often overlooked in this infection, such as treatment options for managing fatigue. Plainly stated, this book is a must-have for patients and health care providers who deal with Lyme disease and its co-infections. Dr. Schaller's many years in clinical practice give the book a practical angle that many other similar books lack. Don't miss this user-friendly resource!

Paperback book, 7 x 10", 374 pages, $55

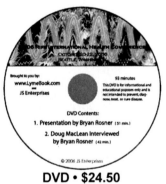

DVD • $24.50

Rife International Health Conference Feature-Length DVD (93 Minutes)

Bryan Rosner's Presentation and Interview with Doug MacLean

The Official Rife Technology Seminar Seattle, WA, USA

If you have been unable to attend the Rife International Health Conference, this DVD is your opportunity to watch two very important Lyme-related presentations from the event:

Presentation #1: Bryan Rosner's Sunday morning talk entitled *Lyme Disease: New Paradigms in Diagnosis and Treatment - the Myths, the Reality, and the Road Back to Health*. (51 minutes)

Presentation #2: Bryan Rosner's interview with Doug MacLean, in which Doug talked about his experiences with Lyme disease, including the incredible journey he undertook to invent the first modern rife machine used to fight Lyme disease. Although Doug's journey as a Lyme disease pioneer took place 20 years ago, this was the first time Doug has ever accepted an invitation to appear in public. This is the only video available where you can see Doug talk about what it was like to be the first person ever to use rife technology as a treatment for Lyme disease. Now you can see how it all began. Own this DVD and own a piece of history! (42 minutes)

Lymebook.com has secured a special licensing agreement with JS Enterprises, the Canadian producer of the Rife Conference videos, to bring this product to you at the special low price of $24.50. Total DVD viewing time: 1 hour, 33 minutes. We have DVDs in stock, shipped to you within 3 business days.

Price Comparison (should you get the DVD?)

Cost of attending the recent Rife Conference (2 people):
　Hotel Room, 3 Nights = $400
　Registration = $340
　Food = $150
　Airfare = $600
　Total = $1,490

Cost of the DVD, which you can view as many times as you want, and show to family and friends:
　DVD = $24.50

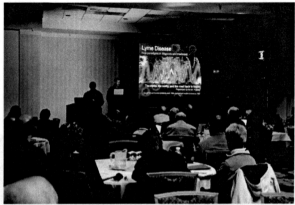

Bryan Rosner Presenting on Sunday Morning In Seattle

DVD
93 Minutes
$24.50

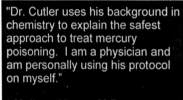

Book • $35

Amalgam Illness, Diagnosis and Treatment: What You Can Do to Get Better, How Your Doctor Can Help

By Andrew Cutler, PhD

This book was written by a chemical engineer who himself got mercury poisoning from his amalgam dental fillings. He found that there was no suitable educational material for either the patient or the physician. Knowing how much people can suffer from this condition, he wrote this book to help them get well. With a PhD in chemistry from Princeton University and extensive study in biochemistry and medicine, Andrew Cutler uses layman's terms to explain how people become mercury poisoned and what to do about it. Mercury poisoning can easily be cured with over-the-counter oral chelators – this book explains how.

In the book you will find practical guidance on how to tell if you really have chronic mercury poisoning or some other problem. Proper diagnostic procedures are provided so that sick people can decide what is wrong rather than trying random treatments. If mercury poisoning is your problem, the book tells you how to get the mercury out of your body, and how to feel good while you do that. The treatment section gives step-by-step directions to figure out exactly what mercury is doing to you and how to fix it.

> "Dr. Cutler uses his background in chemistry to explain the safest approach to treat mercury poisoning. I am a physician and am personally using his protocol on myself."
>
> **- Melissa Myers, M.D.**

Sections also explain how the scientific literature shows many people must be getting poisoned by their amalgam fillings, why such a regulatory blunder occurred, and how the debate between "mainstream" and "alternative" medicine makes it more difficult for you to get the medical help you need.

This down-to-earth book lets patients take care of themselves. It also lets doctors who are not familiar with chronic mercury intoxication treat it. The book is a practical guide to getting well. Sample sections from the book:

- Why worry about mercury poisoning?
- What mercury does to you – symptoms, laboratory test irregularities, diagnostic checklist.
- How to treat mercury poisoning easily with oral chelators.
- Dealing with other metals including copper, arsenic, lead, cadmium.
- Dietary and supplement guidelines.
- Balancing hormones during the recovery process.
- How to feel good while you are chelating the metals out.
- How heavy metals cause infections to thrive in the body.
- Politics and mercury.

This is the world's most authoritative, accurate book on mercury poisoning.

Paperback book, 8.5 x 11", 226 pages, $35

Hair Test Interpretation: Finding Hidden Toxicities

By Andrew Cutler, PhD

Hair tests are worth doing because a surprising number of people diagnosed with incurable chronic health conditions actually turn out to have a heavy metal problem; quite often, mercury poisoning. Heavy metal problems are easy to correct. Hair testing allows the underlying problem to be identified – and the chronic health condition often disappears with proper detoxification.

Hair Test Interpretation: Finding Hidden Toxicities is a practical book that explains how to interpret **Doctor's Data, Inc.** and **Great Plains Laboratory** hair tests. A step-by-step discussion is provided, with figures to illustrate the process and make it easy. The book gives examples using actual hair test results from real people.

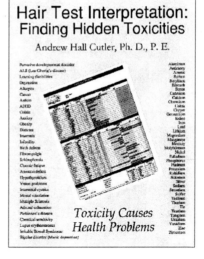

Hair Test Interpretation: Finding Hidden Toxicities
Andrew Hall Cutler, Ph. D., P. E.

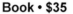

Toxicity Causes Health Problems

Book • $35

One of the problems with hair testing is that both conventional and alternative health care providers do not know how to interpret these tests. Interpretation is not as simple as looking at the results and assuming that any mineral out of the reference range is a problem mineral.

Interpretation is complicated because heavy metal toxicity, especially mercury poisoning, interferes with mineral transport throughout the body. Ironically, if someone is mercury poisoned, hair test mercury is often low and other minerals may be elevated or take on unusual values. For example, mercury often causes retention of arsenic, antimony, tin, titanium, zirconium, and aluminum. An inexperienced health care provider may wrongfully assume that one of these other minerals is the culprit, when in reality mercury is the true toxicity.

> "This new book of Andrew's is the definitive guide in the confusing world of heavy metal poisoning diagnosis and treatment. I'm a practicing physician, 20 years now, specializing in detoxification programs for treatment of resistant conditions. It was fairly difficult to diagnose these heavy metal conditions before I met Andrew Cutler and developed a close relationship with him while reading his books. In this book I found his usual painful attention to detail gave a solid framework for understanding the complexity of mercury toxicity as well as the less common exposures. You really couldn't ask for a better reference book on a subject most researchers and physicians are still fumbling in the dark about."
> **- Dr. Rick Marschall**

So, as you can see, getting a hair test is only the first step. The second step is figuring out what the hair test means. Andrew Cutler, PhD, is a registered professional chemical engineer with years of experience in biochemical and healthcare research. This clear and concise book makes hair test interpretation easy, so that you know which toxicities are causing your health problems.

Paperback book, 8.5 x 11", 298 pages, $35

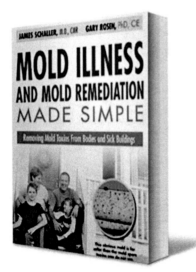

Book • $32.95

Mold Illness and Mold Remediation Made Simple: Removing Mold Toxins from Bodies and Sick Buildings

By James Schaller, M.D. and Gary Rosen, Ph.D.

Indoor mold toxins are much more dangerous and prevalent than most people realize. Visible mold in and around your house is far less dangerous than the mold you cannot see. Indoor mold toxicity, in addition to causing its own unique set of health problems and symptoms, also greatly contributes to the severity of most chronic illnesses.

In this book, a top physician and experienced contractor team up to help you quickly recover from indoor mold exposure. This book is easy to read with many color photographs and illustrations.

Dr. Schaller is a practicing physician in Florida who has written more than 15 books. He is one of the few physicians in the United States successfully treating mold toxin illness in children and adults.

Dr. Rosen is a biochemist with training under a Nobel Prize winning researcher at UCLA. He has written several books and is an expert in the mold remediation of homes. Dr. Rosen and his family are sensitive to mold toxins so he writes not only from professional experience, but also from personal experience.

Together, the two authors have certification in mold testing, mold remediation, and indoor environmental health. This book is one of the most complete on the subject, and includes discussion of the following topics:

- Potential mold problems encountered in new homes, schools, and jobs.
- Diagnosing mold illness.
- Mold as it relates to dryness and humidity.
- Mold toxins and cancer treatment.
- Mold toxins and relationships.
- Crawlspaces, basements, attics, home cleaning techniques, and vacuums.
- Training your eyes to discern indoor mold.
- Leptin and obesity.
- Appropriate/inappropriate air filters and cleaners.
- How to handle old, musty products, materials and books, and how to safely sterilize them.
- A description of various types of molds, images of them, and their relative toxicity.
- Blood testing and how to use it to find hidden health problems.
- The book is written in a friendly, casual tone that allows easy comprehension and information retention.

> "A concise, practical guide on dealing with mold toxins and their effects."
>
> **- Bryan Rosner**

Many people are affected by mold toxins. Are you? If you can find a smarter or clearer book on this subject, buy it!

Paperback book, 8.5 x 11", 140 pages, $32.95

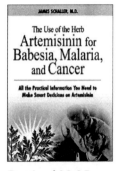

Book • $32.95

The Use of the Herb Artemisinin for Babesia, Malaria and Cancer

By James Schaller, M.D.

This book is the only patient book written in English offering practical, clear, and carefully researched help on Artemisinin medications. Artemisinin herbals are powerful treatments for red blood cell infections like Malaria and Babesia.

Artemisinin can be used as an alternative to pharmaceutical treatments for Babesia and similar infections—or it can be used synergistically with prescription drugs. This book is a must-have for all patients and physicians seeking an artemisinin education.

Paperback book, 7x10", 160 pages, $32.95

Bartonella: Diagnosis and Treatment

By James Schaller, M.D.

2 Book Set • $99.95

In the summer of 2008, Dr. James Schaller wrote another excellent book on Lyme disease co-infections—this time, a book on Bartonella. This book is an ideal complementary resource to his recently published Babesia textbook (see catalog page 4).

Bartonella infections occur throughout the entire world, in cities, suburbs, and rural locations. It is found in fleas, dust mites, ticks, lice, flies, cat and dog saliva, and insect feces.

This 2-book set provides advanced treatment strategies as well as detailed diagnostic criteria, with dozens of full-color illustrations and photographs.

Both books in this 2-part set are included with your order.

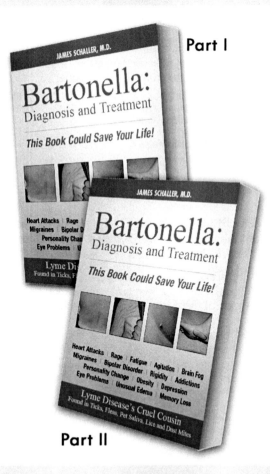

Part I

Part II

2 paperback books, 7 x 10", 500 pages, $99.95

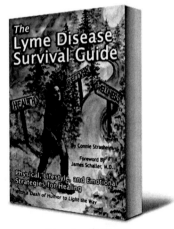

Book • $25.95

The Lyme Disease Survival Guide: Physical, Lifestyle, and Emotional Strategies for Healing

By Connie Strasheim

Author Connie Strasheim is an accomplished health care journalist. This book offers not only a new perspective on Lyme disease diagnosis and treatment, but also much-needed wisdom for dealing with the disease on an emotional and lifestyle level.

Connie skillfully analyzes many new, cutting-edge Lyme disease treatments and healing approaches not addressed anywhere else in available Lyme disease literature. Topics include:

Author Connie Strasheim

- MMS – Miracle Mineral Supplement
- Cellular Behavior & Quantum Techniques
- Ehrlichia Treatment Options
- Colloidal Silver
- Romantic Relationships & Chronic Illness
- Latest Lyme Disease Testing Methods
- Employment Options for Lyme Sufferers
- Dietary Considerations
- Spirituality and Healing
- Hormone Irregularities & Treatments

Paperback book, 7x10", 269 Pages, $25.95

The Stealth Killer: Is Oral Spirochetosis the Missing Link in the Dental & Heart Disease Labyrinth? *By William D. Nordquist, BS, DMD, MS*

Can oral spirochete infections cause heart attacks? In today's cosmopolitan urban population, more than 51 percent of those with root canal–treated teeth probably have infection at the apex of their root. Dr. Nordquist, an oral surgeon practicing in Southern California, believes that any source of bacteria with resulting chronic infection (including periodontal disease) in the mouth may potentially lead to heart disease and other systemic diseases. With more than 40 illustrations and x-ray reproductions, this book takes you behind the scenes in Dr. Nordquist's research laboratory, and provides many tips on dealing with Lyme-related dental problems. A breakthrough book in dentistry & infectious disease!

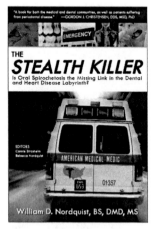

Paperback Book • $25.95

Paperback book, 6x9", 161 pages, $25.95

Marshall Protocol 4-DVD Set

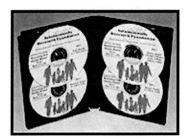

4-DVD Set • $45

Recent Chicago Conference:
"Recovering from Chronic Disease"
Recent Hartford Conference:
"30th Anniversary of Lyme"

The Marshall Protocol is not just important, but believed by some to be critical in Lyme disease recovery. It addresses a part of the Lyme disease complex that no other treatment, protocol, diet, or supplement can touch: infection by cell-wall-deficient bacteria.

Borrelia burgdorferi, the causative bacteria in Lyme disease, comes in three forms: spirochete, cyst, and cell-wall-deficient. All forms must be addressed to achieve a complete recovery. It is thought that spirochetes are successfully killed by rife technology. Cysts can be killed by certain antibiotics (including 5-nitromidizoles and hydroxychloroquine). Cysts can also be exposed and killed by rife therapy with proper treatment timing and planning. However, until the Marshall Protocol, there was not an effective treatment for cell-wall-deficient bacteria.

Conventionally, doctors have tried to use certain types of antibiotics to kill cell-wall-deficient bacteria. Top choices include protein synthesis inhibitors such as the macrolides (Zithromax and Biaxin), the ketolides (Ketek), and the tetracyclines (tetracycline, doxycycline,

> "I believe that the Marshall Protocol fills an important gap in existing Lyme treatment."
>
> **- Bryan Rosner**

and minocycline). Unfortunately, these antibiotics have been ineffective at worst and only moderately effective at best. According to new research and user reports, the Marshall Protocol successfully targets and kills these cell-wall-deficient bacteria.

This 4-DVD set is exclusively offered by lymebook.com. It was assembled for lymebook.com by the founder of the Autoimmunity Research Foundation, Trevor Marshall, PhD, who also invented the protocol. The DVD set includes video recordings from two conferences of particular interest to Lyme sufferers:

- **DVD 1:** 30th Anniversary of Lyme – Hartford, Connecticut
- **DVD 2-4:** Recovering from Chronic Disease – Chicago, Illinois

James P
Kiley, PhD

Leonard
Jason, PhD

Lida H
Mattman, PhD

Janet
Whitley, PhD

Conference Speakers

Andrew
Wright, MD

Trevor G
Marshall, PhD

Meg
Mangin, RN

4-DVD Set

12+ hours of viewing

Coverage of two Conferences

$45

Researching the Marshall Protocol is an Essential Part of Your Lyme Disease Education!

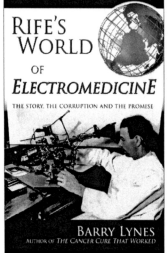

Book • $17.95

Rife's World of Electromedicine: The Story, the Corruption and the Promise

By Barry Lynes

The cause of cancer was discovered in the early 1930's. It was a virus-sized, mini-bacteria or "particle" that induced cells to become malignant and grow into tumors. The cancer microbe or particle was given the name BX by the brilliant scientist who discovered it: Royal Raymond Rife.

Laboratory verification of the cause of cancer was done hundreds of times with mice in order to be absolutely certain. Five of America's most prominent physicians helped oversee clinical trials managed by a major university's medical school.

Sixteen cancer patients were brought by ambulance twice a week to the clinical trial location in La Jolla, California. There they were treated with a revolutionary electromedicine that painlessly, non-invasively destroyed only the cancer-causing microbe or particle named BX. After just three months of this therapy, all patients were diagnosed as clinically cured. Later, the therapy was suppressed and remains so today.

In 1987, Barry Lynes wrote the classic book on Rife history (*The Cancer Cure That Worked*, see catalog page 14). *Rife's World* is the sequel, published in 2009.

Paperback book, 5.5 x 8.5", 90 pages, $17.95

Physicians' Desk Reference (PDR) Books (opposing page)

Most people have heard of *Physicians' Desk Reference* (PDR) books because, for over 60 years, physicians and researchers have turned to PDR for the latest word on prescription drugs.

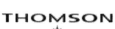

You may not know that Thomson Healthcare, publisher of PDR, offers PDR reference books not only for drugs, but also for herbal and nutritional supplements. No available books come even close to the amount of information provided in these PDRs—*PDR for Herbal Medicines* weighs 5 lbs and has over 1300 pages, and *PDR for Nutritional Supplements* weighs over 3 lbs and has more than 800 pages.

> "I relied heavily on the PDRs during the research phase of writing my books. Without them, my projects would have greatly suffered."
>
> **- Bryan Rosner**

We carry all three PDRs. Although PDR books are typically used by physicians, we feel that these resources are also essential for people interested in or recovering from chronic disease. For the supplements, herbs, and drugs included in the books, you will find the following information: Pharmacology, description and method of action, available trade names and brands, indications and usage, research summaries, dosage options, history of use, pharmacokinetics, and much more! Worth the money for years of faithful use.

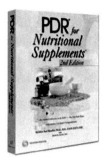

PDR for Nutritional Supplements *2nd Edition!*

This PDR focuses on the following types of supplements:

- Vitamins
- Minerals
- Amino acids
- Hormones
- Lipids
- Glyconutrients
- Probiotics
- Proteins
- Many more!

Book • $69.50

"In a part of the health field not known for its devotion to rigorous science, [this book] brings to the practitioner and the curious patient a wealth of hard facts."

- Roger Guillemin, M.D., Ph.D., Nobel Laureate in Physiology and Medicine

The book also suggests supplements that can help reduce prescription drug side effects, has full-color photographs of various popular commercial formulations (and contact information for the associated suppliers), and so much more! Become educated instead of guessing which supplements to take.

Hardcover book, 11 x 9.3", 800 pages, $69.50

PDR for Herbal Medicines *4th Edition!*

PDR for Herbal Medicines is very well organized and presents information on hundreds of common and uncommon herbs and herbal preparations. Indications and usage are examined with regard to homeopathy, Indian and Chinese medicine, and unproven (yet popular) applications.

In an area of healthcare so unstudied and vulnerable to hearsay and hype, this scientifically referenced book allows you to find out the real story behind the herbs lining the walls of your local health food store.

Use this reference before spending money on herbal products!

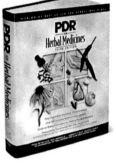

Book • $69.50

Hardcover book, 11 x 9.3", 1300 pages, $69.50

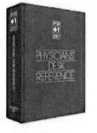

PDR for Prescription Drugs *Current Year's Edition!*

With more than 3,000 pages, this is the most comprehensive and respected book in the world on over 4,000 drugs. Drugs are indexed by both brand and generic name (in the same convenient index) and also by manufacturer and product category. This PDR provides usage information and warnings, drug interactions, plus a detailed, full-color directory with descriptions and cross references for the drugs. A new format allows dramatically improved readability and easier access to the information you need now.

Book • $99.50

Hardcover book, 12.5 x 9.5", 3533 pages, $99.50

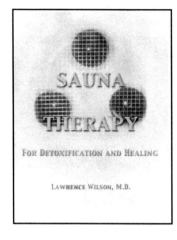

Book • $22.95

Sauna Therapy for Detoxification and Healing

By Lawrence Wilson, MD

This book is the single most authoritative source on sauna therapy. It includes construction plans for a low-cost electric light sauna. The book is well referenced with an extensive bibliography.

Sauna therapy, especially with an electric light sauna, is one of the most powerful, safe and cost-effective methods of natural healing. It is especially important today due to extensive exposure to toxic metals and chemicals.

Fifteen chapters cover sauna benefits, physiological effects, protocols, cautions, healing reactions, and many other aspects of sauna therapy.

Dr. Wilson is an instructor of Biochemistry, Hair Mineral Analysis, Sauna Therapy and Jurisprudence at various colleges and universities including Yamuni Institute of the Healing Arts (Maurice, LA), University of Natural Medicine (Santa Fe, NM), Natural Healers Academy (Morristown, NJ), and Westbrook University (West Virginia). His books are used as textbooks at East-West School of Herbology and Ohio College of Natural Health.

Paperback book, 8.5 x 11", 167 pages, $22.95

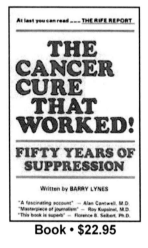

Book • $22.95

Over 50,000 Copies Sold!

The Cancer Cure That Worked: Fifty Years of Suppression

At Last You Can Read... The Rife Report

By Barry Lynes

Investigative journalism at its best. Barry Lynes takes readers on an exciting journey into the life work of Royal Rife. **In 2008, we became the official distributor for this book. Call or visit us online for wholesale terms.**

"A fascinating account..."
-Alan Cantwell, MD

"This book is superb."
-Florence B. Seibert, PhD

"Barry Lynes is one of the greatest health reporters in our country. With the assistance of John Crane, longtime friend and associate of Roy Rife, Barry has produced a masterpiece..." -Roy Kupsinel, M.D., editor of *Health Consciousness Journal*

Paperback book, 5 x 8", 169 pages, $22.95

Rife Video Documentary
2-Part DVD Set, Produced by
Zero Zero Two Productions

Must-Have DVD set for your Rife technology education!

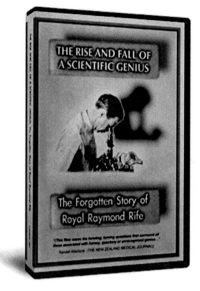

In 1999, a stack of forgotten audio tapes was discovered. On the tapes were the voices of several people at the center of the events which are the subject of this documentary: a revolutionary treatment for cancer and a practical cure for infectious disease.

The audio tapes were over 40 years old. The voices on them had almost faded, nearly losing key details of perhaps the most important medical story of the 20th Century.

But due to the efforts of the Kinnaman Foundation, the faded tapes have been restored and the voices on them recovered. So now, even though the participants have all passed away...

...they can finally tell their story.

2-part DVD Set • $39.95

"These videos are great. We show them at the Annual Rife International Health Conference."
-Richard Loyd, Ph.D.

"A mind-shifting experience for those of us indoctrinated with a conventional view of biology."
-Townsend Letter for Doctors and Patients

In the summer of 1934 at a special medical clinic in La Jolla, California, sixteen patients withering from terminal disease were given a new lease on life. It was the first controlled application of a new electronic treatment for cancer: the Beam Ray Machine.

Within ninety days all sixteen patients walked away from the clinic, signed-off by the attending doctors as cured.

What followed the incredible success of this revolutionary treatment was not a welcoming by the scientific community, but a sad tale of its ultimate suppression.

The Rise and Fall of a Scientific Genius documents the scientific ignorance, official corruption, and personal greed directed at the inventor of the Beam Ray Machine, Royal Raymond Rife, forcing him and his inventions out of the spotlight and into obscurity. **Just converted from VHS to DVD and completely updated.**

Do not miss this opportunity to educate yourself about the history of rife technology!

Includes bonus DVD with interviews and historical photographs! Produced in Canada.

2 DVD-set, including bonus DVD, $39.95

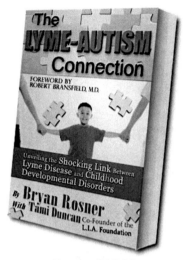

Book • $25.95

The Lyme-Autism Connection:
Unveiling the Shocking Link Between
Lyme Disease and Childhood
Developmental Disorders

By Bryan Rosner & Tami Duncan

Did you know that Lyme disease may contribute to the onset of autism?

This book is an investigative report written by Bryan Rosner and Tami Duncan. Duncan is the co-founder of the *Lyme Induced Autism (LIA) Foundation*, and her son has an autism diagnosis.

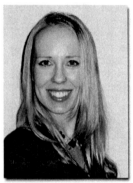

Tami Duncan, Co-Founder of the Lyme Induced Autism (LIA) Foundation

Awareness of the Lyme-autism connection is spreading rapidly, among both parents and practitioners. *Medical Hypothesis*, a scientific, peer-reviewed journal published by Elsevier, recently released an influential study entitled *The Association Between Tick-Borne Infections, Lyme Borreliosis and Autism Spectrum Disorders*. Here is an excerpt from the study:

> *"Chronic infectious diseases, including tick-borne infections such as Borrelia burgdorferi, may have direct effects, promote other infections, and create a weakened, sensitized and immunologically vulnerable state during fetal development and infancy, leading to increased vulnerability for developing autism spectrum disorders. An association between Lyme disease and other tick-borne infections and autistic symptoms has been noted by numerous clinicians and parents."*

—**Medical Hypothesis Journal.**
Article Authors: Robert C. Bransfield, M.D., Jeffrey S. Wulfman, M.D., William T. Harvey, M.D., Anju I. Usman, M.D.

Nationwide, 1 out of 150 children are diagnosed with Autism Spectrum Disorder (ASD), and the LIA Foundation has discovered that many of these children test positive for Lyme disease/Borrelia related complex—yet most children in this scenario never receive appropriate medical attention. This book answers many difficult questions: How can infants contract Lyme disease when autism begins before birth, precluding the opportunity for a tick bite? Is there a statistical correlation between the incidences of Lyme disease and autism worldwide? Do autistic children respond to Lyme disease treatment? What does the medical community say about this connection? Do the mothers of affected children exhibit symptoms? **Find out in this book.**

Paperback book, 6x9", 287 pages, $25.95

Renegade Patient: The No-Nonsense, Practical Guide to Getting the Health Care You Need   By Tedde Rinker, D.O.

Includes Patient Templates & Medical Forms

Stop! Before you pick up the phone to make an appointment with your local Lyme-literate doctor, take a few deep breaths, and ask yourself: "Am I an empowered patient who knows what I need from my physician and how to get it? Am I in control of my health care, and if not, who is?"

Why do you need to ask these questions? Unfortunately, many patients are not in control of their own health care. Physicians, politicians, pharmaceutical and insurance companies, and other third-party organizations are usually in the driver's seat—especially when it comes to controversial Lyme disease.

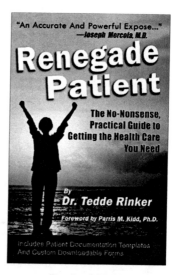

Book • $22.95

Dr. Rinker, an experienced osteopathic physician practicing medicine in Redwood City, California, believes that all patients should become empowered and responsible, equipped with the necessary education and knowledge to navigate the maze of modern medical services. This book includes tools for dealing with all aspects of the medical industry, from insurance companies and physicians' offices to requesting your medical chart and monitoring treatment progress. **This is a hands-on workbook with document templates and forms that you can actually use.**

Paperback book, 6x9", 245 pages, $22.95

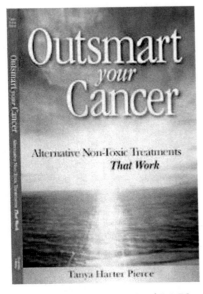

Book and Audio CD • $24.50

**Outsmart Your Cancer:
Alternative Non-Toxic Treatments
That Work   By Tanya Harter Pierce**

Why BLUDGEON cancer to death with common conventional treatments that can be toxic and harmful to your entire body?

When you OUTSMART your cancer, only the cancer cells die — NOT your healthy cells! *OUTSMART YOUR CANCER: Alternative Non-Toxic Treatments That Work* is an easy guide to successful non-toxic treatments for cancer that you can obtain right now! In it, you will read real-life stories of people who have completely recovered from their advanced or late-stage lung cancer, breast cancer, prostate cancer, kidney cancer, brain cancer, childhood leukemia, and other types of cancer using effective non-toxic approaches.

Plus, *OUTSMART YOUR CANCER* is one of the few books in print today that gives a complete description of the amazing formula called "Protocel," which has produced incredible cancer recoveries over the past 20 years! **A supporting audio CD is included with this book.** Pricing = $19.95 book + $5.00 CD.

Paperback book, 6 x 9", 437 pages, with audio CD, $24.95

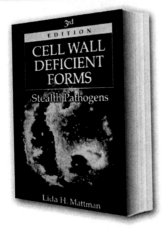

Hardcover Book • $169.95

Cell Wall Deficient Forms: Stealth Pathogens

By Lida Mattman, Ph.D.

Simply put, this is perhaps the most influential infectious disease textbook of the century. Dr. Mattman, who earned a Ph.D. in immunology from Yale University, describes her discovery that a certain type of pathogen lacking a cell wall is the root cause of many of today's "incurable" and mysterious chronic diseases. Dr. Mattman's research is the foundation of our current understanding of Lyme disease, and her work led to many of the Lyme protocols used today (such as the Marshall Protocol, as well as modern LLMD antibiotic treatment strategy). Color illustrations and meticulously referenced breakthrough principles cover the pages of this book. A must have for all serious students of chronic, elusive infectious disease.

Hardcover book, 7.5 x 10.5", 416 pages, $169.95

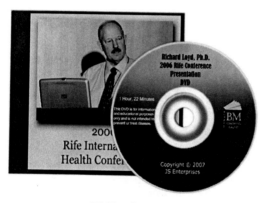

DVD • $24.50

Richard Loyd, Ph.D., presents at the Rife International Health Conference in Seattle

Watch this DVD to gain a better understanding of the technical details of rife technology.

Dr. Loyd, who earned a Ph.D. in nutrition, has researched and experimented with numerous electrotherapeutic devices, including the Rife/Bare unit, various EMEM machines, F-Scan, BioRay, magnetic pulsers, Doug Machine, and more. Dr. Loyd also has a wealth of knowledge in the use of herbs and supplements to support Rife electromagnetics.

By watching this DVD, you will discover the nuts and bolts of some very important, yet little known, principles of rife machine operation, including:

- Gating, sweeping, session time
- Square vs. sine wave
- DC vs. AC frequencies
- Duty cycle
- Octaves and scalar octaves

- Voltage variations and radio frequencies
- Explanation of the spark gap
- Contact vs. radiant mode
- Stainless vs. copper contacts
- A unique look at various frequency devices

DVD, 57 minutes, $24.50

The 2008 Lyme Disease Annual Report, by Bryan Rosner and Contributing Writers

This book serves as Bryan Rosner's annual newsletter.

The 2008 report covers numerous topics, including glyconutrient supplementation, updates on rife machine treatment planning and machine options, evidence supporting the existence of chronic Lyme disease as a real medical condition, statistics indicating the presence of Lyme disease on all continents of the planet,

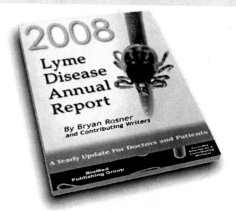

Paperback Book • $19.95

and much more. Includes articles by 6 contributing writers: **James Schaller, M.D., Richard Brand, M.D., Sue Vogan, Ginger Savely, FNP-C, Tami Duncan, Susan Williams, and Richard Loyd, Ph.D. Stay up to date!**

Paperback book, 7 x 10", 168 pages, $22.95

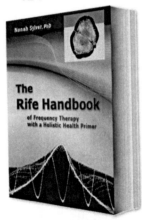

Book • $99.95

The Rife Handbook of Frequency Therapy, With a Holistic Health Primer

New Revised Edition!   By Nenah Sylver, PhD

This is the most complete, authoritative Rife technology handbook in the world. A hardcover book, it weighs over 2 lbs. and has more than 730 pages. A broad range of practical, hands-on topics are covered:

- New Revised Edition released in 2009 is twice as long as original book! Now with a complete index!
- Royal Raymond Rife's life, inventions, and relationships. Recently discovered data explaining how Rife's original machines worked.
- Frequently Asked Questions about Rife sessions and equipment, with extensive session information.
- Ground-breaking information on strengthening and supporting the body.
- A 200-page, cross-referenced Frequency Directory including hundreds of health conditions.
- Bibliography, Three Appendices, Historical Photos, Complete Index, AND MUCH MORE!
- DVD available at www.LymeBook.com with author's recent Rife Conference presentation.

Hardcover book, 8.5 x 11", 730 pages, $99.95

Ordering Options...

Phone: Toll Free (866) 476-7637
Online: www.LymeBook.com

Call today to place an order or request additional catalogs. Detailed product information and secure online ordering is available on our website.

Do you have a book inside you? We are looking for new authors of books on Lyme Disease, alternative medicine, and related topics. Find out more and submit your book proposal online at www.LymeBook.com/submit-book-proposal.

Join Lyme Community Forums (www.lymecommunity.com), a new online discussion group, to communicate for FREE with fellow Lyme sufferers!

DISCLAIMER

This disclaimer is in reference to all books, DVDs, websites, flyers, and catalogs published by Bryan Rosner, DBA BioMed Publishing Group.

Our products are for informational and educational purposes only. They are not intended to prevent, diagnose, treat, or cure disease. Bryan Rosner is a layperson, not a medical professional, and he is not qualified to dispense medical advice.

These books and DVDs are not intended to substitute for professional medical care. Do not postpone receiving care from a licensed physician. Please read our full disclaimer online at: www.lymebook.com/homepage-disclaimer.pdf.

A

AAEM (American Academy of
Environmental Medicine)   366
ABC news   56
Abdominal ultrasound   90
AC Contact Machine   406
ACAM (American College for the
Advancement in Medicine)   366
Accident, motor vehicle   146
Achillodynia   184
Acid
  alpha-lipoic   42, 277, 371
  caprylic   44, 370
  folic   255, 296
  folinic   109
  gamma-aminobutyric   104
  humic   109
  hyaluronic   295
  malic   295
  organic   36
  pantothenic   157
  quinolinic   109
  stomach   294
Acidic blood   45
Acidity   344-5
Acidophilus   164, 295
Ackermann College of Chiropractic   175
Actos   233
Acupuncture   55-6, 61-2, 70-2, 96, 98,
  110, 234
Adaptogens   41, 108
Addictions   105, 185, 393
ADHD   248
Adrenal   69, 73, 157, 257, 279, 293-4,
  300-1, 318-9, 321-2, 330, 371-2
  depletion   75-6, 157, 226, 276-7,
  293, 318, 328, 371
  extract   321
  function   59, 69, 70, 75, 230, 276,
  318-9
  gland status tests   90
  glands   41, 46, 76, 252, 276, 293,
  318-9, 321-2, 349, 361, 376
  weak   330
  glandular formulas   41
  insufficiency   69, 230
  supplements   41

tonic   377
Adrenaline   171, 257, 322
Advanced Cell Training   352
Agents
  chelating   370
  nitrating   111
  oxidizing gaseous   93
Agrobacteria   82
Air Hunger   408
Air pollution   342
Alcohol   166, 209, 340
Alinia   35, 287
Alka Seltzer Gold   97
Alkaline state   300
Alkalinizing nutrients   300
Alkaloids, toxic   84
Allergens   44, 226, 265, 267
Allergies   xiii, 36, 56, 70, 73, 80-1, 90,
  99, 111, 129, 184-5, 193, 215,
  223, 225-8, 230
Allergists   226
Allergy Research Group   42
Allium
  cepa   99
  sativum   99
Allopathic medical profession   203, 219
Aloe vera   94, 101-2, 294
Alpha lipoic acid   103, 109, 112, 279,
  298, 327, 332
ALS   33, 112, 137, 248, 259
Alternative Medicine Definitive Guide to
  Cancer   145
Alternative Medicine Guide to Heart
  Disease   146
Alzheimers   33, 40, 112
Amalgam dental fillings   208, 231, 242,
  410
Amalu, William   42
Amantilla   158, 163
Ambien   71, 105, 376
American Academy
  of Acupuncture   55
  of Anti-Aging Medicine   55
  of Environmental Medicine (AAEM)
  366
  of Family Practice Board Certified
  Member   23

American Board of Holistic and
  Integrative Medicine 247
American College of Family Practice 55
Amino acid xiv, 43, 47, 104, 268-9,
  296, 317, 320, 362, 371, 417
  essential 269
  glycine 224
  levels 269
  L-theanine 377
  lysine 94
  non-essential 269
  phenylalanine 269
  plasma 36
Ammonia 43, 47
Amoxicillin 287
Amphotericin 94-5
Anaerobic microbes 110
Anaerobic-type exercises 46
Anaplasma vii, 36, 39, 82, 386
Andrographis 41, 63, 100, 227, 235,
  237, 340-1
Anger 138, 166-7, 234, 320, 399
  harboring 50
  healing 138
Annual Rife International Health
  Conference 419
Anthroposophy 112
Anti-aging medicine 55, 57
Anti-analgesic 72
Anti-depressants 241, 296, 377
Anti-fungal 338
Anti-inflammatory 72, 206, 241, 291,
  317, 321, 326, 338-9, 349, 407
  pathways 305
  substances 295, 377
    natural 128, 346
Anti-oxidative support 317
Anti-parasitic 338
Antibiotics
  bactericidal 368
  categories 406
  combination of 92, 123, 237, 288,
    368
  cyst busters, synthetic 385
  dosing 125, 236
  double intracellular 34
  effectiveness 392
  intracellular 264
  intramuscular 124, 368
  intravenous 63, 121-2, 236, 239,
    368

long-term 188
lower dose 125
oral 36, 64, 121, 124, 368, 406
overuse 206
protocols viii, 35-7, 57, 62, 64, 122,
  138, 150-1, 172, 188, 206-7, 215,
  261, 263, 266-7, 307
pulsing 138
quinolone 123
resistant coagulase, multiple 95
Antibodies 66, 72, 95, 178-9, 200,
  202, 229-30, 232, 238, 252, 265,
  267, 273, 314, 386-8
Anticoagulant 408
Antigen-antibody response 261
Antihistamines 225-6, 408
Antioxidants 112, 127, 254, 340
Anxiety vii, xiii, xvii, 38, 47, 71, 130,
  140, 158-9, 226, 240, 295-6, 303,
  348, 366, 377-8
APN (Applied Psycho-Neurobiology)
  354, 399
Apple pectin 109
Apples 43, 342, 375
Applied Kinesiology 218, 251, 267,
  336-7
Applied Psycho-Neurobiology (APN)
  354, 399
Argiletz clay 42
Arsenic 410-1
Artemisia 38, 41, 325, 340, 369
  derivatives 394
Artemisinin 103, 122-3, 132, 152,
  237, 288-9, 324, 385, 394, 413
Arterial vasculature 95
Artesunate 385, 387
Arthritis 33, 40, 45, 72, 103, 213,
  248, 258-9, 269, 282, 361, 366
Arthrostim 361
Artificial flavors 250
ASD (Autism Spectrum Disorder) ix,
  33, 38, 107, 112, 145, 261, 335,
  420
Ashwagandha 41, 69, 107, 293, 377
ASO titers 239
Aspergillus 232
Astragalus 94, 99, 291-2
Atkins Center for Complementary and
  Alternative Medicine 365
Atkins diet 366

Atovaquone   35, 122-3, 237, 287, 289, 369
ATP   316, 373
   formation   316
   increased   317
   production   316, 321, 346
   synthesis   321
Australia   285, 299
Autism Spectrum Disorder (ASD)   ix, 33, 38, 107, 112, 145, 261, 335, 420
Autohemotherapy   94
Autoimmune
   conditions   68-9, 90, 98, 101, 178, 226, 229, 258, 260, 265, 332, 336, 372, 415
   inflammatory response   200
Autonomic Response Testing   335-6, 401
Avea   159
Azelaic acid   104
Azithromycin   35, 64, 122, 263-4, 287, 368-9

B

B-12
   deficiencies   373
   hydroxy   48
   methyl   160, 298
   supplements   109
Babesia   vii, x, xi, xv, 26, 35-6, 38-40, 122-3, 149, 152, 236-7, 266, 287-9, 384-8, 393-4, 408, 413
   die-off   388
   duncani   123-4, 387
   killing medications   387
   medications   122, 289
   microti   123-4, 387-8
   species   35, 149, 152
      treatment-resistant   150
   stealth   387
   strains   237
   symptoms   110, 408
   WA-1   123
Bacteria   64, 129, 146, 164-5, 176, 178, 184, 188, 205, 214-5, 222-5, 228, 263-5, 373, 414
   cell-wall-deficient   415
Barrier, blood-brain   46, 107, 111
Bartonella   vii, x, xi, xv, 35-6, 38-40, 65-6, 89, 101-2, 110, 123-4, 150-

2, 237, 289-90, 384-8, 393-4, 413
   strains of   149, 151, 290
Bastyr University in Seattle   79, 80, 99, 285
Baylor College of Medicine   221
B-cells   68
Beam Ray Machine   419
Beans   158, 375
   dried   158
Bedroom   160, 163-4, 348, 376
   circuit breaker   164
Bedtime   127, 159, 170-1, 224, 295, 330, 348, 376
Bee
   propolis   291
   venom   47
Beef   128
   grass-fed   375
Behavior modification   x, 139
Belief   22, 85, 92, 101, 247, 329, 343, 353-4
   healthier   353
   subconscious   353
   systems, personal   20, 87, 353
Benadryl   97, 100, 107
Benzodiazepines   105
Berg, David   109-10
Beta glucan   292
Betaine HCL   273
Biaxin   122, 235, 237, 287, 368, 415
Bicillin injections   121-2, 263-4, 391
Bicom   179
Bilberry   338, 342
Binders, mold biotoxin   233
Biofilms   ix, 93, 96-7, 337, 343-4, 392
Bioflavonoids   97, 112, 277
Bioidentical
   hormone replacement   371
   thyroid hormone   293
Biologo Detox   328
BioMed Publishing Group   iii, iv, 394
Bionic 880   xii, 176-7, 180-1, 184, 186-7, 191-2, 194, 313, 315-7, 332
Biophotons   xii, 175-8, 180-90, 192-4, 315-7, 321, 325-8
BioPure   38, 41
Bioresource's homeopathic molds   41
Biotensor   181, 318
Biotoxins   32-3, 94-5, 155, 271-2, 390
   load   32

mold's 126
surface 390
theory 68
Biotransformation xiv, 253-5
Black cohosh 323
Black Currant 349
Black Poplar 342
Black walnut 40, 94, 273
Bladder 154
Bland, Jeffrey 260, 272
Blier, Gary 352
Blood xii, 20, 48, 92, 94, 109-10, 186-7, 225, 229, 251, 261, 270, 278, 315, 325-6, 388
  cells
    red 148, 386
    white 95, 157
  cortisol tests 230
  fibrin 278
  flow 42, 399
  pressure 126, 130, 253, 278, 366, 374
  stagnation 109-10
  sugar 102, 294, 300
  tests, antibody 311
Blood type diets 45
Boluoke 48, 97, 110
Bone necrosis 186
Boneset 38, 40, 340
Borrelia nosodes 179-81, 187
Borrelogen 41
Boswellia 103, 241, 324, 377
Bovine source immunoglobulins 44
Bowel 102, 154, 260, 300, 345, 375
  cleanses 407
  irritable 81
  movements 105
    regular 376
Boxed cereals 225
Brain 27-8, 42, 46, 79, 84, 88, 97, 99, 104-5, 111-2, 139, 269, 279, 289, 305-6, 353
  aging 258
  allergies 99, 106
  cells 111
  fog vii, 20, 48, 81, 100, 106, 109, 111, 130, 135, 155, 182, 185, 225, 232, 243
  function, restoring normal 100, 112
  Herxes 289
Brand, Richard 423

Bransfield, Robert C., M.D. 420
Breads 233, 370, 375
  white 128-9, 225
Breast cancer 275, 422
Breasts 69, 161
Brimhall, John 335
Bronchitis 96, 186, 310
Buhner, Stephen 41
Buhner's herbal protocol xvi, 340-1
Burbur Detox 155
Burgdorfer, Willy 407
Burning pain 39
Burrascano, Joseph, M.D. 32, 62, 91-2, 124, 138, 366
Burrascano's Pulse Protocol x, 46, 138
Butterfly Effect 262
Butyrate 44
  rectal 44
B-vitamins 277, 317
Byproducts
  clear amino acid 160
  oxidative 253

C

Cadmium 93, 410
Caffeine 73, 113, 225, 268-9, 296, 299
CALDA (California Lyme Disease Association) 31, 114, 120
California Lyme Disease Association (CALDA) 31, 114, 120
California poppy 295
Canada 20, 22-3, 44, 287, 297, 419
Canadian Lyme Disease Foundation 23
Canadian patients 23
Cancer 65, 108, 113, 143, 145, 186, 199, 205, 251, 265, 275, 312, 339, 416, 418-9, 422
Candida x, xv, 32, 36, 41, 44, 48, 126, 206-7, 222-4, 228, 261, 265-6, 286-7, 299, 300, 369-70
Candy bar 250
Cantwell, Alan 418
Carbamazepine 47
Carbohydrates 104, 128-9, 251, 253, 299, 330, 344, 365, 370
Carrot juice 109
Casein 96, 102, 344
Castor oil packs 42, 343
Cat Scratch Fever 38, 89
Catabolic state 331

Index

Catheter   368
Cat's claw   41, 63, 237, 325, 340
CBC and TSH levels   223
CD-57   36, 90, 98, 134, 178, 185-6,
   391
CD4   337
CD8 cells   337
Cefdinir   121, 287, 368
Ceftin   368, 385
Ceftriaxone   64, 121
Cell
   phones   188, 398
   wall   34, 263-4, 322, 327, 415, 422
Cells
   cancerous   275
   damaged   178
   darkened   177
   density   96
   diseased   327
   healthy   422
   human   326
   immune   68, 178, 327
   induced   416
   membranes   264, 400
   nerve   269
   symbiosis   312, 314
Cellular Effects of Photon Therapy   xii,
   177
Cellulase   44
Cephalosporins   35, 264
Charcoal   109, 342-3
Chelation therapy   42, 56, 92-3, 231,
   248, 328, 341
Chelator   298
Chelex   42
Chemical odors   163
Chemotherapy   65
Cheney, Paul   265, 283
Chest x-ray   90
Chi   110
Childhood leukemia   422
Children   39, 53, 99, 175, 390, 408,
   412, 420
Chills   20, 408
Chinese
   herb rehmannia   69
   medicine   56, 58-9, 61, 69, 71, 76,
   110, 270
   sarsaparilla   296
Chiropractors   183, 280, 360-1
Chlamydia pneumoniae   68, 90, 191,

   228, 238, 314, 326, 367
Chlorella   42, 48, 67, 109, 183, 231,
   328, 342-3
Cholestyramine   42, 126, 156, 233,
   390
Chromium picolinate   102
Chronic Fatigue Syndrome (CFS)   viii,
   x, 22, 56, 75, 120-1, 135, 145,
   222, 248, 264-5, 324, 332
Chronic Lyme disease   22, 29, 32, 78,
   98, 105, 109-10, 113, 115-6, 136,
   233, 281, 324, 331, 339, 367-8
Chronic recurrent lumbar spine pain
   184
Chronic strep   228
Cilantro   42, 67, 342
Cilley, Marla   351
Cinnamon   110, 230
Ciprofloxacin   123, 235, 237
Circuit breakers   163-4
Circulation   89, 110, 250, 301, 322,
   378
Clarithromycin   121, 235, 237, 287,
   368
Clay   84, 342
   baths   343
   bentonite   67, 109, 376
   green   42
   plaster   155
Clinical diagnosis of co-infections   viii,
   65
Clinical observations   81, 97, 99, 148,
   260
Clinical Response Formulas   40
Clover, red   323
Co-infections   viii, ix, xi, xiii, 19, 20,
   22-3, 35-7, 39, 40, 65-6, 89-92,
   110, 147-8, 236-7, 266, 286-8,
   368-9, 386
Co-Q10   317, 332, 373
Celiac Disease   282
Cognitive Behavior Therapy   x, 140
Coil Machine   406
Colds, frequent   304
Collagen, regenerating   362
Colonics   49, 98, 102, 104, 342
Colorado   403
Colors   84, 154, 159, 166
Condura   161-2
Conjugated equine estrogen   275
Constipation   101-2, 275

Constitution   199, 201-2, 270, 272, 339
Cordless phones   187, 398
Cordyceps mushroom   41, 69, 293, 372
Core Energetics   60
Coriolus Mushroom   134
Corson, Ann   21
Cortef   108
Cortisol   70, 108, 158, 226, 230, 252, 257-8, 274, 276-7, 294, 321, 323, 349, 367, 371
    allergies   230
    bioidentical   158, 372
    circadian rhythms   315
    levels   70, 158, 276-7, 279, 293-4, 315, 318, 322, 330, 371
        low   265, 294, 371
    low dose   157
    pattern   269, 277
    pharmaceutical   277
    replacement   226, 230
    saliva   264
    synthetic   158, 349
Cortisone   349
    natural   349
Cortrosyn stimulation test   371
Costerton, William   96
Coughing   408
Coughing, dry   38
Counseling   53, 98, 106, 211, 303
Cousins, Norman   117
Cowden, Lee, MD   xi, 145-7, 149, 151, 153, 155, 157, 159, 161, 163, 165, 167, 169, 171-3, 271, 335
Cramps   192
    menstrual   269
Crane, John   418
Cravings   268-9
Creatine monohydrate   160
Crook, William   129
Cryptolepsis   38, 40
Cumanda   40, 151, 158, 164, 385
Curcumin   47, 96, 103, 241, 295, 317, 324, 377
Cutler, Andrew, Ph.D.   410-1
Cyst-targeting antibiotics   406
Cysts   153, 236, 287, 391, 415
Cytokines   95, 323
Cytomegalovirus   90, 228, 290
Cytomel   229

D

Dairy   45, 103, 158, 299, 301, 330-1, 345, 375
    cow   301
    goat   301
Darkfield microscopy   148, 152
Death   146, 180, 222, 306, 347, 422
    cellular   254
    programmed cell   327, 339
Deer antler velvet   157
Deficiencies   47, 75-6, 100, 130-1, 160, 170, 230, 240, 269, 293, 303, 317, 321, 378
    hormonal   275, 294, 377
Degenerative diseases   361, 365-6
Dementia   122, 261
Dental work   34
Denver   403
Depression   vii-ix, xi, xiii, xv, xvii, 47, 71, 106, 130, 158-61, 184, 192, 240-1, 296, 347-8, 377
Derksen, Amy, N.D.   37
Detox Factors   42
Detox footbaths   109
Detox footpads   42
Devil's claw   341
DHEA   69, 157, 256, 274, 277, 294, 322-3, 350
DHEAS   90, 108, 229, 371
Diabetes   186, 251, 253, 366
Diagnosis
    differential   248
    labs support   243
    physical   167
    positive   178
    rheumatoid arthritis   258
Diagnosis and Treatment of Bartonella book   387
Diagnostic
    checklist   410
    criteria   413
    dilemmas   200
    disaster   386
Diagnostic Hints and Treatment Guidelines for Lyme   282
Diagnostic laboratories   89
Diarrhea   101, 132, 265
Diary   169
DiCaprio, Leonardo   85
Diet   xiii-xvii, 43-5, 72-3, 96-7, 127-9, 206-8, 223-5, 240-2, 250-2, 261-

2, 267-9, 330-2, 343-5, 365-7, 373-5, 414-7
  anti-inflammatory 96
  gluten-free 129
  low-carbohydrate 317
  vegetarian 208
  yeast-free 45
Diflucan 94-5, 286, 292, 370
Disability
  benefits 141
  lawyers 141
  payments 141
Disclaimer iv, vii, 424
Diseases
  anaerobic 108
  autoimmune 215, 251, 313, 319, 332, 370
  cardiovascular 248, 261
  immunological 333
  infectious 213-5, 414, 419, 422
  inflammatory bowel 215, 259
  joint 259, 282
  liver 261
  neurodegenerative 111-2
  periodontal 414
  terminal 419
  vascular 145
  zoonotic 83
Disturbance, visual 88
Dizziness 408
DMPS 42, 298, 342
DMSA 42, 67, 109, 231, 298, 342, 370-1
DMSO 105, 377
DNA 97, 111, 156, 176, 251, 253-6, 258, 262, 385
Doctor's Data Laboratories 411
Dogs 139
Doloryx 47
Dopamine 99, 319-20, 347
Doxycycline 26, 35-6, 64, 121, 123-4, 235, 287, 289-90, 310, 368, 385, 415
Drainage remedies 342
Dreams 38, 159, 312, 332
D-ribose 48, 279
Drinking alkaline water 342, 345
Drug proving 198-9
Duncan, Tami 107, 420, 423
Dust mites 386, 413

E

East-West School of Herbology and Ohio College 418
EBV 68-9, 228, 290
Eczema 304, 310
EDTA 67, 297-8, 328, 370-1
EEG 90
EFT techniques 303, 353
Egg whites 128
Ehrlichia vii, xv, 35-6, 39, 65, 82, 237, 290, 367, 384-6
Electric shock 88
Elimination Diet 243, 342
ELISA test 66, 383
EMEM Machine 406, 423
EMF 93, 163-4, 169, 188, 398
  high-frequency 164
  levels, low 188
  pollution 168
  readings 163
  sources, removing 187
Emotional Freedom Technique (EFT) xv, 22, 303, 352-3
Emotions vi, xiii, xiv, 21, 25, 48, 60-1, 154, 165-8, 209-12, 234, 257-8, 282, 352-7, 377, 379, 399, 400
Endocrine system 44, 98, 256, 264-5, 323, 344
Endometriosis 221-2
Endorphins 107, 177
Energy ix, 27, 60, 62, 78, 87, 93, 107-8, 153-4, 177, 183, 251-4, 279, 316, 360-2, 372
Enula 38, 40, 150, 152, 164
Environmental medicine 55, 80, 175, 365
Enzymes 62, 97, 110, 159, 178, 254-5, 260, 269, 278, 301, 392
  digestive 42, 224, 273, 372
  high liver 39
  proteolytic 96
Epigenetics 156, 343
Epinephrine 296, 319, 347
Epsom salts 131
Epstein-Barr virus 33, 68, 90, 191, 228, 238, 290, 324, 367
Estradiol 157, 371
Estrogen 69, 70, 228-9, 256, 274-6, 293-4, 323
Evaluative Kinesiology technique 145
EVOX system 165

Exam   121, 168, 208, 309
  oral   309
  physical   22, 91, 200, 216, 380
Excessive nitric oxide output   331
Excessive Th2 response   266
Excretion   102, 109, 186, 271-2, 328, 341
Exercise   vii, xi, xiii, xv-xvii, 20, 46, 141, 166, 169-71, 183, 230-1, 250, 277, 301, 331, 359
  aerobic   46, 109, 301, 331, 359
  moderate   74, 108, 141, 250
  regular   19, 250
  stretching   42, 46
Exhaustion   110, 318
Extracts
  adrenal organ   322
  broccoli   327
  chlorella algae   328
  embryonic herbal   337
  mangosteen   42
  olive leaf   41
  thymus   322
Eye twitch   357
EZOV   159

F

Faass, Nancy   56
Fallon, Brian, M.D.   115
Fat cells   109, 275
Fat-free milk products   128
Fatigue   vii, xiv, 39, 40, 48, 56, 61, 65, 72, 81, 89, 95, 108, 142, 179, 253, 279
Fatty acids   88, 104, 300, 330
  high dose omega-3   322
  long-chain   273
  omega-3   128, 281, 317, 322, 327
  short-chain   273
Feder, Henry   178
Fermented milk product   233, 301
Fevers   39, 89, 310, 386, 408
  fatal   386
  heavy   311
Fiber   128, 156
  non-absorbable   164
  soluble   375-6
Fibrinogen degradation products   109
Fibroblasts   400
Fibromyalgia   20, 22, 59, 120-1, 145, 222-3, 232, 241, 248, 259, 346, 403
Fingers   161-2
Fish   128, 270, 300, 375
  oil   96, 372, 377
Flagyl   38, 122, 236, 287, 368
  pulsing   122
Flame retardants   398
Flavocoxid   241
Flax oil   300
Flaxseeds   128
Flea   386, 413
  feces   386
  preventing   393
Floaters   88
Flour   129, 225, 250, 331
Flowers   113, 154, 166, 348
Food
  allergies   44, 46, 129, 224-5, 227, 238, 241, 243, 260, 267, 350
  intolerances   330
Foot baths, ionic cleanse   42, 342-3, 358, 371
Forehead   181
  patient's   106, 161
Forsgren, Scott   iv, xviii, 395, 401
Free radicals   ix, 98, 111-2, 127
Free T3   371
Free T4   371
Frontal lobe, impaired   389
Fruits   107, 128-9, 158, 208, 251, 300, 345, 375
  citrus   375
  concentrated   300
  fresh   300
  juices, concentrated   42, 158
  low glycemic index   375
  mangosteen   407
  non-organic   345
  organic   225
Fry Laboratories in Scottsdale   89
Fry, Stephen   89, 117
F-Scan   423
FSH   70, 371
Fungal problems   94, 155-6, 184, 266, 273

G

GABA   46, 71, 104-5, 268, 296, 320, 347, 376-7
  pathways   46
  receptor sites   347

Gabapentin   47
Gaby, Alan   117
Gall bladder   154
   attack   49
GALT (gut-associated lymphoid tissue)
   252, 260, 273
Garlic   41, 45, 94, 99, 300
Gastrointestinal problems   xiv, 35, 67,
   95, 101, 260, 273
Gateway Press   283
Gauss readings   164
Gene expression   250
Genes   75, 94, 156, 172, 251, 271,
   327
Genetic coding   254-5, 343, 379
Genomes   214
Genova Diagnostics   101, 225
Germany   146, 164, 175-6, 191, 194-
   5, 309, 311-2, 314, 320-4, 375,
   401
Gillham, Peter   131
Ginko biloba   48, 104, 112, 338
Glands   45, 319, 328
   endocrine   45
   lymph   65
   pineal   172
Glass vial   153
Glutathione   42, 48, 67-8, 109, 233,
   297-8, 313, 317, 327
   intracellular   315
   lipoceutical   297-8
   nebulized   111
   suppositories   297
Gluten   44, 72, 81, 96, 102, 241, 267-
   8, 273, 299, 344
   sensitivity   129, 224-5, 238, 268,
   272-3, 282, 378
Glycemic diet, low   224, 230
Glycine   46, 224
Glyconutrient   417, 423
Glycosaminoglycans   400
God   iv, 101, 167, 304
Goji berry   42
Gonzalez, George   335, 345
Government   23, 240
Grains   128, 158, 208, 250-1, 299,
   345, 375
Grape alcohol   340-1
Grapefruit   287, 342, 370
Grapevine   339, 342
Growth hormone   108, 157, 230, 256,

345, 367, 371
Guaiacum   291-2
Guilford College in Greensboro   79
Guillemin, Roger   417
Guilt   52, 140, 399
Gulf War Syndrome   248
Gurvich, Alexander G.   176
Gut
   dysbiosis   27, 101, 164, 184
   infections   273
   problems   38
   symptoms   243
Gut-associated lymphoid tissue, *see*
   GALT
Gym   230-1
Gynecology   221

H

Hair   ix, 103, 411
   loss   275
Hair Mineral Analysis   418
Hair test interpretation   411
Halos around lights   88
Hamburg   309-10, 312
Harmony Women's Health in Los Altos
   221
Harris, Steven, M.D.   vii, 31, 33, 35,
   37, 39, 41, 43, 45, 47, 49, 51, 53,
   285
Harvey, William T.   420
Hashimoto's thyroiditis   182, 229
Hass, Sally   258
Haye, Louise   116
HBOT (Hyperbaric Oxygen Treatments)
   xv, 305, 384, 406
Head   65, 106-7, 139, 154, 161-3,
   182-3, 233, 244, 311, 329
Headaches   ix, xv, 19, 38, 61, 65, 70,
   77, 81, 89, 105, 130-1, 162, 296-
   7, 387, 408
   migraine   105
   rebound   105
   withdrawal   73
Healing crisis   235, 356
Health Consciousness Journal   418
Health insurance   52, 106, 122-3, 140,
   219, 230, 287, 289, 421
Heart disease   146, 414
Heat   106-7
Heavy metals   21, 33, 36, 42, 47, 67-
   8, 90, 126, 146, 154, 231, 297-8,

324, 327-8, 342-3, 411
Heilpraktiker xvi, 309-13, 315, 317,
   319, 321, 323, 325, 327, 329,
   331, 333
Hemex laboratories 109
HemoBartonella 82, 89
Hepar comp 182
Heparin 48, 110
   sublingual 110, 278
Hepol 42
Herbal Gem 337, 340
   and PSC Plant Stem Cells xvi, 340
Herbs xv, xvi, 40-1, 63, 65, 69, 71-2,
   97-8, 147-53, 159, 216-7, 235-7,
   291-2, 325-6, 337-8, 340-1, 416-7
Herpes virus 33, 90, 290-1, 324
Herxers, permanent 137
Herxheimer reactions 21, 36-7, 76,
   97, 125, 134, 137, 155, 212-3,
   217, 235, 264, 272, 288-91, 300,
   302
Hesse-Sheehan, Elizabeth, DC xvi,
   335, 337, 339, 341, 343, 345,
   347, 349, 351, 353, 355, 357,
   359, 361, 363
HGH 157, 371
HHV-6 68-9, 228, 238, 290-1, 367
High nighttime cortisol levels 279
High starting doses of antibiotics 390
Histamine 99, 100, 107
Histamine 99, 100, 107
Histoplasmosis 239-40
Hittleman, Richard 142
HLA patterns 94, 390
Homeopathic
   Borrelia nosodes 316
   nosodes 179, 181, 186, 315, 325-6
Homeopathic aggravations 213, 217
Homeopathic Pharmacopoeia (HPCUS)
   198
Homeopaths 198, 205, 207, 212
Homeopathy xiii, 41, 55, 63, 65, 71,
   87, 98, 153, 161, 166, 198-9,
   201-8, 210-4, 216-9, 271
   classical 201, 203, 218, 220, 271
Hormone allergies 226-7
Hormones ix, xiii, 44, 69-71, 108,
   156-7, 225-9, 250-1, 256-7, 271-
   2, 274, 276, 293-4, 319-23, 349-
   50, 371-2
   bioidentical 45, 275, 323, 372

catabolic 294
compounded 229
female 108
fight-or-flight 319
follicle-stimulating 70, 371
grandmother 294
luteinizing 70, 371
minor anabolic 256
pituitary 70, 371
prescription 127
relaxing 71
replacement 229, 257, 371
stress response 257
synthetic 323
Horowitz, Richard, M.D. 20-1, 32, 34,
   91, 117, 150, 153, 248, 271
Hot baths 295
Houttuynia 151
HPCUS (Homeopathic Pharmacopoeia)
   198
HSV-1 290-1
HSV-2 291
5-HTP 71, 160, 268, 295-6, 376-7
Hug 142-3
Humor x, 139-40
Husband 21, 306-7, 329
Hydrocortisone 41, 70, 294
Hydrotherapy 96, 98, 189
Hydroxycobalamin 332
Hydroxychloroquine 38, 235, 415
5-Hydroxytryptophan 105
Hyper-alert immune systems 226
Hyperactivity 185
Hyperbaric Oxygen Treatments, *see*
   HBOT
Hypercoagulation xiv, 109, 277-8
Hyperthyreosis 192
Hypnosis 48, 211
Hypochondriacs 113, 224
Hypochondriasis 248
Hypoperfusion 399
Hypothalamus 95, 98-9
Hypothyroidism 275
Hypoxia ix, 110-1

I

IBS (irritable bowel syndrome) 159,
   213
ICHT Italian treatment 406
IDSA 29, 32
IgA 232

low secretory   101
IgE   232
IGeneX labs   20, 82, 89, 383, 388
IgG   186, 232
  allergy tests   300
  antibodies   226, 291
  subtypes   367
IgM   186
IL-6   387-8
IL-10   315
IL-1B   315, 387-8
ILADS (International Lyme and
    Associated Diseases Society)   20,
    23, 29, 32, 55, 57, 62, 64, 80, 91,
    114, 117, 120, 150, 247, 285
Illness
  biotoxin   ix, 91, 94-5, 102
  mold toxin   412
  psychosomatic   88, 184
Imitrex   105
Immune surveillance   33, 398-9
Immune system suppression   258, 350
Indoor mold spores   342
Industrialized foods   250
Infections
  chronic   93-4, 96, 107, 110, 239,
    313-4, 344, 414
  dental   34
  high fever   186
  intracellular   314, 331
  low-grade   403
  opportunistic   32, 68, 204, 238, 266,
    313, 367, 369
  oral Herpes   186
  parasitic   38, 367
  pylori   224
  strep   239
  untreated Babesiosis   305
  urinary tract   207
Infectious Disease Society of America
    (IDSA)   29, 32
Infertility   221
Inflammation   ix, xiv, xvi, 36, 44, 72-
    3, 95-6, 223-6, 252-3, 261, 264,
    274-9, 296, 323-5, 338-9, 389-90
Injections   70, 121, 157, 227, 229,
    320, 322, 332, 368, 372
Injury   259, 346
Insect
  bites   94
  feces   413

Insecticides   343, 398
Insomnia   vii-xi, xiv, xv, xvii, 46, 59,
    71, 81, 105, 126, 159, 163, 179,
    279, 295, 318, 347-8
Institute of Functional Medicine   267,
    282
Insulin   73, 102, 108, 250
  resistance   73, 102, 230, 253, 277
IntegraMed Academy   xi, 146, 168,
    172-3
Interferon gamma   315, 323
Interleukin   323
International Lyme and Associated
    Diseases Society, *see* ILADS
Internet   20-1, 25-6, 29, 50, 60, 86,
    112, 114, 133, 136-7, 150-1, 168,
    172, 222, 355, 392
  support groups   26, 136
Intestimax   44
Intestine   44, 67, 97, 101, 131, 189,
    224, 232, 252, 260, 399
Intracellular glutathione levels   90
Iodine   69, 157, 293
Ions   93
Iron   130
  glycinate   372
  levels, low   373
Irritability   130
Irritable bowel syndrome (IBS)   159,
    213
Irritable immune system   81
Isolation   393

J

Jefferson Medical College   365
Jemsek, Joseph G.   62, 86
Jernigan, David   41-2
Job   22, 106, 120, 132, 140, 143, 151,
    199, 203, 207, 209, 231, 242,
    244, 323, 358
  full-time   120
Joints   20, 97, 103, 130, 170-1, 259,
    295, 311
Jones, Charles Ray, M.D.   80, 82, 91,
    97, 117, 124, 248, 282
Joseph Burrascano's Lyme Disease
    Treatment Guidelines   91
Juice   132
  beet   42
  drinking lemon   300
  fresh vegetable   109

Juniper 342

K

Kane, Patricia 104
Kaprex 46
Kava kava 159
Kavinase 347
Kefir 294, 301
Ketek 121-2, 415
Ketoprofen cream 46
Key and Wellness Pharmacies 47
Ki Therapy 161-3
Kidneys 33, 36, 97-8, 154, 207, 375, 399
Kids 33, 47, 53, 304
Kinnaman Foundation 419
Klein, Karin 195
Klinghardt Axiom 396-7
Klinghardt, Dietrich, M.D., Ph.D. iii, xviii, 32, 335, 354, 395-6, 399, 401
Knees 171
Konner, Melvin 107
Kryptopyrrole 100
Kunold, Marlene xvi, 309, 311, 313, 315, 317, 319, 321, 323, 325, 327, 329, 331, 333
Kupsinel, Roy 418

L

Lab4More 320
LabCorp 290
Lability 106, 111
Lactic acidosis 159
Lactoferrin 97, 99
Lakato 158, 164
Lamasil 94
Lamaze childbirth instructor 119
Lamictol 106
Lariam 35, 123, 289
LarreaPlus 291
Laser 153-4, 156, 160, 166, 343, 345-7, 362
Latex allergies 111
Lavender 105
L-carnitine 277, 332
Leaky Gut 44, 256
Lecithin 72, 327
Ledum 203
Leg pain 21-2

Legs 171
Lemon water 97
Lemons 158
Leptin 73, 412
    resistance 102
Lethargy 253
Leukocytes 178, 186, 190
Levaquin 123, 289-90, 385
Levofloxacin 123, 237, 289, 369
Levoxyl 229
LIA (Lyme Induced Autism) Foundation 420
Libido 53, 294
Lice 86, 413
Licorice 45, 94, 99, 103, 110, 277, 293, 321, 372
Ligaments 361
Light 93, 102, 121, 153-4, 157, 160, 163, 177, 231, 321, 324, 329, 332, 346, 362, 396
    bulb 233
    infrared 178
    photonic 177, 315
    red 163
    therapy 93, 335, 343, 345-6
Limbic Stress Assessment (LSA) 267
Limbic system 139
Linden Tree 342, 348
Lipoprotein 109
Lipped mussels, green 99
Lipton, Bruce 343
Lithium orotate 160, 407
Liver ix, 33, 36, 42, 67, 97, 103, 154, 207, 272, 291-2, 327, 343-4, 360, 375, 399
    cleanses 407
    detoxification process 37, 67, 255, 271
Liver Extende 42
Liver's cytochrome P450 system 103
LiZyme-Forte 161
L-lysine 291
Lombard, Robert 384
Longevity Healthcare for New Medicine 248, 282
Love 77-8, 224, 384
    unconditional 167
Low-dose Naltrexone 44, 72, 377
Low-frequency Gauss meter 163-4
Loyd, Richard, Ph.D. 406, 419, 423
LSA (Limbic Stress Assessment) 267

L-theanine 46, 296
L-tryptophan 268, 296
L-tyrosine 268, 296
Lumbrokinase 48
Lunesta 105
Lyme-Autism Connection 420
Lyme disease
    conferences 52, 56
    infants contracting 420
Lyme Disease Solution, by Ken
        Singleton, M.D. 96
Lyme disease support groups 114, 305
Lyme Disease Survival Guide vi, 19,
        25, 403, 414
Lyme Induced Autism (LIA) 107, 420
Lyme-Literate Medical Doctor iii, 20,
        26-7, 57, 62, 151, 239, 242-3,
        271, 281, 285, 290, 298, 354,
        361, 366
Lyme-literate psychiatrist 47, 105-6
Lyme, neurological 264
Lyme Nosode 203
Lyme support groups 26
Lymebook.com 409, 415
Lymphatic 33, 42, 68
    drainage problems 155, 227, 343,
        375
    system 76, 154, 182, 227
Lymphocyte 178, 180, 185-6, 190
    activity 190
    differentiation 185, 190
    sub-populations 337
    subset tests 336
    transformation test 311-2, 314
Lymphoma 65
Lymphomyosot 182
Lynes, Barry 416, 418

M

MacDonald on Borrelia biofilm research
        96
Macrolides 34, 415
Macrophages 178
Mag Malate 132
Magnesium x, xvii, 41, 47, 93, 105,
        127, 130-2, 182, 292, 295-6, 317,
        332, 348, 367, 372-4
    deficiencies 130-1, 293, 373
    dosing 132
    elemental 131
    glycinate 372

levels, intracellular 131, 373-4
MagTab SR 132
Malaria 394, 413
Malarone 35, 123, 289, 369, 387
MALT (mucosa-associated lymphoid
        tissue) 260
Mannatech glyconutrient products 48
MARCoNS 95
Marra, Susan L. ix, 79, 81, 83, 85, 87,
        89, 91, 93, 95, 97, 99, 101, 103,
        105, 117
Marshall Protocol xi, 172, 406-7, 415,
        422
Massage 96, 98, 227, 306
Mattman, Lida, Ph.D. 415, 422
Mayo Clinic 20
McFadzean, Nicola, N.D. xv, 37, 285,
        287, 289, 291, 293, 295, 297,
        299, 301, 303, 305, 307
McJeffries, William 158
MCS 332
Mcshane, Maureen iii, vii, 19-23
Meal 168, 170, 344
Meat 45, 107, 158, 345
Medications
    antiviral 228, 369
    diabetic 183, 230
    oral 36, 122, 289, 368
    prescription 21, 224, 360
Meditation 50, 60, 98, 304-5, 378
Mediterranean-based diet 208, 251
Mefloquine 123, 289
Melanocyte stimulating hormone (MSH)
        95
Melatonin 55, 71, 105, 163, 172, 224,
        295, 330, 348, 376
Memories 48, 170, 269, 354, 372
    cellular 354
    releasing traumatic 48
Memory changes 370
Memory Loss 258, 408
Mepron 35, 122-3, 237, 287, 289,
        369, 373, 385, 387
    depletes Co-Q10 373
Mercury 68, 93, 189, 231, 298, 343,
        367, 370, 375, 406, 410-1
    poisoning, chronic 410
Metabolism 69, 99, 176, 183, 191,
        253, 270, 293-4
Metagenics 42, 46-7, 299
Methyl-B12 297

Methylation pathway problems   45, 343
Methylcobalamin   104, 297
Metronidazole   34-5, 122, 236, 287, 368
Metzger, Deborah   xiii, 221, 223, 225, 227, 229, 231, 233, 235, 237, 239, 241, 243, 245
Micro-currents   280
Microbes, intracellular   311, 317, 325, 331-2
Migraines   ix, 105, 269, 296-7, 390, 394
Milk   126-7, 131, 330
  almond   300
  goat   301
  thistle   103, 407
Mind, subconscious   48, 165, 303, 353-4, 356
Mineral baths   407
Minerals   43, 71, 129, 131, 159, 292-3, 322, 342, 362, 374, 392, 411, 417
  trace   99, 292, 298
Minocycline   35, 263-4, 415
Miracle Mineral Supplement   51, 414
Mitochondria   75, 107, 214, 279, 316, 331, 349
Mold   21, 32-3, 50, 68, 94, 126, 156, 169, 184, 208, 226, 232-3, 272, 389-90, 398, 412
  antibody   36
  detoxification problems   68
  indoor   389
Money   23, 114, 136, 217, 219, 224, 243-4, 303, 305, 359, 380, 416
Morgellons   82, 120, 131
Morrison, Jeffrey, M.D.   xvii, 365, 367, 369, 371, 373, 375, 377, 379, 381
Mosquitoes   86, 164
Multiple Sclerosis (MS)   40, 109-10, 122, 179, 239, 248, 332, 341, 414
Muran, Peter J., M.D.   xiv, 247-9, 251, 253, 255, 257, 259, 261, 263, 265, 267, 269, 271, 273, 275, 277
Muscle
  aches   243
  cramping   95, 373
  groups   259
  relaxant   296
  spasms   295
  strength   318

Mushrooms   69, 99, 233, 336
Mycobutin   385
Mycoplasma   vii, xv, 33, 36, 39, 68, 82, 191, 228, 238, 278, 290
Mycotoxins   21, 156, 398
Myelin sheath   88, 322
Myers, Melissa   410
Myofascial release   227

N

NAC   67, 297-8
N-acetyl cysteine   67, 97, 297
NAET   267
NaHCO3   182
NanoGreens   300
Nanotech Chitosan   42, 156
Narby, Jeremy   84
Nasal cannula   111
Nasal spray   95
Natural Calm   127, 131
Natural Healers Academy   418
Natural Health Research Clinic   80
Natural killer (NK)   316, 370, 372
Natural remedies   46, 56, 70-1, 287, 295-6
Naturopathic physicians   37, 45, 80-4, 99, 101, 285, 288, 309
NatuRx   155
Nerve pain   243
Nerves   88, 170, 322, 346, 360
Nervous system   69, 80, 88, 127, 177, 295, 297, 328, 341, 345, 348, 360-2, 377
Neuro-Antitox   42
Neuroborreliosis   99, 104, 106, 320
Neuroinflammation   106
Neurological symptoms   121-2, 289, 296
  increased   65
  strong   35, 263, 292
Neurontin   72, 377
Neuropathy   38, 346
Neurotoxins   47, 67, 93, 327
Neurotransmitter   xvi, 99, 104, 160, 177, 225, 227, 256, 262, 268-9, 286, 317, 319-20, 347-8
  allergies   226, 240
  communications   62
  desensitization   240
  imbalances   xiv, 76, 256, 320
  inhibitory   296

panel, complete 347
precursors 160, 320, 348
replacement 71
Neurotropic behavior 88
New York Medical College 55
Niacinamide 103-4
Nicola's Lyme Formula 291
Nitazoxanide 34-5, 287
Nitric
  oxide xvi, 111, 319, 331
    levels, elevated 331
  stress
    cycle 332
    levels 315, 317
Nizoral 370
NK (natural killer) cells 178, 316, 370, 372
NMT 21-2
Non-pharmaceutical antibiotics 406
Nosodes 180-2, 187, 193, 325-6, 328
Notatum 41
NutraMedix 38, 40-2, 146, 161
NutrEval 225
Nutrient absorption 101-2
Nutrients 43, 57, 67, 96-8, 100, 106, 108, 110-2, 127-8, 160, 224-5, 240, 250-2, 292-3, 371-3, 400
Nuts 91, 107, 423
  raw 300
  roasted soy 128
Nystatin 94, 286-7, 292, 370

O

Obesity 251, 258, 269, 366, 412
  adolescent 253
Ohio College of Natural Health 418
Oil
  clove bud 151
  emu 105
  linseed 322
  ozonated castor 325
  rizol 38
Olive leaf 291, 325
Ondamed 62, 270-1
Open Eye Pictures 86
Operative Gynecologic Laparoscopy 222
Oral chelators 298, 410
Oregano 41, 44, 94, 99, 110, 273
Organs ix, 36, 91, 97-8, 170, 176-8, 207, 271, 292, 312, 343, 346,
360, 375, 399, 400
Oxidative stress xiv, 36, 251-3, 256, 331
Oxygen 74, 93, 100, 110-1, 155, 278, 305, 316, 348, 399, 406
  stabilized 313, 315, 317
Ozone 93, 98, 182, 311, 325, 406

P

Pacemakers 192
Pain vii, viii, xi, xiii-xvii, 20, 46-7, 72, 161-2, 183-4, 193, 241-2, 269, 280, 295-7, 323-4, 345-7, 377
  joint 56, 65, 77, 81, 89, 103, 130, 163, 239, 265, 346
Pancreatin 102, 104
Parasites 33, 38, 164, 222-3, 228, 260, 265, 272-3, 388
Parkinson's disease 145, 254, 269
Parsley Detox 41, 155, 162
Pectins 342-3
Pelvic
  bone 162
  pain 222
    chronic 221-2
Penicillins 121, 264, 368
Perimenopause 71, 228, 295
Peristalsis 102
Peroxynitrite ix, 111-2, 319, 331
Peru 146
Pesticides 178, 208, 254, 343, 375
PET scan 90
Petadolex 105
Pfeiffer, Carl 99, 107
PH 45, 131, 342
Phenomena 32, 86, 190, 218
Phenylalanine 269
Phyllanthus amarus 103
Physical activities 60, 230-1
Phytochemicals 338-9, 341
PICC 368
Pinella 42, 48, 155, 162
Plant stem cells xvi, 44, 337-43, 345, 348, 361-2
Plants 84-5, 176, 323, 337-8, 340-1
  embryonic 337-8
PMS 61, 70, 226, 294
Pollens 129, 225-6
Positive Lyme tests 201-2
Post-Lyme Syndrome 179
Prayer 50, 167, 304-5, 352, 354

Preceptorship   21, 91
Pregnenolone   69, 108, 157, 277, 294, 371
Princeton University   410
Pro-inflammatory cytokines   95
Proanthocyanidins   110
Probiotics   50, 101, 164, 214, 224, 260, 287, 292, 294-5, 302, 317, 372, 417
Progesterone   69-71, 157, 226, 228-9, 274, 276, 294-5, 323, 371
Proguanil   123, 289, 369, 387
Prophylaxis   203-4
Protein powder   300
Proteins
  animal   45, 331
  low-fat   128-9
Protocel   422
Provera   275
Provigil   48
Psychological/psychiatric problems   39, 48, 79, 119, 193, 211
Psyllium   67, 102, 156, 164, 375
PTSD   136, 332
Pyridoxine   100, 104
Pyrole   100
Pyroluria   100, 240

Q

Quantum Neurology   343, 345-6, 350, 358, 361
Quercetin   97, 100, 107, 338
Questran   67
QXCI   311

R

Rage   106-7, 393
Rapid Eye Therapy   354
Rashes   66, 383
Raxlen, Bernard   81
Recall Healing   167
Reflex Sympathetic Dystrophy   38, 346-7
Reflexes   38, 121, 130, 346
Reiki   98
Relapse   138, 148, 151, 204-5, 222
Relationships   53, 60, 93, 102, 107, 210, 215, 217, 219-20, 396-7, 399, 412, 424
Remission   138, 180, 188, 259, 316, 339
Researched Nutritionals   42, 292, 294-5, 302
Resveratrol   41, 279, 340-1
Rheumatoid factor   36, 238-9
Rheumatologists   57, 59, 77, 259, 282
Rhodiola   41, 69, 107, 293, 377
Rice   128, 158
  brown   129, 299, 375
  mucil   156, 164
  white   129, 225, 375
Rickettsia   191
Rifampin   35, 103, 123-4, 290, 369, 385
Rife machines   51, 92-3, 311, 385, 406-7
Right Spin Glutathione   155, 162
Rocephin   64, 121, 263-4
Root   42, 101, 167, 224, 329, 354, 414
  burdock   42
  butter   105
  canals   242
  dandelion   102, 109, 299
  marshmallow   101, 156, 164
  red   40, 42
  stephania   41
  valerian   158, 295, 376
  yucca   43, 48
Rosen, Gary   412
Rosner, Bryan   iv, 406-7, 409, 412, 415-6, 420, 423-4
RSD (reflex sympathetic dystrophy)   38, 346-7

S

Saccharomyces boulardii   102, 295
S-Adenosyl-L-methionine   103, 160
Saliva   230, 276, 293, 319, 349, 413
  hormone tests   229
Salt   51, 407
Samento   235, 237, 291-2, 406
Saunas   98, 231, 342-3, 358, 371, 406-7, 418
  electric light   418
  infrared   109, 155
Savely, Ginger   x, 119, 121, 123, 125, 127, 129, 131, 133, 135, 137, 139, 141, 143, 423
SCENAR   183
Schaller, James, M.D., M.A.R.   iii, xviii, 151, 383, 394, 407-8, 412-3, 423

Sciatica problem, long-standing   347
Seaweed   375
Selenium citrate   103
Sensitivities
   multiple chemical   81, 111, 252
   sun   235
Serotonin   71, 99, 160, 177, 226, 320, 347
Serrapeptase   48
Serum leptin levels   102
Sesquiterpene   348
Sex hormones   95, 371
Shellfish allergies   156
Shoemaker, Ritchie, M.D.   126, 156, 271, 379
Siberian Ginseng   108, 321
Sick Buildings   412
Silymarin   103
Skin   ix, 33, 38, 52, 86, 103, 156, 161, 170, 177, 206-7, 226, 231, 243, 343, 357
Sleep   xiii, 20, 46, 62, 71, 73, 99, 105, 126-7, 162-3, 171-2, 223-4, 295-6, 318, 376, 391
   apnea   224
   cycles   105, 127
   disordered   223-4
Slippery elm bark   156, 164
Smilax   38, 40, 291-2, 302
Smilax   296
Smoking   128, 185
Smoothies   128, 132
Snake oil   281
Solar plexus   181, 315-6
Solvents   327, 343
Sour cherry   241
Soybean   323
Spina bifida   255
Spine, lumbo-sacral   171
Spirituality   viii, xv, 50, 85, 167, 303-4, 414
Spirochetes   84, 93, 98, 104, 115, 148, 152-3, 264, 383, 392, 398, 415
Sporanox   94
Stem cells   xvi, 339-41, 348-9
Stool tests   36, 243
Stools   102, 128, 132, 367
Strasheim, Connie   iii, iv, vi, vii, 19, 25-30, 248, 262, 403, 414
Streptococci   399

Stress   33, 50, 53, 59, 73-4, 98, 101, 103, 127, 139-40, 209, 253, 276, 318-9, 323, 349-51
Stricker, Raphael, M.D.   90, 247
Sugar
   craving   128
   white   73, 129, 209, 225, 299, 331
Sulfate, vanadyl   102
Sunlight   xi, 46, 49, 50, 172, 301, 321, 350
Symptoms
   autistic   420
   bi-polar   38
   chronic   22
   classic magnesium deficiency   131
   diabetic   186
   joint   375
   musculoskeletal   121
   neuropathic   39
   rheumatoid   265
   severe   187, 288
Symptoms, adrenal fatigue   318
Synthroid   372
Syntrion   101
SyRegule   101

T

T3   229, 274-5, 322
   sustained release   229
T4, free   229
Tabebuia species   94
Taurine   103-5
T-cells   46
Tea   113
   chamomile   376
   green   112
   kombucha   294
   tree   94
Teasel   40, 291-2, 302
   cream   38
Tendon pain   290
Testosterone   69, 157, 228-9, 256, 274, 276, 294, 367, 371
Tests   36-9, 66-8, 72-3, 89, 90, 129, 178-81, 183, 190, 200, 226, 228-31, 272-4, 311, 314-5, 318-24, 391-2
   antibody   314, 387
   co-infection   337
   energetic   159, 190
   laboratory   91-2, 108, 202, 251,

253, 263, 336
saliva   274, 315, 347
serologic   178-9
symptom   89
Tetracyclines   35, 415
Th1   68, 190, 265-6, 283, 326
Th2   265, 283
Thick blood   ix, 109-10
Thomson Healthcare   416
Thoring, Tod   32, 38, 40
Thorne Research   372
Thyroid   69, 76, 90, 98, 108, 157, 181-
    2, 226, 229, 253, 256-7, 274, 293,
    319, 322, 371-2
Tick bites   22, 113, 304, 367, 393, 420
Ticks   19, 22, 86, 113, 146, 310, 386,
    388-9, 391, 393, 406, 408, 413
Tinidazole   34, 236, 287-8
Titers   69, 134
TMJ   34
TNF alpha   315, 323-4
Tobacco   209, 237
Tongue   155, 161-2
Townsend Letter   419
Toxin binders   42, 95, 232, 327, 343,
    376
Toxins   61, 64, 67-8, 75-6, 109, 146,
    153-7, 176-7, 181-2, 189, 208,
    225, 231-2, 254-6, 327-8, 395-
    400
  emotional   165, 189
  physical   154, 165-6, 189, 360
  stored   327, 398
Transdermal
  neuropathy creams   47
  remedies   46, 229
Transfer factor   43, 68, 99, 227, 286,
    292, 302
Traumas   74-5, 146, 154, 166, 234,
    353-4, 399
TravaCor   347
Treatment
  failures   383-5, 387
  fatigue   391
Tremors   20, 370
TSH   229, 274, 319, 371
Tuberculosis   33, 199, 238, 278
Tularemia   82
Tumors   312, 416
Tuna fish   375
Turkey   300, 375

Turmeric   47, 94, 110, 159, 377

U

Ultra Clear   42, 299
UltraInflamX   47
Ultraviolet blood irradiation   94
Underweight   318
University
  of Colorado   403
  of Connecticut Health Center   221
  of Guayaquil   163
    in Ecuador   159
  of Heidelberg in Heidelberg   175
  of Natural Medicine   418
  of Rochester   365
  of Texas Medical School   221
Urinary tract   206
Urination   108
  frequent   127
Urine tests   319, 331, 370
  24-hour   274
  organic acid   349
  provoked heavy metal   370

V

Vaginal
  insufflations   93
  tablets   229
Valcyte   94, 291
Valproic acid   47
Valtrex   94, 291, 360
Vascular
  endothelial growth factor (VEGF)   95,
    387-8
  endothelium   89
Vasoconstriction   89, 159, 399
Vasodilation   89
Vasopressin   108
Vega device   181
Vegetables   107, 128-9, 158, 208,
    225, 251, 300, 344-5, 373
VEGF (vascular endothelial growth
    factor)   95, 387-8
Vertebrae   170
  upper lumbar   171
  upper thoracic   171
Vertebral segments   361
Vincent's Hospital   197
Vinegar   233, 370
Vinpocetine   104

Index

Viral infections 69, 134, 214
   chronic 291
Viral titers 134
Viruses 32, 41, 68, 94, 176, 178, 184,
      222-3, 225-6, 228, 238, 265, 290-
      1, 324, 342, 357
   opportunistic xv, 290-1
   re-activated 228, 238
Visual FISH exams 387
Vitalzym 42
Vitamin
   buffered 98
   intravenous 68, 332, 372
Vitamin, 25-hydroxy 367
Vitamin B-5 41, 157, 293, 321, 372
Vitamin B-6 69, 100, 104
Vitamin B-12 90, 105, 127, 160, 292,
      295-7, 332, 367, 372-3
Vitamins 73, 92, 94, 98, 104, 112,
      129-30, 183, 189, 255, 272, 281,
      292, 302, 315, 317

W

Waistline, pronounced 253
Washington State University 111
Water 61, 81, 94, 96, 110-1, 113,
      128, 132, 162, 166, 205, 232,
      270, 300, 325, 389
   alkaline 342
   cold 88
   green 342
   sea 61
Wavelength 194, 316
Weeping eyes 80
Weight loss viii, 20, 65, 76, 268
Wellbutrin 241
Wellness Medical Center of Integrative
      Medicine 366
Wellness Pharmacies 47
Westbrook University 418
Western Blot Test 20, 383
Wheat 103, 107, 126, 330-1, 341
White Willow 342
Whitley, Janet 415
Whitmont, Ronald, M.D. xii, 197, 199,
      201, 203, 205, 207, 209, 211,
      213, 215, 217, 219
William McK Jefferies 277
Williams
   Linda 105
   Louisa 335

Susan 423
Wilson
   Andy Abramson 86
   Lawrence 418
Wobenzym 42
Woodland Essence 40
Wounds 184

X

Xenobiotics 68
Xymogen 42, 44, 47
Xyrem 46, 376

Y

Yale University 422
Yang, Therese 32
Yasko protocol 43
Yoga 142, 233-4, 301, 359, 378
Yogurt 301, 375

Z

Zeolites 42, 109, 327
Zhang, Dr. 41, 46, 385
Zinc 93, 99, 100, 104, 182, 291, 293,
      314, 322
   deficiencies 240
   supplementation 322
Zithromax 35, 38, 64, 122-3, 237,
      287-9, 385, 415
Zoonotic diseases report 88
Zyactinase 97
Zyto 149, 165, 267

LaVergne, TN USA
24 February 2011

217711LV00002B/2/P